T0259477

Genitourinary Pathology

Editor

MING ZHOU

SURGICAL PATHOLOGY CLINICS

www.surgpath.theclinics.com

Consulting Editor
JASON L. HORNICK

December 2022 • Volume 15 • Number 4

ELSEVIER

1600 John F. Kennedy Boulevard • Suite 1800 • Philadelphia, Pennsylvania, 19103-2899

http://www.theclinics.com

SURGICAL PATHOLOGY CLINICS Volume 15, Number 4
December 2022 ISSN 1875-9181, ISBN-13: 978-0-323-91975-3

Editor: Taylor Hayes
Developmental Editor: Diana Grace Ang

Surgical Pathology Clinics (ISSN 1875-9181) is published quarterly by Elsevier Inc., 360 Park Avenue South, New York, NY 10010. Months of issue are March, June, September, and December. Business and Editorial Office: Elsevier Inc., 1600 John F. Kennedy Blvd., Ste. 1800, Philadelphia, PA 19103-2899. Accounting and Circulation Offices: Elsevier Inc., 3251 Riverport Lane, Maryland Heights, MO 63043. Periodicals postage paid at New York, NY and at additional mailing offices. Subscription prices are $237.00 per year (US individuals), $376.00 per year (US institutions), $100.00 per year (US students/residents), $283.00 per year (Canadian individuals), $395.00 per year (Canadian Institutions), $284.00 per year (foreign individuals), $395.00 per year (foreign institutions), and $120.00 per year (international students/residents), $100.00 per year (Canadian students/residents). Foreign air speed delivery is included in all *Clinics'* subscription prices. All prices are subject to change without notice. **POSTMASTER:** Send address changes to *Surgical Pathology Clinics*, Elsevier, 3251 Riverport Lane, Maryland Heights, MO 63043. **Customer Service: 1-800-654-2452 (US). From outside the United States, call 1-314-447-8871. Fax: 1-314-447-8029. E-mail: JournalsCustomerServiceusa@elsevier.com (for print support)** and JournalsOnlineSupport-usa@elsevier.com **(for online support)**.

Reprints. For copies of 100 or more, of articles in this publication, please contact the Commercial Reprints Department, Elsevier Inc., 360 Park Avenue South, New York, NY 10010-1710. Tel. 212-633-3874; Fax: 212-633-3820; E-mail: reprints@elsevier.com.

Surgical Pathology Clinics of North America is covered in *MEDLINE/PubMed (Index Medicus)*.

Contributors

CONSULTING EDITOR

JASON L. HORNICK, MD, PhD
Director of Surgical Pathology and
Immunohistochemistry, Brigham and Women's
Hospital, Professor of Pathology, Harvard
Medical School, Boston, Massachusetts, USA

EDITOR

MING ZHOU, MD, PhD
Professor and Chair, Department of Anatomic
and Clinical Pathology, Tufts University School
of Medicine, Chair and Pathologist-in-Chief,
Department of Pathology and Laboratory
Medicine, Tufts Medical Center, Boston,
Massachusetts, USA

AUTHORS

MAHMUT AKGUL, MD
Assistant Professor, Division Chief,
Genitourinary Pathology, Department of
Pathology and Laboratory Medicine, Albany
Medical Health System, Albany, New York,
USA

DILARA AKHOUNDOVA, MD
Department for BioMedical Research,
University of Bern, Department of Medical
Oncology, Inselspital, University Hospital of
Bern, Bern, Switzerland

HIKMAT AL-AHMADIE, MD
Department of Pathology, Memorial Sloan
Kettering Cancer Center, New York, New York,
USA

KHALEEL I. AL-OBAIDY, MD
Department of Pathology and Laboratory
Medicine, Henry Ford Health, Detroit,
Michigan, USA

MAHUL AMIN, MD
Department of Pathology and Laboratory
Medicine, University of Tennessee Health

Science, Memphis, Tennessee, USA;
Department of Urology, Keck School of
Medicine, University of Southern California,
Los Angeles, California, USA

MANJU ARON, MD
Professor of Clinical Pathology and Urology,
Departments of Pathology and Urology, Keck
School of Medicine, University of Southern
California, Los Angeles, California, USA

EZRA BARABAN, MD
Departments of Pathology, Urology, and
Oncology, Johns Hopkins Medical Institutions,
Baltimore, Maryland, USA

DANIEL M. BERNEY, FRCPath
Department of Cellular Pathology, Barts Health
NHS Trust, Department of Molecular
Oncology, Barts Health Cancer and Barts
Health NHS Trust, London, United Kingdom

QI CAI, MD
Assistant Professor, Department of Pathology,
The University of Texas Southwestern Medical
Center, Dallas, Texas, USA

JIE-FU CHEN, MD
Department of Pathology, Memorial Sloan
Kettering Cancer Center, New York, New York,
USA

BENJAMIN L. COINER, MD
Vanderbilt University School of Medicine,
Nashville, Tennessee, USA

EVA COMPÉRAT, MD
Department of Pathology, General Hospital of
Vienna, Medical University of Vienna, Vienna,
Austria; Department of Pathology, Sorbonne
University, Assistance Publique-Hôpitaux de
Paris, Hôpital Tenon, Paris, France

BOGDAN CZERNIAK, MD, PhD
Professor, Department of Pathology, The
University of Texas MD Anderson Cancer
Center, Houston, Texas, USA

ABHISHEK DASHORA, MD, FRCPath
Department of Cellular Pathology, Barts Health
NHS Trust, London, United Kingdom

JONATHAN EPSTEIN, MD
Departments of Pathology, Urology, and
Oncology, Johns Hopkins Medical Institutions,
Baltimore, Maryland, USA

FELIX Y. FENG, MD
Department of Radiation Oncology, University
of California, San Francisco, San Francisco,
California, USA

JATIN S. GANDHI, MD
Assistant Professor, Department of Pathology
and Laboratory Medicine, Emory University
School of Medicine, Seattle, Washington, USA

JENNIFER B. GORDETSKY, MD
Department of Pathology, Microbiology, and
Immunology, Vanderbilt University Medical
Center, Vanderbilt University School of
Medicine, Professor, Department of Urology,
Vanderbilt University Medical Center,
Nashville, Tennessee, USA

CHARLES C. GUO, MD
Professor, Department of Pathology, The
University of Texas MD Anderson Cancer
Center, Houston, Texas, USA

ONDREJ HES, MD, PhD
Department of Pathology, Charles University in
Prague, Faculty of Medicine in Plzeň,
University Hospital Plzeň, Pilsen, Czech
Republic

MUHAMMAD T. IDREES, MD
Department of Pathology, Indiana University
School of Medicine, Indianapolis, Indiana, USA

MARTIN J. MAGERS, MD
IHA Pathology and Laboratory Medicine, Ann
Arbor, Michigan, USA

MEHDI MANSOOR, MD, FRCPC
Department of Pathology and Laboratory
Medicine, Cumming School of Medicine,
University of Calgary, Rockyview General
Hospital, Calgary, Alberta, Canada

SAMBIT K. MOHANTY, MD
Director of Surgical and Molecular Pathology,
Surgical and Molecular Pathology, CORE
Diagnostics (India), Advanced Medical
Research Institute, Gurugram, Haryana,
India

ANDRÉ OSZWALD, MD
Department of Pathology, General Hospital of
Vienna, Medical University of Vienna, Vienna,
Austria

ANIL V. PARWANI, MD, PhD, MBA
Professor of Pathology and Biomedical
Informatics, Vice Chair and Director of
Anatomic Pathology, Director of the Digital
Pathology Shared Resource, Department of
Pathology, The Ohio State University Wexner
Medical Center, Cooperative Human Tissue
Network (CHTN) Midwestern Division,
Columbus, Ohio, USA

**ANKUSH URESH PATEL, MBBCh, BAO,
LRCP & SI**
Research Fellow, Department of Laboratory
Medicine and Pathology, Mayo Clinic,
Rochester, Minnesota, USA

COLIN C. PRITCHARD, MD, PhD
Department of Laboratory Medicine and
Pathology, University of Washington, Seattle,
Washington, USA

SOROUSH RAIS-BAHRAMI, MD
Department of Urology, Department of
Radiology, O'Neal Comprehensive Cancer
Center, University of Alabama at Birmingham,
Birmingham, Alabama, USA

MARK A. RUBIN, MD
Department for BioMedical Research,
University of Bern, Bern Center for Precision
Medicine, Inselspital, University Hospital of
Bern, Bern, Switzerland

RAJAL B. SHAH, MD
Dr. Charles T. Ashworth Professor of
Pathology, The University of Texas
Southwestern Medical Center, Dallas, Texas,
USA

SHAHROKH SHARIAT, MD
Department of Urology, Comprehensive
Cancer Center, Medical University of Vienna,
Vienna, Austria

FARSHID SIADAT, MD, FRCPC
Department of Pathology and Laboratory
Medicine, Cumming School of Medicine,
University of Calgary, Rockyview General
Hospital, Calgary, Alberta, Canada

KIRIL TRPKOV, MD, FRCPC
Department of Pathology and Laboratory
Medicine, Cumming School of Medicine,
University of Calgary, Rockyview General
Hospital, Calgary, Alberta, Canada

THOMAS WAGNER, MD
Department of Pathology, Copenhagen
University Hospital, Rigshospitalet,
Department of Oncology, Copenhagen
University Hospital, Rigshospitalet,
Copenhagen, Denmark

GABRIEL WASINGER, MD
Department of Pathology, General Hospital of
Vienna, Medical University of Vienna, Vienna,
Austria

SEAN R. WILLIAMSON, MD
Department of Pathology, Robert J. Tomsich
Pathology and Laboratory Medicine Institute,
Cleveland Clinic Foundation, Director,
Genitourinary Pathology, Vice Chair,
Education, Professor of Pathology, Cleveland
Clinic and Cleveland Clinic Lerner College of
Medicine, Cleveland, Ohio, USA.

MING ZHOU, MD, PhD
Professor and Chair, Department of Anatomic
and Clinical Pathology, Tufts University School
of Medicine, Chair and Pathologist-in-Chief,
Department of Pathology and Laboratory
Medicine, Tufts Medical Center, Boston,
Massachusetts, USA

Contents

> The Gleason scoring system and Grade Group systems facilitate accurate grading and reporting of prostate cancer, which are essential tasks for surgical pathologists. Gleason Pattern 4 is critical to recognize because it signifies a risk for more aggressive behavior than Gleason Pattern 3 carcinoma. Prostatic adenocarcinoma with radiation or androgen therapy effect, with aberrant P63 expression, or with Paneth cell–like differentiation represent pitfalls in prostate cancer grading because although they display architecture associated with aggressive behavior in usual prostatic adenocarcinoma, they do not behave aggressively and using conventional Gleason scoring in these tumors would significantly overstate their biologic potential.

> Cribriform lesions of the prostate represent an important and often diagnostically challenging spectrum of prostate pathology. These lesions range from normal anatomical variation, benign proliferative lesions, premalignant, suspicious to frankly malignant and biologically aggressive entities. The concept of cribriform prostate adenocarcinoma (CrP4) and intraductal carcinoma of the prostate (IDC-P), in particular, has evolved significantly in recent years with a growing body of evidence suggesting that the presence of these morphologies is important for clinical decision-making in prostate cancer management. Therefore, accurate recognition and reporting of CrP4 and IDC-P architecture are especially important. This review discusses a contemporary diagnostic approach to cribriform lesions of the prostate with a focus on their key morphologic features, differential diagnosis, underlying molecular alterations, clinical significance, and reporting recommendations.

> Historically, the detection of prostate cancer relied upon a systematic yet random sampling of the prostate by transrectal ultrasound guided biopsy. This approach was a nontargeted technique that led to the under detection of cancers at biopsy and the upgrading of cancers at radical prostatectomy. Multiparametric MRI-targeted prostate biopsy allows for an image-directed approach to the identification of prostate cancer. MRI-targeted biopsy of the prostate is superior for the detection of clinically significant prostate cancer. As this technique has become more

prevalent among urologists, pathologists need to recognize how this development impacts cancer diagnosis and reporting.

Prostate cancer (PCa) is characterized by profound genomic heterogeneity. Recent advances in personalized treatment entail an increasing need of genomic profiling. For localized PCa, gene expression assays can support clinical decisions regarding active surveillance and adjuvant treatment. In metastatic PCa, homologous recombination deficiency, microsatellite instability-high (MSI-H), and CDK12 deficiency constitute main actionable alterations. Alterations in DNA repair genes confer variable sensitivities to poly(ADP-ribose)polymerase inhibitors, and the use of genomic instability assays as predictive biomarker is still incipient. To date there is a lack of consensus as to testing standards.

The reporting recommendations on "flat and papillary urothelial neoplasia," published in 2 position articles by the Genitourinary Pathology Society in July 2021, was a collective contribution of 38 multidisciplinary experts aiming to clarify nomenclature, classification of flat and papillary urothelial neoplasia and controversial issues. In this review, we discuss some of these recommendations including nomenclature, practical approaches, and their importance for clinical practice.

Urothelial carcinoma (UC) is known to encompass a wide spectrum of morphologic features and molecular alterations. Approximately 15% to 25% of invasive UC exhibits histomorphologic features in the form of "divergent differentiation" along other epithelial lineages, or different "subtypes" of urothelial or sarcomatoid differentiation. It is recommended that the percentage of divergent differentiation and or subtype(s) be reported whenever possible. Recent advances in molecular biology have led to a better understanding of the molecular underpinning of these morphologic variations. In this review, we highlight histologic characteristics of the divergent differentiation and subtypes recognized by the latest version of WHO classification, with updates on their molecular and clinical features.

Staging and reporting of cancers of the urinary tract have undergone major changes in the past decade to meet the needs for improved patient management. Substantial progress has been made. There, however, remain issues that require further clarity, including the substaging of pT1 tumors, grading and reporting of tumors with grade heterogeneity, and following NAC. Multi-institutional collaborative studies with prospective data will further inform the accurate diagnosis, staging, and reporting of these tumors, and in conjunction with genomic data will ultimately contribute to precision and personalized patient management.

Bladder cancer is a heterogeneous disease, which exhibits a wide spectrum of clinical and pathologic features. Recent genomic studies have revealed that distinct molecular alterations may underlie the diverse clinical behaviors of bladder cancer, leading to a novel molecular classification. The intrinsic molecular subtypes exhibit distinct gene expression signatures and different clinicopathologic features. Genomic alterations also underlie the development of bladder cancer histologic subtypes. Genomic characterization provides new insights to understanding the biology of bladder cancer and improves the diagnosis and treatment of this complex disease. Biomarkers can aid the selection of patients for immune checkpoint therapy.

In recent years, several emerging diagnostic entities have been described in renal cell carcinoma (RCC). However, our understanding of well-known and established entities has also grown. Clear cell papillary RCC is now relabeled as a tumor rather than carcinoma in view of its nonaggressive behavior. Renal tumors with a predominantly infiltrative pattern are very important for recognition, as most of these have aggressive behavior, including fumarate hydratase-deficient RCC, SMARCB1-deficient medullary carcinoma, collecting duct carcinoma, urothelial carcinoma, and metastases from other cancers.

This review summarizes current knowledge on several novel and emerging renal entities, including eosinophilic solid and cystic renal cell carcinoma (RCC), RCC with fibromyomatous stroma, anaplastic lymphoma kinase-rearranged RCC, low-grade oncocytic renal tumor, eosinophilic vacuolated tumor, thyroidlike follicular RCC, and biphasic hyalinizing psammomatous RCC. Their clinical features, gross and microscopic morphology, immunohistochemistry, and molecular and genetic features are described. The diagnosis of most of them rests on recognizing their morphologic features using immunohistochemistry. Accurate diagnosis of these entitles will further reduce the category of "unclassifiable renal carcinomas/tumors" and will lead to better clinical management and improved patient prognostication.

This article reviews the recent advances and potential future changes in the classification of testicular germ cell and sex cord stromal tumors, highlighting changes in the classification system and terminology with description on newer entities. A discussion on approaching difficult areas and diagnostic pitfalls is also included along with the utility of ancillary investigations. Areas with limited knowledge are highlighted to providing direction for future studies and a bulleted summary in the form of critical care points is provided.

Khaleel I. Al-Obaidy, Martin J. Magers, and Muhammad T. Idrees

Testicular tumors are the most common solid tumors in young men, the vast majority of which are of germ cell origin. The staging of human cancers is paramount to correct patient management. Staging systems have passed through several developments leading to the release of the most recent 8th edition of the American Joint Committee for Cancer (AJCC) staging manual, which is based on the current understanding of tumor behavior and spread. In this review, the authors summarize the current AJCC staging of the germ cell tumors, highlight essential concepts, and provide insight into the most important parameters of testicular tumors.

Ankush Uresh Patel, Sambit K. Mohanty, and Anil V. Parwani

As machine learning (ML) solutions for genitourinary pathology image analysis are fostered by a progressively digitized laboratory landscape, these integrable modalities usher in a revolution in histopathological diagnosis. As technology advances, limitations stymying clinical artificial intelligence (AI) will not be extinguished without thorough validation and interrogation of ML tools by pathologists and regulatory bodies alike. ML solutions deployed in clinical settings for applications in prostate pathology yield promising results. Recent breakthroughs in clinical artificial intelligence for genitourinary pathology demonstrate unprecedented generalizability, heralding prospects for a future in which AI-driven assistive solutions may be seen as laboratory faculty, rather than novelty.

SURGICAL PATHOLOGY CLINICS

SERIES OF RELATED INTEREST

Clinics in Laboratory Medicine
http://www.labmed.theclinics.com/
Medical Clinics
https://www.medical.theclinics.com/

THE CLINICS ARE AVAILABLE ONLINE!
Access your subscription at:
www.theclinics.com

Dedication

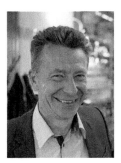

Ondrej Hes, MD, PhD

This issue is dedicated to our friend and colleague, Dr Ondrej Hes, who was fondly known by those close to him as Ondra. Sadly, he passed away suddenly on July 2, 2022. Ondra was a coauthor of the article entitled, "Kidney Tumors: New and Emerging Kidney Tumor Entities," in this issue and was a world-renowned pathologist and an eminent figure in the international urologic pathology community. He was a great scholar and pathologist, credited for the recognition of many renal tumor entities and subtypes that have reshaped the understanding and diagnosis of contemporary renal tumor pathology. He was an excellent teacher, educator, and mentor to many students and colleagues. He was also an environmentalist, who devoted much of his time to the protection of nature and wildlife habitats. Although many attributes can be ascribed to him, probably the truest one is that Ondra was a great human being. He was kind, modest, humble, and always eager to help anyone in need. He was most generous in sharing his time, knowledge, and wisdom with everyone he met. He would not say "no" or "can't" to anyone, and he made everyone feel respected and special in his presence. Ondra's humanity and exemplary work ethic will live on as an inspiration, a celebrated memory, and a fine example of a life well lived.

Kiril Trpkov, MD
Department of Pathology and
Laboratory Medicine
Cumming School of Medicine
University of Calgary
Rockyview General Hospital
7007 14 Street, Calgary
Alberta T2V 1P9, Canada

Ming Zhou, MD, PhD
Department of Anatomic and
Clinical Pathology
Tufts University School of Medicine
Department of Pathology and Laboratory
Medicine
Tufts Medical Center
800 Washington Street, #115
Boston, MA 02111, USA

E-mail address:
mzhou3@tuftsmedicalcenter.org

Surgical Pathology 15 (2022) xiii
https://doi.org/10.1016/j.path.2022.09.002
1875-9181/22/© 2022 Published by Elsevier Inc.

Preface

Towards Precision Genitourinary Pathology

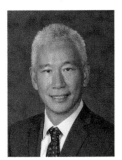

Ming Zhou, MD, PhD
Editor

Precision medicine requires precision pathology, that is, precise and clinically relevant histopathologic classification, grading, staging, and reporting of cancer. Genitourinary Pathology Society (GUPS), an international organization aiming to advance the science and practice of urologic pathology, recently convened experts to review new and evolving concepts and controversial topics in prostate, bladder, and kidney cancer pathology in an effort to advance precision genitourinary pathology. Six position papers ensued.[1-6] Many of the recommendations were incorporated in the recently published World Health Organization (WHO) Classifications of Tumors of the Urinary System and Male Genital Organs.[7] It is imperative for pathologists to keep abreast of these changes in order to generate diagnoses and reports that meet contemporary patient management needs.

Grading continues to play a critical role in prostate cancer (PCa) management and therapy planning. Baraban and Epstein provided an overview of recent updates and key concepts related to Gleason grading and Grade Groups and discussed both common and unusual morphologic challenges with each Gleason pattern and strategies for addressing them. Malignant cribriform lesions, including cribriform cancer and intraductal carcinoma, have emerged recently as one of the most important morphologic patterns for PCa management. Cai and Shah presented a contemporary diagnostic approach to cribriform lesions and addressed the controversies pertaining to whether intraductal carcinoma should be graded. New diagnostic tools, including MR imaging and

targeted biopsies, genomic testing, and artificial intelligence-enabled diagnostic algorithms, have significantly reshaped pathologists' roles in PCa diagnosis. Coiner and colleagues reviewed the benefits of MR imaging and targeted biopsies and recommendations for reporting such biopsies. Molecular tumor profiling has gained relevance in personalized clinical management and precision oncology treatment of localized and metastatic PCa. Akhoundova and colleagues reviewed the role of gene expression assays for genomic risk stratification to support decision algorithm regarding active surveillance or indication of intensification of therapy in localized cancer, and tumor molecular characterization by next-generation sequencing as well as by assays assessing HRD and MSI status to predict benefit from molecularly targeted therapies. Patel and colleagues summarized the recent breakthroughs in clinical artificial intelligence, especially in the deployment in the diagnosis of PCa, and laid out the prospects for a future with artificial intelligence–driven assistive solutions in genitourinary pathology.

Regarding urothelial neoplasia, there has been continuous debate and discussion on the classification of papillary and flat neoplasia. Comperat and colleagues presented the recent reporting recommendations by GUPS on "flat and papillary urothelial neoplasia" and offered diagnostic tips for such lesions. Gandhi and colleagues highlighted the histologic characteristics of subtype histology and divergent differentiation recognized by the WHO classification, with updates on their

Surgical Pathology 15 (2022) xv–xvi
https://doi.org/10.1016/j.path.2022.09.001
1875-9181/22/© 2022 Published by Elsevier Inc.

molecular and clinical features. Aron and Zhou argued for additional modifications of the pTNM staging, including T1 and T2 substaging, for better risk stratification. Not yet used in clinical practice, the molecular classification of bladder cancer, however, has gained momentum. Guo and Czerniak emphasized the distinct molecular alterations underlying the diverse clinical behaviors of bladder cancer that have led to novel molecular classifications, and have improved diagnosis and treatment of this complex disease. They also discussed biomarkers to aid the selection of patients for immune checkpoint therapy that has changed the therapeutic landscape of bladder cancer.

The classification of renal neoplasia has changed significantly in the WHO classification, 5th edition, with new entities added, including several oncocytic tumors (eosinophilic, solid, and cystic renal cell carcinoma). Several tumors with distinct morphology and molecular changes, such as low-grade oncocytic tumors and eosinophilic vacuolated tumor, were also included as emerging entities. Much of the credit goes to GUPS renal neoplasia working groups, who published two position papers, one on new developments in the existing WHO kidney tumor entities and one on new and emerging kidney tumor entities. These topics were reviewed by Akgul and Williamson, and Siadat and colleagues, respectively.

The classification and staging of testicular germ cell neoplasms have not changed significantly. However, the nuance of classification and staging that are important for clinical management may not be fully comprehended due to the infrequency of these tumors in the clinical practice. Dashora and colleagues reviewed the recent advances and potential future changes in the classification of testicular germ cell and sex cord stromal tumors, with a discussion on practical approaches to difficult diagnostic areas and pitfalls, along with utility of ancillary investigations. Al-Obaidy and colleagues summarized the current AJCC staging of the germ cell tumors, highlighted essential concepts, and provided insight into the most important parameters of testicular tumors staging.

I am very fortunate to have assembled a panel of renowned genitourinary pathologists to review and bring to you the most recent updates, which are important for the precision and personalized management of prostate, bladder, kidney, and testis tumors. It is my hope that the changes outlined in these reviews will bring us a step closer to precision genitourinary pathology.

Ming Zhou, MD, PhD
Department of Anatomic and Clinical Pathology
Tufts University School of Medicine
Department of Pathology and Laboratory Medicine
Tufts Medical Center, 800 Washington Street
Boston, MA 02111, USA

E-mail address:
mzhou3@tuftsmedicalcenter.org

REFERENCES

1. Epstein JI, Amin MB, Fine SW, et al. The 2019 Genitourinary Pathology Society (GUPS) White Paper on Contemporary Grading of Prostate Cancer. Arch Pathol Lab Med 2021;145(4):461–93.

2. Fine SW, Trpkov K, Amin MB, et al. Practice patterns related to prostate cancer grading: results of a 2019 Genitourinary Pathology Society clinician survey. Urol Oncol 2021;39(5):295.e1–8.

3. Trpkov K, Hes O, Williamson SR, et al. New developments in existing WHO entities and evolving molecular concepts: the Genitourinary Pathology Society (GUPS) update on renal neoplasia. Mod Pathol 2021;34(7):1392–424.

4. Trpkov K, Williamson SR, Gill AJ, et al. Novel, emerging and provisional renal entities: the Genitourinary Pathology Society (GUPS) update on renal neoplasia. Mod Pathol 2021;34(6):1167–84.

5. Compérat E, Amin MB, Epstein JI, et al. The Genitourinary Pathology Society update on classification of variant histologies, T1 substaging, molecular taxonomy, and immunotherapy and PD-L1 testing implications of urothelial cancers. Adv Anat Pathol 2021;28(4):196–208.

6. Amin MB, Comperat E, Epstein JI, et al. The Genitourinary Pathology Society update on classification and grading of flat and papillary urothelial neoplasia with new reporting recommendations and approach to lesions with mixed and early patterns of neoplasia. Adv Anat Pathol 2021;28(4):179–95.

7. WHO Classification of Tumours Editorial Board. Urinary and male genital tumours [Internet]. Lyon (France): International Agency for Research on Cancer; 2022 [cited YYYY Mmm D]. WHO classification of tumours series, 5th ed.; vol. 8. Available from: https://tumourclassification.iarc.who.int/chapters/36 (Accessed September 12, 2022).

Prostate Cancer
Update on Grading and Reporting

Ezra Baraban, MD[a],*, Jonathan Epstein, MD[a,b,c],*

KEYWORDS

- Prostate cancer • Gleason scoring • Grade groups • Intraductal carcinoma
- Prostatic adenocarcinoma with aberrant P63 expression
- Prostatic adenocarcinoma with Paneth cell–like differentiation

---

Key points

- Prostatic adenocarcinoma shows a broad range of morphology and clinical behavior, and pathologic features play an essential role in avoiding overtreatment for indolent tumors while facilitating early, definitive therapy for high-risk lesions.
- Gleason Pattern 4 is critical to recognize and quantify in pathology reports because it signifies the potential for more aggressive clinical behavior and thus may significantly alter clinical management.
- Grade Groups have simplified and recalibrated the Gleason scoring system such that the least aggressive tumors composed exclusively of Gleason Pattern 3 are designated Grade Group 1, with successively more aggressive tumors designated Grade Groups 2 to 5 as the prognosis worsens.
- Extraglandular mucin, tangential sectioning, mucinous fibroplasia, and intraductal carcinoma represent important considerations that may lead to either underdiagnosis or overdiagnosis of Gleason Pattern 4. Recognition of intraductal carcinoma is most important in the absence of invasive Gleason pattern 4 or 5 carcinoma because it signifies a high risk of unsampled high-grade carcinoma.
- Prostate cancer with androgen or radiation therapy effect, with aberrant P63 expression, and with Paneth cell–like differentiation typically show architectural patterns that would qualify for Gleason Patterns 4 and 5. However, these tumors are biologically indolent, and are excluded from Gleason scoring. Failure to recognize these special tumor variants and treatment effect may lead to significant overestimation of their biologic potential and overtreatment.

ABSTRACT

The Gleason scoring system and Grade Group systems facilitate accurate grading and reporting of prostate cancer, which are essential tasks for surgical pathologists. Gleason Pattern 4 is critical to recognize because it signifies a risk for more aggressive behavior than Gleason Pattern 3 carcinoma. Prostatic adenocarcinoma with radiation or androgen therapy effect, with aberrant P63 expression, or with Paneth cell–like differentiation represent pitfalls in prostate cancer grading because although they display architecture associated with aggressive behavior in usual prostatic adenocarcinoma, they do not behave aggressively and using conventional Gleason scoring in these tumors would significantly overstate their biologic potential.

INTRODUCTION

Prostatic adenocarcinomas exhibit a broad spectrum of morphology and clinical behavior, ranging

---

[a] Department of Pathology, Johns Hopkins Medical Institutions, 401 North Broadway, Weinberg Building, Room 2242, Baltimore, MD 21287, USA; [b] Department of Urology, Johns Hopkins Medical Institutions, 401 North Broadway, Weinberg Building, Room 2242, Baltimore, MD 21287, USA; [c] Department of Oncology, Johns Hopkins Medical Institutions, 401 North Broadway, Weinberg Building, Room 2242, Baltimore, MD 21287, USA

* Corresponding author. Department of Pathology, Johns Hopkins Medical Institutions, 401 North Broadway, Weinberg Building, Room 2242, Baltimore, MD 21287, USA

E-mail addresses: ebaraba1@jhmi.edu (E.B.); jepstein@jhmi.edu (J.E.)

Surgical Pathology 15 (2022) 579–589
https://doi.org/10.1016/j.path.2022.07.008

surgpath.theclinics.com

from low-volume, biologically inert tumors to high-grade, aggressive malignancies. This striking variety creates both challenges and opportunities; precise grading and quantification of prostate cancer facilitates early, definitive clinical intervention for high-risk tumors, and, just as importantly, enables avoidance of overtreatment in patients with tumors unlikely to cause morbidity or mortality. The pathologist's accurate diagnosis and grading of prostate cancer along with the assessment of tumor volume on biopsy plays a critical role in patient management and therapeutic planning. In this review, an overview of recent updates and key concepts related to Gleason scoring and Grade Groups (GGs) is followed by a discussion of both common and unusual morphologic challenges that arise with each Gleason pattern alongside strategies for addressing them. Finally, selected rare but clinically important situations are highlighted where Gleason scoring should be deliberately avoided.

RECENT DEVELOPMENTS AND KEY CONCEPTS IN GLEASON SCORING AND GRADE GROUPS

The Gleason scoring system serves as the foundation for prognosticating prostatic adenocarcinoma, and it has continued to evolve in recent years. Importantly, the lowest grade patterns of adenocarcinoma diagnosed in routine practice, corresponding to the most biologically indolent forms of prostate cancer, have drifted upward, with Gleason patterns 1 and 2 no longer diagnosed, with Gleason pattern 3 thus the lowest possible pattern of low-grade adenocarcinoma. GGs represent a major recent development that translate traditional, entrenched histopathologic terminology (Gleason patterns 3 to 5 and the resulting 9 possible Gleason scores) into an unambiguous, clinically oriented, and prognostically validated scoring scheme, which assigns each of the 9 possible Gleason scores to a single GG ranging from 1 to 5.[1] GGs therefore unequivocally convey to patients and clinicians that a carcinoma composed of pure Gleason pattern 3 (Gleason score 3 + 3 = 6) is the most indolent form of prostate cancer, and such tumors are therefore designated as GG 1. An additional benefit of assigning GGs in addition to Gleason scores in all prostate cancer cases is the condensation of the 9 possible Gleason scores into 5 discrete prognostic groups. GGs 1 to 3 are synonymous with Gleason scores 3 + 3 = 6, 3 + 4 = 7, and 4 + 3 = 7, respectively, whereas GGs 4 (4 + 4 = 8, 3 + 5 = 8, and 5 + 3 = 8) and 5 (4 + 5 = 9, 5 + 4 = 9, and 5 + 5 = 10) each aggregate 3 prognostically

similar Gleason scores together. This system has been widely endorsed and adopted,[2] with pathology reports for prostate biopsies now routinely mentioning not only the traditional Gleason score (the most abundant pattern of carcinoma followed by the highest grade pattern) but also the corresponding GG of the tumor.

A clinically critical threshold is the distinction between Gleason pattern 3 and pattern 4. By definition, any amount of pattern 4 excludes a patient from the very-low and low-risk groups of the National Comprehensive Cancer Network guidelines.[3] These patients may qualify for the favorable-intermediate risk group and potential candidacy for active surveillance, depending on the percentage of the tumor showing pattern 4 and various clinical and imaging considerations. Because the presence and amount of Gleason pattern 4 is such a crucial parameter, recent recommendations emphasize uniformity and precision in its definition and reporting.[4] Specifically, the major genitourinary pathology societies GUPS and ISUP recommend reporting the percentage of Gleason pattern 4 in biopsies containing 3 + 4 = 7 (GG2) or 4 + 3 = 7 (GG3) carcinoma because the prognosis and therapeutic outlook may differ significantly between patients with GG2 carcinoma with a small amount of pattern 4, versus a GG2 tumor bordering on GG3.[5] Uptake of this recommendation by practicing pathologists is currently variable but increasing. To maximize the amount of actionable information in the pathology report, while minimizing unnecessary tasks for the pathologist, it is not necessary or recommended to report the percentage of Gleason pattern 4 in cases with any GG5 carcinoma in any part of the case; in such patients reporting the percentage of Gleason pattern 4 in cores with GG2 or GG3 carcinoma will not affect clinical decision-making. However, in the majority of cases with GG2 and/or GG3 carcinoma, GG5 tumor is not present elsewhere and reporting the percentage of pattern 4 in each specimen involved by GG2 or GG3 carcinoma provides an extra degree of important information to clinicians, which would otherwise be lost, particularly regarding patients whose tumors may exist near the boundary between two GGs. For instance, reporting the percent Gleason pattern 4 enables pathologists to succinctly convey that a GG3 tumor with 90% pattern 4 in multiple biopsy cores may be expected to behave more closely to a GG4 tumor. This information could then be logically integrated with other clinical and pathologic features to inform a more nuanced treatment plan more tailored to the true nature of the patient's tumor. Conversely, it may be quite reasonable for an individual patient (depending on life expectancy, comorbidities, personal risk tolerance) to elect for active surveillance if biopsies demonstrate a small volume of GG2 carcinoma with less than 5% Gleason pattern 4. Routinely reporting percent Gleason pattern 4 also reduces the apparent magnitude of interobserver disagreement when pathologists disagree on borderline cases, which may straddle GG2 and GG3. If the percent Gleason pattern 4 is not reported, such a discrepancy may be alarming to patients and clinicians but it should be straightforward to understand that 2 pathologists may occasionally but reasonably disagree between GG2 with 40% Gleason pattern 4 and GG3 with 60% Gleason pattern 4. In general, when dealing with borderline cases, for example, cases with roughly equal amounts of Gleason patterns 3 and 4, where the percent Gleason pattern 4 approaches but is not definitively beyond 50%, a conservative approach is warranted because even ostensibly subtle changes in interpretation and reporting may trigger significant changes in management clinically. For patients opting for radical prostatectomy, the distinction between GG2 and GG3 in a biopsy will likely not alter management, and a definitive Gleason score and GG will be rendered at the time of radical prostatectomy. However, for patients electing radiation therapy, the distinction between whether or not to recommend androgen deprivation therapy may hinge on the specific percentage of Gleason pattern 4; specifically, patients with GG2 carcinoma typically forgo androgen deprivation, whereas GG3 patients are routinely considered for androgen deprivation therapy in addition to radiation.[6] Thus, even subtle changes in percent Gleason pattern 4 can have potentially dramatic clinical consequences, which reinforce the importance of a conservative approach when confronting borderline cases.

Because the percentage of Gleason pattern 4 in GGs 2 and 3 has potentially high clinical importance, we recommend using standardized reporting terminology. To balance the goal of reporting precise, granular data while maximizing interobserver agreement, we report percentage of Gleason pattern 4 in all cases without GG5 carcinoma elsewhere as either less than 5%, 10%, and in succeeding increments of 10% up to 90%; by convention greater than 95% Gleason pattern 4 (assuming a reasonable volume of carcinoma is present) is regarded as 4 + 4 = 8 (GG 4). In a biopsy with a small focus of carcinoma (ie, occupying 5% or less of an individual core) that is predominantly composed of Gleason pattern 4, it is recommended to err toward a diagnosis of 4 + 3 = 7 rather than 4 + 4 = 8 if there are even

a few glands of Gleason pattern 3 present. Occasionally, very small foci of carcinoma are encountered that comprise a mixture of Gleason patterns 3 and 4. In such cases, the percentage of Gleason pattern 4 or even the GG may differ radically depending on the level examined or the interpretation of a few borderline glands as either Gleason pattern 3 or 4. Again, a conservative approach is recommended, and in rare instances, it may be reasonable to refrain from reporting percentage Gleason pattern 4 in such cases given that the percentage is so likely to be artifactually inflated (or deflated) by the minute size of the focus of carcinoma.[7] In such cases, it is helpful to explain with a comment clarifying that the focus is too small to accurately assign a percent of Gleason pattern 4.

It is not uncommon to encounter a tumor composed of a combination of Gleason patterns 3 to 5. The recommended approach to integrating this mixture of patterns into a Gleason score varies depending on whether this situation is encountered in a biopsy or a prostatectomy specimen. In a biopsy, it is imperative to clearly communicate the presence of even a minimal amount of pattern 5 even if there are far greater amounts of pattern 3 and 4, as the presence of any pattern 5 likely signifies the presence of a high-risk tumor that requires definitive therapy.[8] Therefore, when reporting biopsies containing carcinoma with all 3 patterns, the approach to grading is consistent; by definition, the most abundant pattern is the primary pattern of the Gleason score, and regardless of the relative amounts of the other 2 patterns, the highest grade pattern is designated the secondary pattern of the Gleason score. Therefore, any Gleason pattern 5 encountered on a biopsy, even if it is vastly outnumbered by patterns 3 and 4, by definition becomes part of the Gleason score; if it is the most abundant pattern, it becomes the primary pattern, and even if it is the least abundant pattern, it is regarded as the secondary pattern of either 3 + 5 = 8 (GG4) or 4 + 5 = 9 (GG5). Conversely, when evaluating a prostatectomy, one has a global view of the tumor and can reasonably judge if there is a truly minute amount of Gleason pattern 5 in an otherwise GG2 or GG3 tumor. In this situation, one could reasonably argue that a very small amount of Gleason pattern 5 is insufficient to justify the significant upgrade from GG2 or GG3 to GG4 or GG5 if the Gleason pattern 5 is significantly outnumbered by patterns 3 and 4. Therefore, in a prostatectomy, a tumor nodule composed predominantly of Gleason patterns 3 and 4 with less than 5% Gleason pattern 5 is designated as Gleason score 3 + 4 = 7 or 4 + 3 = 7 with a minor tertiary pattern 5; the GG is based on the Gleason score and not affected by the minor tertiary pattern 5. Available data[9] suggest that reporting minor tertiary pattern 5 essentially fine-tunes the prognostic power of the Gleason system such that a GG2 tumor with minor tertiary pattern 5 has a prognosis intermediate between GG2 and GG3, and a GG3 tumor with minor tertiary pattern 5 has a prognosis intermediate between GG3 and GG4.

Cribriform prostate cancer has recently emerged to be a Gleason pattern 4 subpattern that connotes adverse clinical outcomes. Readers are referred to the article "Cribriform Lesions of the Prostate Gland" for a detailed discussion. Another common issue that arises when evaluating prostate biopsies is the diagnosis and reporting of intraductal carcinoma. Intraductal carcinoma is an important mimicker of invasive high-grade prostatic adenocarcinoma that in the vast majority of cases represents retrograde colonization or cancerization of preexisting prostatic ducts and acini by high-grade invasive prostatic adenocarcinoma.[10] If there is already overtly invasive high-grade prostatic adenocarcinoma present in the same or other biopsy cores (which is often the case), intraductal carcinoma becomes less crucial to recognize because it will not alter the prognosis or management of these patients. However, recognition becomes far more critical in biopsies lacking concurrent high-grade invasive tumor. When intraductal carcinoma is identified in a biopsy in the absence of invasive carcinoma or only in the presence of GG1 tumor, it signifies a high likelihood of an unsampled aggressive adenocarcinoma, thereby radically altering the prognosis and clinical approach for such patients.[11] Therefore, on biopsy in the absence of invasive high-grade tumor, distinguishing intraductal carcinoma from Gleason pattern 4 or 5 invasive carcinoma, on the one hand, and from the largely clinically insignificant high-grade PIN, on the other hand, becomes imperative. Furthermore, although in the vast majority of cases intraductal carcinoma represents retrograde extension of high-grade invasive adenocarcinoma, a rare subset is purely intraductal where high-grade invasive tumor will not be identified in the radical prostatectomy.[12,13] As long as negative margins are achieved, these "precursor type" intraductal carcinomas would be regarded as essentially cured with a dramatically better long-term prognosis compared with typical cases of intraductal carcinoma, which are typically associated with invasive, aggressive tumors and thus associated with a significant risk for disease recurrence after definitive therapy even if the surgical margins are free of tumor.

Whether IDC-P should be graded and incorporated in the final Gleason score is subject to debate and is discussed in more detail in the article "Cribriform Lesions of the Prostate Gland."

Distinction of intraductal carcinoma from Gleason patterns 4 or 5 adenocarcinoma is often made using immunohistochemical stains for basal cell markers. However, there are several morphologic features on routine hematoxylin & eosin (H&E) stained sections, which if present can be either indicative or highly suggestive of intraductal carcinoma (**Fig. 1**).

However, immunohistochemical stains are not useful for distinguishing intraductal carcinoma from high-grade prostatic intraepithelial neoplasia (HGPIN). This differential diagnosis is resolved solely by strict adherence to the morphologic criteria for intraductal carcinoma,[14] which mandate either solid or dense cribriform architecture where the volume of neoplastic epithelium unequivocally exceeds that of the luminal spaces. In the absence of these features, lesions with loose cribriform architecture but with either comedo necrosis or frankly anaplastic cytological features that are far beyond the morphologic spectrum of HGPIN qualify for the diagnosis. Noninvasive lesions with some but not all of the criteria for intraductal carcinoma should be labeled as atypical intraductal proliferations (AIP).[15] Many of these lesions likely represent incipient or undersampled intraductal carcinoma and merit distinction from HGPIN, the latter, a diagnosis, which currently has lost clinical significance.[16] Lesions previously diagnosed as cribriform HGPIN should now be considered as either AIP or intraductal carcinoma depending on the degree of epithelial density, cytological atypia, and/or necrosis.[17]

MORPHOLOGIC ISSUES IN GLEASON SCORING

Gleason pattern 3 consists of individual, well-formed, discrete glands with patent lumina (ie, not fused or poorly formed). As long as adjacent well-formed glands can be discerned from each other, an architecture consisting of back-to-back glands should be regarded as Gleason pattern 3.

The presence of mucin associated with neoplastic epithelium in a prostate biopsy raises a number of potential issues. First, one should at least consider the possibility of a metastasis before assuming a prostatic primary and proceeding with grading. Specifically, intracellular mucin in the form of signet ring cells or goblet cells is vanishingly rare in prostatic adenocarcinoma, and this finding should raise suspicion for involvement by adenocarcinoma from another primary site such as colon, bladder, or urethra.[18,19] The rare myxoid/mucinous variant of urothelial carcinoma is also a potential consideration but if one

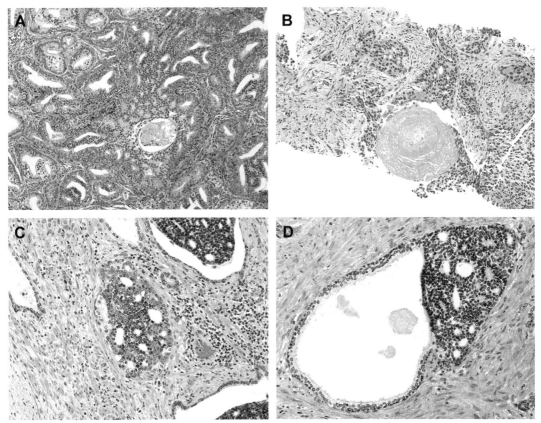

Fig. 1. Intraductal carcinoma of the prostate. (*A*) Large, dense cribriform glands with branching contours should raise the possibility of intraductal carcinoma versus invasive cribriform, Gleason pattern 4 adenocarcinoma. (*B*) The presence of corpora amylacea in association with a dense cribriform glandular proliferation is suspicious for colonization of preexisting benign glands by high-grade carcinoma. (*C*) A somewhat subtle example of intraductal carcinoma showing partial involvement of a preexisting benign gland where the intraductal carcinoma has nearly entirely replaced a benign gland, with only a small strip of residual nonneoplastic epithelium at left. (*D*) A more overt example from the same case showing partial glandular involvement with an abrupt transition from benign glandular epithelium (left) to intraductal carcinoma at right. Partial involvement of benign glands is the most definitive morphologic feature that a dense cribriform proliferation represents intraductal carcinoma rather than invasive cribriform carcinoma.

subtracts the extracellular material, these tumors show typical cytologic features of urothelial carcinoma and are usually admixed with conventional urothelial carcinoma.[20] If necessary, a panel of stains anchored by NKX3.1 and GATA3 can be helpful, with the caveat that a rare subset of GG5 prostatic adenocarcinomas may aberrantly express GATA3.[21] Markers of intestinal differentiation such as CDX2 should be interpreted with caution given that expression may be seen in urothelial carcinoma and prostatic carcinomas in addition to adenocarcinomas of true gastrointestinal origin.[22,23]

However, secreted, extracellular, intraluminal mucin is typical of prostatic adenocarcinoma and although not entirely specific, this can be a useful feature to support the diagnosis of carcinoma in a small focus. Extracellular, extraluminal mucin that is not surrounded by glandular epithelium is pathognomonic for adenocarcinoma if associated with neoplastic prostatic epithelium. When prostatic adenocarcinoma is associated with extracellular, extraluminal mucin, grading has historically been somewhat controversial. Some important concepts to evaluating such tumors are as follows. First, the diagnosis of prostatic mucinous adenocarcinoma can only be made at the time of radical prostatectomy because this designation requires that at least 25% of the tumor mass consists of neoplastic epithelium floating within pools of extracellular, extraglandular mucin. Therefore, in any biopsy or transurethral resection, the terminology prostatic adenocarcinoma with mucinous features is recommended. The Gleason score and GG ultimately drive the prognosis of these tumors rather than the presence or extent of the extra-glandular mucin.[24,25] Therefore, the key tasks of the pathologist when encountering a mucinous tumor in the prostate are to consider and exclude metastasis, and to avoid being distracted by the extracellular material and focus on grading the tumor based on the underlying architecture of the neoplastic epithelium. As with nonmucinous tumors, individual, well-formed glands are graded as Gleason pattern 3, with fused or cribriform glands representing Gleason pattern 4.

Related to the issue of extraglandular, extracellular mucin is mucinous fibroplasia, which is also quite useful in establishing a malignant diagnosis in limited material[26,27] but can make grading challenging due to the architectural distortion of the associated epithelium. In effect, mucinous fibroplasia artifactually inflates the architectural complexity of neoplastic glands, leading to potential overdiagnosis of Gleason pattern 3 carcinoma as higher grade tumor. It is critical to recognize mucinous fibroplasia before grading prostatic adenocarcinoma because this finding should significantly raise one's threshold for diagnosing pattern 4. In areas of mucinous fibroplasia, pattern 3 should be the default diagnosis and in order to assign Gleason pattern 4 or 5, patterns that are unattributable to distortion from mucinous fibroplasia are required.[28] Specifically, one cannot rely on the presence of poorly formed or fused glands in the setting of mucinous fibroplasia because these can easily be the result of tissue distortion rather than the presence of true Gleason pattern 4. Typically, overtly cribriform glands that cannot be ascribed to mucinous fibroplasia should be present to diagnose Gleason pattern 4 in this setting.

Key considerations to note before assigning Gleason pattern 4 are to ensure that one is not overdiagnosing a few tangentially cut, poorly formed glands at the periphery of a focus of otherwise Gleason pattern 3 tumor; examination of sequential levels with resolution of such a focus into well-formed glands helps to avoid this pitfall, as does requiring a minimum number of at least a discrete cluster of several poorly formed glands before considering a focus as a minimal amount of Gleason pattern 4.[29] Although the pattern of poorly formed glands is susceptible to overinterpretation due to tangential sectioning, a single bona fide cribriform gland should be regarded as pattern 4 because this architecture cannot be ascribed to tangential sectioning of a pattern 3 gland. A comprehensive discussion of the key differential diagnoses to consider when encountering cribriform glands are addressed in a separate article in this issue and include AIP as well as IDCP as discussed above.

Before diagnosing Gleason pattern 5, particularly in the absence of adjacent Gleason pattern 3 and/or 4, a variety of entities should be systematically considered and excluded. Two common entities that frequently mimic pattern 5 prostatic adenocarcinoma are small cell carcinoma and urothelial carcinoma. Prominent mitotic and apoptotic activity, high nuclear-to-cytoplasmic ratio, nuclear molding, geographic necrosis, and the absence of prominent central nucleoli are features that should trigger further studies to exclude small cell carcinoma.[30] Expression of neuroendocrine markers alone without appropriate morphologic features is insufficient to warrant the diagnosis of small cell carcinoma because acinar adenocarcinoma of various grades is known to express neuroendocrine markers.[31] In the appropriate morphologic context, the absence of significant expression of all markers of prostatic acinar differentiation including NKX3.1, P501S, and PSA, is much more compelling evidence of small cell carcinoma than expression of neuroendocrine markers such as synaptophysin, chromogranin, or INSM1.[32] Immunohistochemical loss of Rb is emerging as a useful marker to support the diagnosis of small cell carcinoma as part of a panel of immunostains in the differential diagnosis with GG5 adenocarcinoma.[33] Small cell carcinoma usually arises during or after androgen deprivation therapy and is therefore considered a form of "treatment-related neuroendocrine prostatic carcinoma." Prominent desmoplasia or tumor-associated inflammation, nuclear pleomorphism, or squamoid features are suggestive of urothelial carcinoma.[34,35] Both benign (xanthoma or nonspecific granulomatous prostatitis [NSGP]) and malignant (hematolymphoid neoplasms) nonepithelial lesions may also merit consideration, and if suspected, immunohistochemical stains should readily resolve the differential diagnosis.[36,37] When the question is fundamentally related to lineage, it is best to use broad spectrum epithelial markers such as CAM5.2 as opposed to prostate-specific markers which can be negative in poorly differentiated tumors. Also recommended is an appropriate panel of markers targeted to the relevant differential diagnosis (CD163 or CD68 for xanthoma or NSGP, CD45 or other lineage-associated markers such as CD20 for hematolymphoid lesions). Particularly when considering a diagnosis of pattern 5 prostatic adenocarcinoma based on the presence of cribriform or solid glands with central comedo type necrosis, intraductal carcinoma should be a strong consideration. Recent evidence suggests that foci previously diagnosed as Gleason pattern

5 based on comedo-necrosis frequently turn out to be intraductal carcinoma when examined by immunohistochemistry for basal cells.[38] In summary, before arriving at a diagnosis of Gleason pattern 5 adenocarcinoma, one should confirm the lesion is truly epithelial, of prostatic origin, glandular rather than neuroendocrine, and invasive.

SELECTED SITUATIONS WHERE PROSTATIC ADENOCARCINOMA SHOULD NOT BE GRADED

Accurate, consistent assignment of the Gleason score and GG is likely the most important task for the pathologist in cases of invasive prostatic adenocarcinoma. However, it is equally important to recognize select rare but specific circumstances, in which Gleason scoring is specifically not recommended and if applied may be misleading or detrimental to patient care. If these situations are not recognized, patients may be exposed to significant overtreatment because applying Gleason scoring would significantly overestimate the biologic potential of the tumor. Two common scenarios in which invasive prostatic adenocarcinoma should not be graded are those in which the morphology has been altered by either radiation and/or androgen deprivation therapy. These interventions result in reproducible morphologic changes to invasive prostatic adenocarcinoma, which cause Gleason scoring to drastically overstate its aggressiveness. Following androgen deprivation or radiation, even GG1 or GG2 tumors may acquire the architecture of Gleason patterns 4 or 5.[39] However, paradoxically when tumors demonstrate radiation or androgen deprivation effect, despite growing with architecture similar to highly aggressive untreated tumors, biologically they are senescent and such changes actually correlate with favorable clinical outcomes. Therefore, such cases should be reported as prostate adenocarcinoma with treatment effect and no Gleason score or GG should be assigned. Histologically, several key features are useful for distinguishing tumors with treatment effect with architectural features of Gleason patterns 4 and 5 from bona fide GG4 or GG5 tumors. Nuclear pyknosis is a hallmark of adenocarcinoma with androgen deprivation effect such that tumor cells may be confused with lymphocytes. Cytoplasmic vacuolization is characteristic of adenocarcinoma with radiation effect such that tumor cells may be confused with histiocytes.[40] Immunohistochemical stains for low molecular weight keratin such as CAM5.2 are the most reliable ancillary study for addressing the differential diagnosis between subtle tumor cells and inflammatory cells. Perhaps the most useful feature is the presence of characteristic therapy-related changes within adjacent benign prostatic epithelium that should raise suspicion for the presence of nearby tumor with androgen deprivation or radiation effect (Fig. 2). Atrophy of secretory cells with concomitant diffuse prominence of basal cells signify successful blockade of androgen signaling.[41] Glands lined by multilayered epithelium streaming parallel to the basement membrane, with large bizarre but degenerative appearing nuclei interspersed among smaller cells are features diagnostic of radiated benign prostate tissue.[42] As mentioned previously, patients receiving radiation often also receive hormonal therapy, and thus, the presence of one effect on either benign or malignant epithelium should raise suspicion for the other. If there is viable carcinoma that shows no evidence of treatment effect, usual Gleason grading and GGs should be applied, and importantly, the absence of therapy effect on the tumor should be explicitly stated. However, if only tumor with treatment effect is identified, prostatic adenocarcinoma with treatment effect should be diagnosed with a note explaining that grading is not applicable.

There are 2 rare variants of prostate cancer, which, if one focused solely on the architectural features, would be often graded as aggressive carcinomas because they frequently display Gleason patterns 4 or 5. However, in stark contrast to usual prostatic adenocarcinoma, their architecture does not reflect their biologic potential, and the available evidence indicates these are quite indolent variants of prostatic adenocarcinoma. Therefore, although prostatic adenocarcinoma with aberrant P63 expression and prostatic adenocarcinoma with Paneth cell–like differentiation frequently show areas unequivocally qualifying for Gleason patterns 4 and 5, conventional Gleason scoring could potentially lead to dramatic overtreatment.[43–46] Thus, the primary significance of these variants for pathologists is to avoid reflexively diagnosing high-grade prostatic adenocarcinoma based on architecture alone; instead, cytological features are the key to their recognition.

Prostatic adenocarcinoma with aberrant P63 expression may seem similar morphologically to usual prostatic adenocarcinoma, in which case it may be graded as such; however, the classic appearance is a combination of basaloid nests composed of atrophic cells, which may even raise the differential diagnosis of basal cell hyperplasia or basal cell carcinoma (Fig. 3).[47] Importantly, although the tumor cells are strongly P63 positive

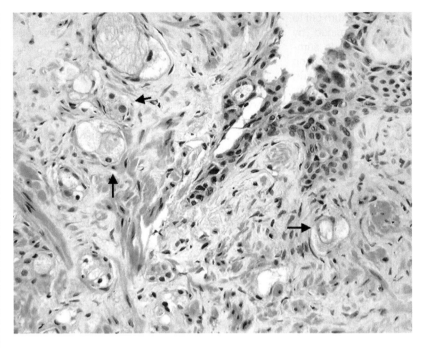

Fig. 2. Benign prostate tissue with radiation effect with adjacent invasive adenocarcinoma with radiation effect. Atrophic glands lined by epithelium, which streams parallel to the basement membrane (upper right) are classic features of benign prostate tissue with radiation effect. These glands are lined by an admixture of smaller cells with interspersed larger nuclei with degenerative features including smudgy chromatin and intranuclear pseudoinclusions. Infiltrating between these benign glands (*arrows*) are nests and clusters of epithelioid cells, some with cytoplasmic vacuolization and abundant eosinophilic cytoplasm, morphology typical of adenocarcinoma with radiation effect.

by definition, staining for high-molecular weight cytokeratin should be absent, in contrast to basal cell proliferations. Prostatic adenocarcinoma with Paneth cell–like differentiation may architecturally resemble either low or high grade usual prostatic adenocarcinoma but usually shows distinctive cytoplasmic granularity, which can be confirmed with diffuse expression of neuroendocrine markers even in a subset of rare cases where the eosinophilic granules may be less prominent or absent morphologically.[43] Prostatic adenocarcinoma with Paneth cell–like differentiation also demonstrates intensely amphophilic, purplish cytoplasm and trabecular or corded architectural patterns reminiscent of well-differentiated neuroendocrine tumors of other sites (**Fig. 4**), and typically lacks

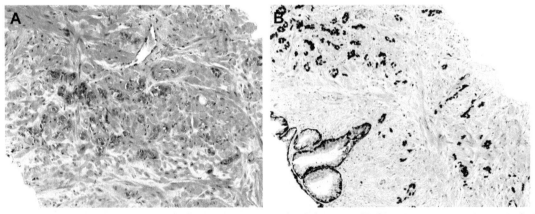

Fig. 3. Prostatic adenocarcinoma with aberrant P63 expression. (*A*). Focus of infiltrating carcinoma composed of nests, cords, and single cells, which immediately suggest the possibility of invasive high-grade prostatic adenocarcinoma. (*B*) PIN4 immunostain confirms the diagnosis, demonstrating diffuse nuclear P63 expression in lesional cells. The absence of high molecular weight cytokeratin staining along with the infiltrative morphologic appearance support the diagnosis of invasive carcinoma. Appropriate basal cell labeling for both cytokeratin and P63 in adjacent benign prostate tissue (bottom left) serves as a useful internal control.

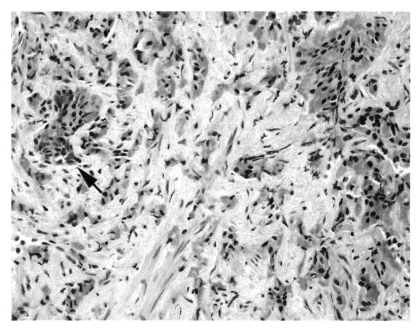

Fig. 4. Prostatic adenocarcinoma with Paneth cell–like differentiation. Infiltrating cords and nests of epithelioid cells with prominent amphophilic to purple cytoplasm is characteristic. This example shows that this tumor can occasionally lack the characteristic bright red to orange cytoplasmic granules, which are focally present at left (arrow) but absent in the remainder of the tumor. The cytoplasmic character and corded, nested architecture reminiscent of well-differentiated neuroendocrine tumors from other sites help to identify cases that lack abundant red cytoplasmic granules.

the high-grade nuclear atypia and prominent nucleoli that would be expected in the vast majority of high grade usual prostatic adenocarcinomas.

SUMMARY

In this review, key concepts related to grading and reporting prostatic adenocarcinoma have been discussed. The extinction of Gleason patterns 1 and 2 and clarification of reporting Gleason scoring using GGs are important developments. The clinical ramifications of distinguishing Gleason patterns 3 and 4 are highlighted, as is the resulting emphasis on reporting the percentage of Gleason pattern 4 on a routine basis in cases lacking GG5 adenocarcinoma. An approach to the recognition and reporting of intraductal carcinoma is provided; particular attention to this entity is warranted in cases lacking concurrent high-grade invasive carcinoma due to its heightened clinical significance in this setting. Selected morphologic issues specific to each Gleason score are discussed, with mucinous fibroplasia and mucinous features potentially complicating the diagnosis of Gleason pattern 3, crowded or tangentially sectioned foci of Gleason pattern 3 potentially leading to overdiagnosis of pattern 4, and small cell carcinoma, intraductal carcinoma, and urothelial carcinoma representing key mimickers of Gleason pattern 5. Although diligent application of Gleason scoring is the most important task of the pathologist in the vast majority of prostatic adenocarcinomas, a rare subset of tumors that deceptively demonstrate high-grade architectural patterns despite biological indolence is highlighted. These tumors should not be graded because the Gleason grading system would overestimate their malignant potential, potentially leading to unnecessary overtreatment.

CLINICS CARE POINTS

- Grade Groups stratify prostatic adenocarcinomas into 5 prognostic distinct groups, enabling pathology reports to clearly communicate that Gleason score 3 + 3 = 6 adenocarcinoma (Grade Group 1) is the lowest grade prostatic adenocarcinoma.

- Gleason Pattern 4 is critical to recognize because it signifies a risk for more aggressive behavior than Gleason Pattern 3 carcinoma, and therefore has major implications for patient management.

- Gleason pattern 3 with mucinous fibroplasia, tangential sectioning, and mucinous features are key patterns to recognize in order to avoid overdiagnosis of Gleason pattern 4.

- Intraductal carcinoma, small cell carcinoma, urothelial carcinoma, xanthoma, and lymphoma are important mimickers of Gleason Pattern 5, and should force one to confirm the tumor is epithelial, invasive, glandular rather than neuroendocrine, and prostatic in origin before diagnosing Gleason Pattern 5.

- Because morphologically unremarkable usual prostatic adenocarcinoma of all grades may express neuroendocrine markers, immunohistochemical expression of neuroendocrine markers in prostatic adenocarcinoma without morphologic features of small cell carcinoma has no clinical significance. Therefore, in the absence of morphologic features concerning for neuroendocrine carcinoma, stains for neuroendocrine differentiation should not be performed on prostatic adenocarcinoma.

- In the appropriate morphologic context, the absence of significant expression of markers of prostatic acinar differentiation, including NKX3.1, P501S, and PSA, is much more compelling evidence of small cell carcinoma than expression of neuroendocrine markers such as synaptophysin, chromogranin, or INSM1.

- Prostatic adenocarcinoma with radiation or androgen therapy effect, with aberrant P63 expression, or with Paneth cell–like differentiation represent pitfalls in prostate cancer grading because although they display architecture associated with aggressive behavior in usual prostatic adenocarcinoma, they do not behave aggressively. Grading these tumors by assigning a Gleason score and corresponding Grade Group would significantly overstate their biologic potential.

DISCLOSURE

The authors have nothing to disclose.

REFERENCES

1. Epstein JI, Zelefsky MJ, Sjoberg DD, et al. A contemporary prostate cancer grading system: a validated alternative to the gleason score. Eur Urol 2016;69(3):428–35.
2. Humphrey PA, Moch H, Cubilla AL, et al. The 2016 WHO classification of tumours of the urinary system and male genital organs-part b: prostate and bladder tumours. Eur Urol 2016;70(1):106–19.
3. Mohler JL, Antonarakis ES, Armstrong AJ, et al. Prostate cancer, version 2.2019, NCCN clinical practice guidelines in oncology. J Natl Compr Canc Netw 2019;17(5):479–505.
4. Epstein JI, Amin MB, Fine SW, et al. The 2019 genitourinary pathology society (GUPS) white paper on contemporary grading of prostate cancer. Arch Pathol Lab Med 2021;145(4):461–93.
5. Cole AI, Morgan TM, Spratt DE, et al. Prognostic value of percent gleason grade 4 at prostate biopsy in predicting prostatectomy pathology and recurrence. J Urol 2016;196(2):405–11.
6. Mohler JL, Antonarakis ES. NCCN guidelines updates: management of prostate cancer. J Natl Compr Canc Netw 2019;17(5):583–6.
7. Sadimin ET, Khani F, Diolombi M, et al. Interobserver reproducibility of percent gleason pattern 4 in prostatic adenocarcinoma on prostate biopsies. Am J Surg Pathol 2016;40(12):1686–92.
8. Trpkov K, Zhang J, Chan M, et al. Prostate cancer with tertiary Gleason pattern 5 in prostate needle biopsy: clinicopathologic findings and disease progression. Am J Surg Pathol 2009;33(2):233–40.
9. Baras AS, Nelson JB, Han M, et al. The effect of limited (tertiary) Gleason pattern 5 on the new prostate cancer grade groups. Hum Pathol 2017;63:27–32.
10. Wobker SE, Epstein JI. Differential diagnosis of intraductal lesions of the prostate. Am J Surg Pathol 2016;40(6):e67–82.
11. Porter LH, Lawrence MG, Ilic D, et al. Systematic review links the prevalence of intraductal carcinoma of the prostate to prostate cancer risk categories. Eur Urol 2017;72(4):492–5.
12. Robinson BD, Epstein JI. Intraductal carcinoma of the prostate without invasive carcinoma on needle biopsy: emphasis on radical prostatectomy findings. J Urol 2010;184(4):1328–33.
13. Khani F, Wobker SE, Hicks JL, et al. Intraductal carcinoma of the prostate in the absence of high-grade invasive carcinoma represents a molecularly distinct type of in situ carcinoma enriched with oncogenic driver mutations. J Pathol 2019;249(1):79–89.
14. Guo CC, Epstein JI. Intraductal carcinoma of the prostate on needle biopsy: Histologic features and clinical significance. Mod Pathol 2006;19(12):1528–35.
15. Miyai K, Divatia MK, Shen SS, et al. Clinicopathological analysis of intraductal proliferative lesions of prostate: intraductal carcinoma of prostate, high-grade prostatic intraepithelial neoplasia, and atypical cribriform lesion. Hum Pathol 2014;45(8):1572–81.
16. Herawi M, Kahane H, Cavallo C, et al. Risk of prostate cancer on first re-biopsy within 1 year following a diagnosis of high grade prostatic intraepithelial neoplasia is related to the number of cores sampled. J Urol 2006;175:121–4.
17. Shah RB, Nguyen JK, Przybycin CG, et al. Atypical intraductal proliferation detected in prostate needle biopsy is a marker of unsampled intraductal carcinoma and other adverse pathological features: a prospective clinicopathological study of 62 cases with emphasis on pathological outcomes. Histopathology 2019;75(3):346–53.
18. Osunkoya AO. Mucinous and secondary tumors of the prostate. Mod Pathol 2018;31(S1):S80–95.

19. Bohman KD, Osunkoya AO. Mucin-producing tumors and tumor-like lesions involving the prostate: a comprehensive review. Adv Anat Pathol 2012; 19(6):374–87.

20. Tavora F, Epstein JI. Urothelial carcinoma with abundant myxoid stroma. Hum Pathol 2009;40(10):1391–8.

21. McDonald TM, Epstein JI. Aberrant GATA3 staining in prostatic adenocarcinoma: a potential diagnostic pitfall. Am J Surg Pathol 2021;45(3):341–6.

22. Leite KR, Mitteldorf CA, Srougi M, et al. Cdx2, cytokeratin 20, thyroid transcription factor 1, and prostate-specific antigen expression in unusual subtypes of prostate cancer. Ann Diagn Pathol 2008; 12(4):260–6.

23. Herawi M, De Marzo AM, Kristiansen G, et al. Expression of CDX2 in benign tissue and adenocarcinoma of the prostate. Hum Pathol 2007;38(1):72–8.

24. Osunkoya AO, Nielsen ME, Epstein JI. Prognosis of mucinous adenocarcinoma of the prostate treated by radical prostatectomy: a study of 47 cases. Am J Surg Pathol 2008;32:468–72.

25. Epstein JI, Egevad L, Amin MB, et al. The 2014 international society of urological pathology (ISUP) consensus conference on gleason grading of prostatic carcinoma: definition of grading patterns and proposal for a new grading system. Am J Surg Pathol 2016;40(2):244–52.

26. Baisden BL, Kahane H, Epstein JI. Perineural invasion, mucinous fibroplasia, and glomerulations: diagnostic features of limited cancer on prostate needle biopsy. Am J Surg Pathol 1999;23(8):918–24.

27. Magi-Galluzzi C. Prostate cancer: diagnostic criteria and role of immunohistochemistry. Mod Pathol 2018; 31(S1):S12–21.

28. Epstein JI, Allsbrook WC Jr, Amin MB, et al. The 2005 International Society of Urological Pathology (ISUP) consensus conference on Gleason grading of prostatic carcinoma. Am J Surg Pathol 2005;29:1228–42.

29. Zhou M, Li J, Cheng L, et al. Diagnosis of "poorly formed glands" gleason pattern 4 prostatic adenocarcinoma on needle biopsy: an interobserver reproducibility study among urologic pathologists with recommendations. Am J Surg Pathol 2015;39(10): 1331–9.

30. Epstein JI, Amin MB, Beltran H, et al. Proposed morphologic classification of prostate cancer with neuroendocrine differentiation. Am J Surg Pathol 2014;38(6):756–67.

31. Kaur H, Samarska I, Lu J, et al. Neuroendocrine differentiation in usual-type prostatic adenocarcinoma: Molecular characterization and clinical significance. Prostate 2020;80(12):1012–23.

32. Nadal R, Schweizer M, Kryvenko ON, et al. Small cell carcinoma of the prostate. Nat Rev Urol 2014; 11(4):213–9.

33. Tan HL, Sood A, Rahimi HA, et al. Rb loss is characteristic of prostatic small cell neuroendocrine carcinoma. Clin Cancer Res 2014;20(4):890–903. Epub 2013 Dec 9.

34. Sanguedolce F, Russo D, Mancini V, et al. Morphological and Immunohistochemical biomarkers in distinguishing prostate carcinoma and urothelial carcinoma: a comprehensive review. Int J Surg Pathol 2019;27(2):120–33.

35. Chuang AY, DeMarzo AM, Veltri RW, et al. Immunohistochemical differentiation of high-grade prostate carcinoma from urothelial carcinoma. Am J Surg Pathol 2007;31(8):1246–55.

36. Chuang AY, Epstein JI. Xanthoma of the prostate: a mimicker of high-grade prostate adenocarcinoma. Am J Surg Pathol 2007;31(8):1225–30.

37. Oppenheimer JR, Kahane H, Epstein JI. Granulomatous prostatitis on needle biopsy. Arch Pathol Lab Med 1997;121(7):724–9.

38. Fine SW, Al-Ahmadie HA, Chen YB, et al. Comedonecrosis revisited: strong association with intraductal carcinoma of the prostate. Am J Surg Pathol 2018;42(8):1036–41.

39. Srigley JR, Delahunt B, Evans AJ. Therapy-associated effects in the prostate gland. Histopathology 2012;60(1):153–65.

40. Gaudin PB, Zelefsky MJ, Leibel SA. Histopathological effects of three-dimensional conformal external beam radiation therapy on benign and malignant prostate tissues. Am J Surg Pathol 1999;23:1021–31.

41. Reuter VE. Pathological changes in benign and malignant prostatic tissue following androgen deprivation therapy. Urology 1997;49(3A Suppl):16–22.

42. Magi-Galluzzi C, Sanderson H, Epstein JI. Atypia in nonneoplastic prostate glands after radiotherapy for prostate cancer: duration of atypia and relation to type of radiotherapy. Am J Surg Pathol 2003;27(2): 206–12.

43. So JS, Gordetsky J, Epstein JI. Variant of prostatic adenocarcinoma with Paneth cell-like neuroendocrine differentiation readily misdiagnosed as Gleason pattern 5. Hum Pathol 2014;45(12):2388–93.

44. Salles DC, Mata DA, Epstein JI. Significance of Paneth cell-like differentiation in prostatic adenocarcinoma: a retrospective cohort study of 80 cases. Hum Pathol 2020;102:7–12.

45. Giannico GA, Ross HM, Lotan T, et al. Aberrant expression of p63 in adenocarcinoma of the prostate: a radical prostatectomy study. Am J Surg Pathol 2013;37(9):1401–6.

46. Tan HL, Haffner MC, Esopi DM, et al. Prostate adenocarcinomas aberrantly expressing p63 are molecularly distinct from usual-type prostatic adenocarcinomas. Mod Pathol 2015;28(3):446–56.

47. Osunkoya AO, Hansel DE, Sun X, et al. Aberrant diffuse expression of p63 in adenocarcinoma of the prostate on needle biopsy and radical prostatectomy: report of 21 cases. Am J Surg Pathol 2008; 32(3):461–7.

Cribriform Lesions of the Prostate Gland

Qi Cai, MD, Rajal B. Shah, MD*

KEYWORDS

- Cribriform • Prostate adenocarcinoma • Intraductal carcinoma • Ductal adenocarcinoma
- Atypical intraductal proliferation • High-grade prostatic intraepithelial neoplasia
- Clear cell cribriform hyperplasia • Central zone gland

Key points

- Cribriform lesions of the prostate gland are of wide-ranging significance from normal anatomical variation, benign proliferative lesions, premalignant, suspicious to frankly malignant and biologically aggressive.

- Both cribriform prostate adenocarcinoma (CrP4) and intraductal carcinoma of the prostate (IDC-P) are independent predictors of aggressive tumor behavior and potentially affect clinical decision making in prostate cancer (PCa) management.

- Due to their shared clinical significance, molecular features, and "cribriform" morphology, contemporary studies have lumped CrP4 and IDC-P as PCa with "cribriform architecture".

- Both the Genitourinary Pathology Society (GUPS) and International Society of Urologic Pathology (ISUP) recommend reporting the presence of CrP4 and IDC-P in prostate biopsy and radical prostatectomy specimens.

- Vast majority of IDC-P represents a "retrograde" spread of associated high-grade and high volume PCa; pure IDC-P without invasive component is rare.

- Whether IDC-P component in the presence of invasive PCa should be graded or not remains controversial.

- The diagnosis of cribriform HGPIN in biopsy setting is not recommended as underlying IDC-P could not be excluded; such lesion should be diagnosed as "atypical intraductal proliferation, suspicious for IDC-P".

ABSTRACT

"Cribriform lesions of the prostate represent an important and often diagnostically challenging spectrum of prostate pathology. These lesions range from normal anatomical variation, benign proliferative lesions, premalignant, suspicious to frankly malignant and biologically aggressive entities. The concept of cribriform prostate adenocarcinoma (CrP4) and intraductal carcinoma of the prostate (IDC-P), in particular, has evolved significantly in recent years with a growing body of evidence suggesting that the presence of these morphologies is important for clinical decision-making in prostate cancer management. Therefore, accurate recognition and reporting of CrP4 and IDC-P architecture are especially important. This review discusses a contemporary diagnostic approach to cribriform lesions of the prostate with a focus on their key morphologic features, differential diagnosis, underlying molecular alterations, clinical significance, and reporting recommendations."

Department of Pathology, 04.449, The University of Texas Southwestern Medical Center, 5323 Harry Hines Boulevard, Dallas, TX 75390, USA
* Corresponding author.
E-mail address: Rajal.Shah@UTSouthwestern.edu
Twitter: @rajalbshah (R.B.S.)

Surgical Pathology 15 (2022) 591–608
https://doi.org/10.1016/j.path.2022.07.001
1875-9181/22/© 2022 Elsevier Inc. All rights reserved.

Abbreviations	
CrP4	Cribriform Prostate Adenocarcinoma
IDC-P	Introductal Carcinoma of the Prostate
PCa	Prostate Cancer
GUPS	Genitourinary Pathology Society
ISUP	Internatiional Society of Urologic Pathology
AIP	Atypical Intraductal Proliferation
HGPIN	High Grade Prostatic Intraepithelial Neoplasia
PTEN	Phosphatase And Tensin Homolog
ERG	ETS Transcription Factor ERG
EPE	Extraprostatic Extension
PNI	Perineural Invasion
RP	Prostatectomy
GG	Grade Group
GS	Gleason Score
mpMRI	Multiparametric Magnetic Resonance Imaging
ADC	Apparent Diffusion Coefficient
NCCN	National Comprehensive Cancer Network
PSA	Prostate Specific Antigen
PSMA	Prostate Specific Membrane Antigen
NKX3.1	NK3 Homeobox 1
CDX2	Caudal Type Homeobox 2
CK	Cytokeratin
GATA3	GATA Binding Protein 3

BACKGROUND

Over the last several years, accumulating evidence suggests that malignant cribriform lesions, specifically cribriform prostate adenocarcinoma (CrP4) and intraductal carcinoma of the prostate (IDC-P), are independent predictors of aggressive tumor behavior and potentially affect clinical decision making in prostate cancer (PCa) management. However, in practice, there are several problem areas that may create difficulty in the diagnosis and reporting of CrP4 and IDC-P. Specifically, the distinction of CrP4 from certain PCa morphologies and the distinction of borderline atypical intraductal proliferations (AIP) from cribriform high grade prostatic intraepithelial neoplasia (HGPIN) can be challenging. In addition, it remains controversial when CrP4 should be distinguished for grading purposes from IDC-P which also typically presents as "cribriform architecture" and connotes adverse outcomes. The Genitourinary Pathology Society (GUPS) and International Society of Urologic Pathology (ISUP) recommend reporting the presence of CrP4 and IDC-P in both prostate biopsy and prostatectomy specimens. These recommendations require practicing pathologists be able to make an accurate and reproducible diagnosis of these clinically significant cribriform lesions. This review focuses on clinically significant cribriform lesions, specifically CrP4, IDC-P, ductal adenocarcinoma, and AIP. Benign cribriform lesions that mimic clinically significant lesions have been addressed in the differential diagnosis section.

DEFINITION OF THE CRIBRIFORM GLAND

The word "cribriform" is derived from the Latin word cribrum ("sieve") which means an object containing many perforations. In pathology, it describes glands composed of sheets of tumor cells that form cohesive rounded or irregularly shaped trabeculae with perforations or multiple "punched out" lumina. The cribriform glands could have a rounded, oblong, or irregular contour.

MORPHOLOGICAL SPECTRUM OF CRIBRIFORM LESIONS

There is a broad spectrum of prostate lesions that display cribriform architecture, including benign, premalignant, suspicious, to frankly malignant, and biologically aggressive entities. Entities within each category are listed in **Table 1**.

A GENERAL DIAGNOSTIC APPROACH TO PROSTATE CRIBRIFORM LESIONS

A general diagnostic approach to cribriform lesions is illustrated in **Fig. 1**.

The first step is a careful evaluation of cytoplasmic and nuclear characteristics of secretory epithelial cells, specifically nuclear enlargement, prominent nucleoli, coarse chromatin, and nuclear pleomorphism. Benign proliferations demonstrate clear or eosinophilic cytoplasm and bland nuclear features while atypical cribriform lesions are characterized by amphophilic cytoplasm and nuclear atypia in secretory cells. Careful low power evaluation of architectural characteristics of atypical cribriform lesions also provides important diagnostic clues. The presence of confluent mass forming or back-to-back atypical cribriform gland growth, the presence of irregular infiltrative borders, perineural invasion, or extraprostatic extension would typically suggest an invasive process (**Fig. 2**). For a lesion that lacks obvious morphologic features of invasion, systemic evaluation of several additional architectural and cytological features (number of glands as a few versus multiple, size of glands in relation to adjacent benign glands, gland contour as regular versus branching, loose versus dense proliferation, degree of cellular pleomorphism, intraluminal necrosis and presence of basal cells) and in some cases Phosphatase And Tensin Homolog (PTEN) and ETS

Table 1

Morphological spectrum of cribriform lesions of the prostate gland

Benign	*Borderline (suspicious)*
• Central zone glands	• Atypical intraductal proliferation (AIP)
• Reactive glands with psuedocribriform architecture	
• Clear cell cribriform hyperplasia	
• Basal cell hyperplasia	

Preneoplastic	*Malignant*
• Cribriform HGPIN	• Intraductal carcinoma (IDC-P)
	• Invasive cribriform carcinoma
	• Ductal adenocarcinoma
	• Basal cell carcinoma

Transcription Factor ERG (ERG) biomarkers may provide additional help in resolving the diagnosis.

CRIBRIFORM PROSTATE ADENOCARCINOMA

CLINICAL SIGNIFICANCE

All CrP4 regardless of its size and shape are currently graded as Gleason pattern 4.[1] There is growing evidence that CrP4 in both biopsies and radical prostatectomies (RP) is associated with adverse clinical outcomes, including worse biochemical recurrence-free, metastasis-free, and cancer-specific survival than those without.[2–6] Specifically, CrP4 carries a much higher risk of disease progression compared to the other Gleason grade 4 patterns.[3,6] Among men with grade group (GG) 2 PCa at biopsy, some studies have demonstrated a higher risk of failure in the presence of cribriform morphology, while patients without cribriform architecture carried the same risk as GG1 cancer, implying that CrP4 diagnosis might affect clinical decision making.[7] Whereas the value of cribriform architecture has mostly been studied for Gleason score (GS) 7 patients, some studies have demonstrated its independent prognostic value in men with GS 8 and GS 9-10 PCa.[8] However, the majority of studies addressing the significance of CrP4 have not distinguished between IDC-P and CrP4 to determine outcomes, and have referred to these lesions collectively as "cribriform growth", limiting assessment of the independent influence of these parameters. Recently, a further modification to the Gleason system by incorporating cribriform morphology to improve its prognostic utility has been proposed.[9] Due to multiple lines of evidence supporting the association with adverse outcomes, both the GUPS and the ISUP recommended reporting of CrP4 in needle biopsy and RP specimen.[10,11]

MORPHOLOGICAL FEATURES

Although the cribriform pattern has the best interobserver reproducibility among genitourinary pathologists (ranging from 54%-79%) compared with other Gleason 4 patterns,[12–15] there is still a significant variability and ambiguity in diagnosing this pattern. Specifically, differentiation of CrP4 from complex fused glands, complex glands with papillary proliferation, glands with partial or Roman bridging, complex "glomeruloid-like" growth pattern, or PCa exhibiting complex cribriform-like morphology but with intra- or extra-glandular mucin or involving a nerve creates significant challenges in classification, diagnostic reproducibility, and reporting of CrP4. Recently, there have been

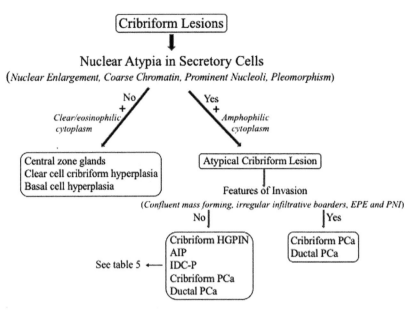

Fig. 1. A simplified diagnostic approach to prostatic cribriform lesions. HGPIN-high grade prostatic intraepithelial neoplasia; AIP-atypical intraductal proliferation; IDC-P-intraductal carcinoma of the prostate; PCa-prostate cancer; EPE-extraprostatic extension; PNI-perineural invasion.

attempts to improve the histological definition of the cribriform gland, specifically pertaining to CrP4. ISUP proposed a consensus definition of CrP4 as "a confluent sheet of contiguous malignant epithelial cells with multiple glandular lumina that are easily visible at low power (objective magnification × 10).[16,17] There should be no intervening stroma or mucin separating individual or fused glandular structures. In a separate interobserver reproducibility study among experienced genitourinary pathologists, Shah and colleagues found that in addition to the lack of intraglandular stroma or mucin, three additional features were associated with reproducibility for CrP4 diagnosis, which included transluminal bridging, a clear luminal space along the periphery of the gland accounting for <50% of the gland circumference and dense cellular proliferation (**Fig. 3**). They also

found reproducible morphological features that were against the CrP4 diagnosis, which included partial bridging, the majority of intraglandular cells in contact with stroma, mucinous fibroplasia, single attachment to the gland border by tumor cells forming glomerulation, and a clear luminal space along the periphery of the gland accounting for >50% of the gland circumference (**Fig. 4**). It is recommended that the diagnosis of CrP4 should be based not only on the presence of the classic definitional features but on the absence of features against the CrP4 diagnosis. **Table 2** summarizes these reproducible morphological features for and against CrP4 diagnosis.[14]

In some studies, CrP4 has been divided into small or large CrP4 based on its size in relation to adjacent benign glands, the number of lumina, and the greatest cross-sectional diameter.[18] Specifically, a

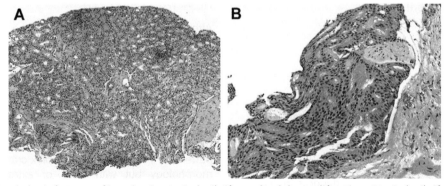

Fig. 2. Morphologic features of invasion in atypical cribriform glandular proliferation. Atypical cribriform glands are confluent in back-to-back arrangement and demonstrate irregular infiltrative borders (*A*) and perineural invasion (*B*).

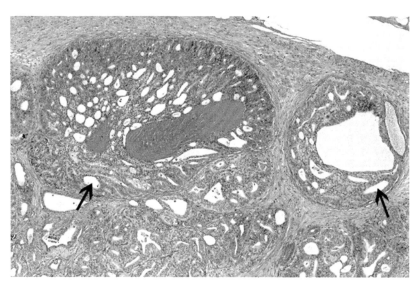

Fig. *3.* Reproducible morphological features for diagnosis of cribriform carcinoma. A dense sheet of tumor cells forms multiple lumens with transluminal bridging, imparting a "sieve-like" architecture. A majority of intraglandular cells are not in direct contact with stroma or mucin, and a clear luminal space along the periphery of the gland (*arrow*) accounts for <50% of the gland circumference.

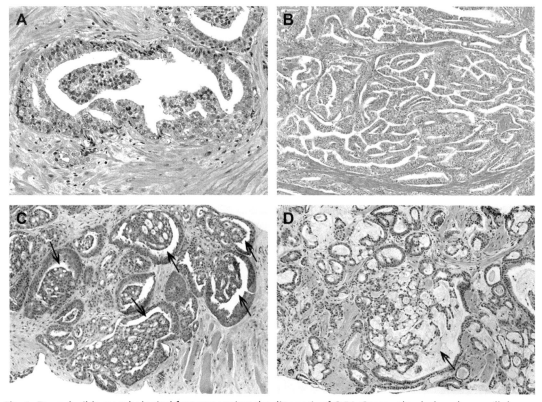

Fig. 4. Reproducible morphological features against the diagnosis of CrP4. Cancer glands show loose cellular proliferation forming multiple incomplete (partial) bridging (*A*). PCa exhibiting complex proliferation of interconnecting tumor cells with well-formed slit-like lumina. However, the majority of tumor cells are in contact with the stroma and blood vessels (*B*). Small to medium cancer glands showing glomeruloid pattern 4 morphology. Intraluminal proliferation is attached to the border of the gland with one attachment and a clear luminal space along gland periphery occupies >50% of gland circumference (*C, arrow*). PCa with intraluminal mucinous fibroplasia (*arrow*), creating a complex architecture mimicking cribriform architecture (*D*).

Table 2
Morphologic features "diagnostic of" and "against" cribriform prostate adenocarcinoma

Features Diagnostic of Cribriform Adenocarcinoma	Features Against Cribriform Adenocarcinoma
• Transluminal bridging • Majority of intraglandular tumor cells not in contact with stroma • Lack of intraglandular mucin • A clear luminal space along the periphery of the gland occupying <50% of the gland circumference • Dense intraglandular tumor cell proliferation	• Partial bridging • Majority of intraglandular tumor cells in contact with stroma • Presence of mucinous fibroplasia • Single attachment to gland border by tumor cells forming "glomeruloid-like" pattern • A clear luminal space along the periphery of the gland occupying >50% of the gland circumference

cribriform gland twice the size of the adjacent benign glands and exhibiting >12 lumina has been proposed as large CrP4. Hollemans and colleagues[3] used the criterion of "twice the size of the diameter of adjacent benign glands" and demonstrated that, in a multivariable analysis, only large CrP4 was an independent predictive factor for biochemical recurrence-free survival in GG2 patients. However, most studies, when assessing for outcomes associations, have neither differentiated CrP4 based on size, nor have utilized varying definitions for the size cut-off. For these reasons, in our opinion, routine reporting of CrP4 as two separate categories (large vs small) requires additional studies to demonstrate the value of such division.

INTRADUCTAL CARCINOMA OF THE PROSTATE

HISTORICAL PERSPECTIVE AND DEFINITION

IDC-P is not a new concept. Its recognition as a separate entity was raised as early as the 1980s.[19] For many years IDC-P was largely considered as one of the architectural patterns of HGPIN. In recent years, there has been a renewed interest in understanding this entity, leading to its recognition as a distinct entity in the 2016 World Health Organization (WHO) classification of PCa.[20] The current definition of IDC-P refers to the expansile proliferation of prostate cancer cells within the preexisting prostatic ducts and acini caused by the retrograde spread of high-grade and high volume invasive PCa cells. However, it has been recognized that a small proportion of IDC-P may in fact arise in patients with no invasive cancer or only GG1 PCa.[21–23] Morphologic and molecular studies suggest that this type of IDC-P arises from adjacent HGPIN and is potentially represented as a precancerous lesion (carcinoma in situ).[24] Therefore, it has been argued that IDC-P

may in fact represent two distinct diseases, one of which is a retrograde spread of adjacent high-grade and high volume disease and the other one truly an in situ disease.[25,26]

CLINICAL SIGNIFICANCE

There is now robust evidence that IDC-P is an adverse pathological feature. Patients with PCa harboring IDC-P would be ineligible for active surveillance. In the setting of invasive cancer, IDC-P remains an independent predictor of various adverse outcomes including earlier biochemical recurrence, distant metastasis, and worse disease-specific survival.[27,28] Most cases of isolated IDC-P in needle biopsies represent IDC-P with an unsampled aggressive invasive PCa but rare cases may represent precursor IDC-P with favorable outcomes. The management of patients whose prostate biopsies show only IDC-P without an associated invasive component is controversial. Some experts recommend radical therapy, while others recommend prompt repeat biopsy. An alternative clinicopathologic approach has been proposed to take into consideration of the extent, morphologic appearance, and location (with respect to any MRI abnormality) of isolated IDC-P in needle biopsies, as well as radiologic features (MRI and bone scan findings).[25]

MORPHOLOGICAL FEATURES AND DIAGNOSTIC CRITERIA

The diagnosis of IDC-P is based on a constellation of major and minor architectural and cytological features (Table 3).[29] Several investigators have proposed diagnostic criteria for IDC-P so that the diagnosis of IDC-P can be reproducible. Guo and Epstein proposed a set of morphologic criteria for IDC-P on needle biopsy,[30] which are currently the most commonly used criteria to diagnose

Table 3
Morphological features of intraductal carcinoma of the prostate

Major Features	Minor Features
Atypical glands with expansile architecture with at least partially preserved basal cells demonstrating one of these four features: • Solid growth filling the glands • Dense cribriform architecture (defined as >50% of the glands is composed of epithelium relative to luminal spaces) • Marked/bizarre nuclei pleomorphism/ nucleomegaly • Non-focal comedonecrosis	• Involvement of many glands (>6) • Involved glands are irregular or branching at right angles • Easily identifiable/frequent mitoses • "Central maturation" with two distinct cell populations consisting of tall pleomorphic, mitotically active cells at the periphery and cuboidal, monomorphic, quiescent cells at the center

IDC-P in all types of prostate specimens. In the setting of enlarged, atypical glands with at least a partially retained basal cell layer, the major criteria include solid growth or dense cribriform architecture (the latter is defined as > 50% of the gland is composed of epithelium relative to luminal spaces); or (2) loose cribriform (<50%) or micropapillary architecture having either marked pleomorphism/nucleomegaly or comedonecrosis. The presence of any one of these features is considered diagnostic for IDC-P. Some uncertainty remains about the definition of "dense" cribriform pattern, with recommendations for both 50% and 70% epithelium relative to luminal spaces existing in the literature.[10] The GUPS has proposed a 50% of cut-off for the definition of "dense" cribriform.[10]

Minor criteria that have been proposed by others include (1) involvement of many glands (>6); (2) involved glands have irregular contour or right-angle branching; (3) easily identifiable/frequent mitoses, and (4) "central maturation"- 2 distinct cell populations consisting of tall, pleomorphic, mitotically active cells at the periphery and cuboidal, monomorphic, quiescent cells at the center.[29,31] Large expansile branching glands with dense cribriform growth with or without intraluminal necrosis is the most common morphological presentation and solid intraluminal growth expanding the gland is the most reproducible feature for IDC-P. Representative examples depicting major and minor features for diagnosis of IDC-P are illustrated in **Fig. 5**.

MOLECULAR FEATURES OF CRIBRIFORM PROSTATE ADENOCARCINOMA AND INTRADUCTAL CARCINOMA OF THE PROSTATE

As CrP4 and IDC-P share cribriform morphology and have a comparable prognostic impact, most molecular and genetic studies have not distinguished them and consider them essentially as PCa with "cribriform architecture". **Table 4** summarizes the most common molecular and protein alterations that have been reported individually or collectively for CrP4 and IDC-P.

GRADING AND REPORTING OF INTRADUCTAL CARCINOMA OF THE PROSTATE

Whether IDC-P should be graded or not remains controversial and debated. In 2014 ISUP recommended IDC-P without invasive carcinoma not be graded.[1] The 2016 WHO GU bluebook stated that 'IDC-P should not be factored into the grading of a carcinoma.[20] However, several recent studies have argued that IDC-P should be incorporated into the final GS with invasive cancer.[9,26,32,33] Most Gleason grade outcome studies published before 2014 ISUP recommendations included cases for which IDC-P were not consciously separated from invasive PCa and therefore IDC-P, if present, was most likely graded and incorporated in the final Gleason grade. In addition, the distinction between IDC-P and invasive PCa is not always possible based on H&E morphology and requires basal cell immunohistochemistry on multiple tissue blocks to confirm in almost all cases,[34–36] a practice that would be impractical or impossible to implement across the world. Recent studies have shown that incorporation of IDC-P into Gleason grade may actually improve its outcome predictions.[37,38] As the result, the 2019 ISUP consensus recommended IDC-P be incorporated in the GS with invasive PCa.[11]

However, in 2019 GUPS recommended not to include IDC-P when rendering the final GS on biopsy and radical prostatectomy[10] for several reasons. IDC-P is rarely found associated with no or minute focus of PCa and may represent a precursor, rather than invasive lesion such that it would be inappropriate to grade a precursor lesion using the grading system for invasive cancer.[23,39] IDC-P is also rarely found with Gleason

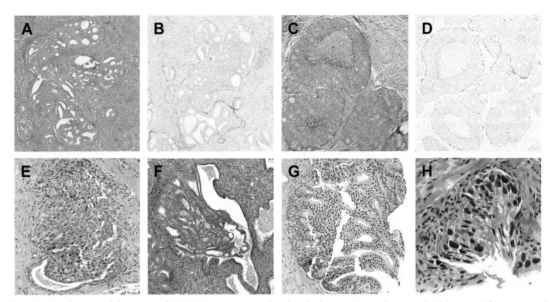

Fig. 5. Morphological features of IDC-P. Large expansile glands demonstrate dense cribriform proliferation and irregular branching contour (*A*). p63 immunohistochemical staining demonstrates the preservation of basal cells (*B*). Expansile glands with dense cribriform proliferation and central comedonecrosis (*C*). Immunohistochemical staining of p63 showing preserved basal cells (*D*). Expansile glands with solid architecture (*E*). IDC-P exhibit partial involvement of a gland (*F*). Dense cribriform with two cell populations (*G*). Pleomorphic bizarre nuclei (*H*).

Table 4
Summary of common genomic and molecular alterations present in cribriform prostate adenocarcinoma /Intraductal carcinoma

Morphological Spectrum Examined	Genomic and Molecular Changes (Frequency)	Reference
Combined CrP4/IDC-P	• Somatic copy number alteration: deletion of 8p, 10q23 • *TMPRSS2:ERG* rearrangements (46.3%) • Loss of tumor suppressor: *PTEN* (16–39%) • Oncogene amplification: *MYC* (24%) • Point mutation: *SPOP* (10–17%), *FOXA1* (5.49–15%), *TP53* (8.54–19%) • Mutation of DNA damage repair gene: *BRCA2* (45.2%), *ATM* (7.32%) • Overexpression of long noncoding RNA: *SChLAP1*	Bottcher et al,[52] 2018 Elfandy et al[53] 2019 Elfandy et al[53] 2019 Bottcher et al,[52] 2018 Elfandy et al,[53] 2019 Bottcher et al,[52] 2018 Elfandy et al[53] 2019 Bottcher et al,[52] 2018 Elfandy et al[53] 2019 Lozano et al,[54] 2021 Elfandy et al[53] 2019 Chua et al[55] 2017
CrP4	• Loss of tumor suppressor: PTEN (38%)	Shah et al[56] 2019
IDC-P	• Loss of tumor suppressor: PTEN (69%) • Loss of heterogeneity (60%) • Loss of tumor suppressor: combined *TP53* and *RB* (52%) • *TMPRSS2:ERG* rearrangements (75%)	Shah et al,[56] 2019 Lotan et al[57] 2013 Dawkins et al[58] 2000 Bettendorf et al[59] 2018 Han et al[50] 2010

6 PCa,[21] the prognostic significance of which is not known. Furthermore, in a recent study, the number of cases whose highest grade would have changed if IDC-P was incorporated in the final grade was very small with only 1.6% of biopsy and 0.6% of radical prostatectomy specimens,[40] although another study found that the GG was increased by 1 or 2 in almost a quarter of cases.[41]

It will require published data to adjudicate these differences. When they choose to use one particular recommendation, pathologists should review and be aware of the data that support that recommendation and communicate with clinicians for potential clinical implications of the recommendation. Our personal preference is not to grade IDC-P when it is an isolated finding without concomitant PCa, or is associated with Gleason 6 (Grade group 1) PCa, but grade and incorporate IDC-P with invasive PCa for grading if it is found with PCa of GS ≥ 3 + 4 = 7 (GG 2). Regardless, it is recommended that basal cell stains should be utilized judiciously, specifically in the setting of "precursor-like" IDC-P when there is no definitive infiltrative carcinoma or a suspicion for IDC-P in the setting of low-grade GG 1 infiltrative carcinoma in order to correctly assign the GS to the case. An example illustrating this point is represented in **Fig. 6.**

DETECTION OF CRIBRIFORM PROSTATE ADENOCARCINOMA/INTRADUCTAL CARCINOMA OF THE PROSTATE BY MULTIPARAMETRIC MRI

Multiparametric MRI (mpMRI) imaging characteristics of PCa is discussed in another article. A few studies have investigated the ability of mpMRI to detect CrP4 and IDC-P, which would be particularly useful in patients with GG1 and 2 PCas on biopsy who may be considering active surveillance. Initial studies have suggested that the visibility of mpMRI for these morphologies is not good.[42] Several recent studies have demonstrated high sensitivity of mpMRI for the detection of cribriform morphology at lesion level although there is a complicated relationship between cribriform histology and region ADC value which is the most important parameter largely determining the visibility of the lesion on mpMRI.[43] In a study by Tonttila and colleagues[44] mpMRI detected cancers with cribriform or intraductal growth with a sensitivity of 90.5%. Prendeville and colleagues[45] found mpMRI with fusion targeted biopsy was significantly associated with increased detection of cribriform/intraductal carcinoma (20/22) compared with systematic sextant biopsy of mpMRI-negative region (3/22). A small mpMRI study of fifteen tumors with IDC-P demonstrated that GG2/3 tumors with IDC-P had lower ADC than

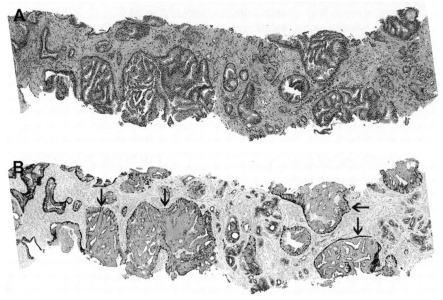

Fig. 6. GG1 Prostate adenocarcinoma with IDC-P. This case demonstrates that the distinction of IDC-P from CrP4 may be clinically relevant. Biopsy shows well-formed discrete and large atypical dense cribriform glands (*A*). PIN4 staining demonstrates the preservation of basal cells in atypical dense cribriform glands (*arrows*), confirming IDC-P, while invasive PCa demonstrates the lack of basal cell staining (*B*). With the use of basal cell staining, the diagnosis is GG 1 PCa with IDC-P. If one includes IDC-P in grading, the final grade would be 4 + 3 = 7, GG3.

matched tumors with a similar percentage of pattern 4 and without IDC-P, which resembled high-risk cancer on mpMRI.[46] These studies further support the National Comprehensive Cancer Network (NCCN) recommendation for performing mpMRI when considering patients for active surveillance.

DIFFERENTIAL DIAGNOSIS

Since CrP4 and IDC-P are related entities, their differential diagnoses are considered jointly in this section. Table 5 summarizes various morphological and immunohistochemical features that are helpful in the differential diagnosis of atypical cribriform lesions.

Clear cell cribriform hyperplasia: Clear cell cribriform hyperplasia is a benign entity that may be confused with CrP4 and IDC-P, particularly when it is florid in presentation. It is typically encountered in the transition zone of the prostate so the presence in the biopsy is rare. At low power, nodular architecture is often appreciated. The involved glands usually have bland cytology without nuclear atypia and prominent nucleoli. Importantly, the cytoplasm is pale or mildly eosinophilic. It lacks amphophilic cytoplasmic characteristics of CrP4 and IDC-P. Frequently, a prominent basal cell layer is appreciated. Another useful feature includes the presence of frequent Roman bridges where nuclei stream parallel to bridges instead of the perpendicular orientation. Stroma surrounding glands are frequently cellular and have benign prostate hyperplasia (BPH)-like spindle cell stroma. A representative example of clear cell cribriform

hyperplasia from a transurethral resection specimen is shown in Fig. 7.

Basal cell hyperplasia: The basal cell hyperplasia sometimes may present with prominent cribriform/psuedocribriform growth and mimic CrP4. Basal cell hyperplasia usually occurs in the transition zone. Therefore, it is less common to see in the prostatic biopsy. Helpful morphologic features for benign changes include nodular architecture at low power magnification, dense luminal calcifications, and cellular BPH-like spindle cell stroma. Glands show nuclear stratification with oval, coffee-bean-like nuclei with frequent central grooves, and have a bland vesicular appearance. The cytoplasm is scant. In addition, immunohistochemical stain shows positivity for basal cell markers p63 and high molecular cytokeratin, and lack of racemase expression. A representative example of basal cell hyperplasia from a transurethral resection specimen is shown in Fig. 8.

Cribriform HGPIN: HGPIN represents the most significant and clinically relevant differential diagnosis specifically for IDC-P, particularly in a prostate biopsy. HGPIN glands are typically smooth with rounded contours, similar in size to the adjacent benign glands. The cells lack marked nuclear atypia and the nuclei are only 2 to 3 times the size of the adjacent benign nuclei, with exceptionally rare mitoses. Micropapillary patterns can be seen in both high-grade PIN and IDC-P. The presence of solid nests, dense cribriform architecture, or comedonecrosis essentially rules out the diagnosis of HGPIN (Fig. 5). Most importantly, significant nuclear atypia (i.e., bizarre pleomorphic nuclei), with nuclei significantly larger than the adjacent benign nuclei, is only seen in IDC-P.

Table 5
Differential diagnosis of atypical cribriform lesions

Cribriform Lesions	Architecture and Cytology	# Of Glands	Basal Cells	PTEN Loss and *TMPRSS2:ERG* Gene Fusions
Cribriform HGPIN	Uniform contour with acinar cytology	Single or few	+	-
AIP	Loose cribriform or markedly atypical nuclei falling short of IDC-P diagnosis with acinar cytology	Few to many	+	+ (Majority)
IDC-P	Solid/dense cribriform ± comedonecrosis/pleomorphic nuclei with acinar cytology	Few to many	+	+ (Majority)
Cribriform PCa	Variable confluent cribriform glands with acinar cytology	Variable	-	Variable
Ductal PCa	Confluent cribriform/papillae with ductal cytology	Variable	-/Focal +	Variable

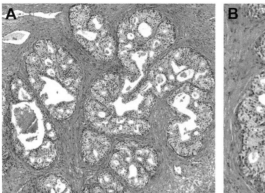
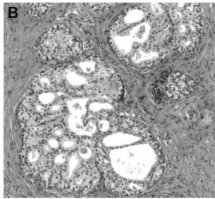

Fig. 7. Clear cell cribriform hyperplasia. At low power, the proliferation of large cribriform glands with pale to mildly eosinophilic cytoplasm demonstrates nodular architecture (*A*). At higher magnification, glands have bland cytology without nuclear atypia and prominent nucleoli. A prominent basal cell layer is appreciated. Roman bridges where nuclei stream parallel to bridges instead of the perpendicular orientation. There is a BPH-like cellular spindle cell stroma (*B*).

CrP4: Cribriform carcinoma lacks basal cell lining. Confluent growth, irregular infiltrative borders, perineural invasion or extraprostatic extension suggests cribriform carcinoma; discrete expansile branching glands suggest IDC-P. Contemporary literature lumps both CrP4 and IDC-P as "cribriform architecture", as both are associated with similar adverse outcomes. However, the distinction between the two is important specifically in two situations: when there is a lack of definitive infiltrative carcinoma with the suspicion for IDC-P and in the setting of low-grade infiltrative carcinoma where documentation of IDC-P is necessary to correctly assign GS to the case (Fig. 6). In the setting of high-grade PCa, the distinction between the two is of little clinical significance.

Ductal adenocarcinoma: The diagnosis of ductal adenocarcinoma is based on strict cytological features, notably the presence of pseudostratified columnar lining epithelium within cribriform and papillary components. Lack of basal cell lining supports ductal adenocarcinoma diagnosis but residual basal cells are frequently present in ductal adenocarcinoma exhibiting intraductal spread. Fig. 9 shows an example of ductal adenocarcinoma with focal preservation of basal cells.

Secondary involvement by colonic adenocarcinoma: The presence of more typical ductal and/or acinar morphology, along with an immunohistochemical panel of PSA, PSMA, NKX3.1, β-catenin, CDX-2, and villin can be helpful. Colorectal tumors often demonstrate luminal dirty necrosis and are negative for PSA, PSMA, and NKX3.1, whereas are often positive for ß-catenin, CDX-2, and villin.

Adenoid cystic (basal cell) carcinoma of the prostate: Rarely adenoid cystic (basal cell)

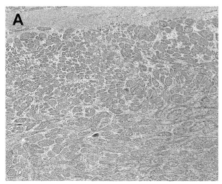
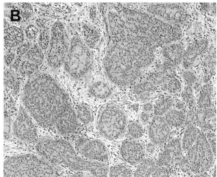

Fig. 8. Basal cell hyperplasia. The basal cell hyperplasia sometimes may present with prominent cribriform/psuedocribriform growth and mimic CrP4. At low power, glands demonstrate nodular growth (*A*). At higher magnification, glands are lined by stratified nuclei with scant cytoplasm. Nuclei are oval, coffee-bean-like with frequent central grooves, and have a bland vesicular appearance. The stroma surrounding glands shows hyalinization. There is a BPH-like cellular spindle cell stroma (*B*).

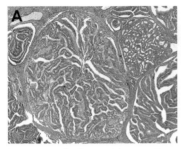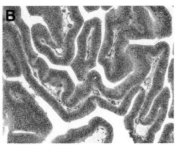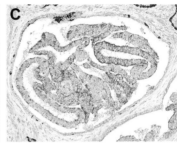

Fig. 9. Ductal adenocarcinoma. Cancer glands exhibiting papillary and cribriform architecture lined by pseudostratified tall columnar cells with abundant amphophilic cytoplasm grow within ducts. The tumor cells have elongated and pseudostratified nuclei (*A* and *B*). PIN-4 staining demonstrates focal preservation of basal cells and overexpression of racemase in cancer cells (*C*).

carcinoma may present with prominent cribriform growth and enter into the differential diagnosis of CrP4. Nuclear features are similar to basal cell hyperplasia characterized by a high N: C ratio, hypochromatic ovoid coffee bean-type nuclei, and nuclear stratification. Stroma around glands has hyalinized appearance. In contrast to basal cell hyperplasia, glands demonstrate infiltrative features including the presence of extraprostatic extension and perineural invasion. Adenoid cystic (basal cell) carcinoma is positive for basal cell markers p63 and high molecular weight cytokeratin, CK903 while prostate-specific markers PSA, NKX3.1, and PSMA are negative. An opposite staining pattern is expected for CrP4. A representative example of basal cell carcinoma in a needle biopsy is shown in **Fig. 10**.

DUCTAL ADENOCARCINOMA

CLINICAL SIGNIFICANCE

Ductal adenocarcinomas are more aggressive than acinar carcinoma, present at more advanced stages (non-organ-confined disease), and are now regarded as Gleason pattern 4 or pattern 5 with necrosis. Pure ductal adenocarcinoma is rare (1.3%); a majority has mixed ductal and acinar morphology (incidence of ~5%). Periurethral or centrally located tumors may manifest with urinary obstruction and hematuria.[47]

MORPHOLOGICAL FEATURES

Ductal adenocarcinoma grows within and expands the prostatic urethra and periurethral ducts or more commonly involves peripheral zone prostatic ducts and acini. A variety of architectural patterns often intermingle, including confluent cribriform, papillary, and solid. Cancer glands are lined by pseudostratified tall columnar cells with abundant amphophilic cytoplasm. In papillary pattern, true fibrovascular cores are seen. In cribriform pattern, lumina are often compressed with slit-like architecture. Ductal adenocarcinoma frequently is found in association with acinar adenocarcinoma. Ductal adenocarcinoma commonly demonstrates intraductal spread into preexisting ducts with the preservation of basal cell layers (**Fig. 9**).

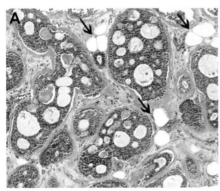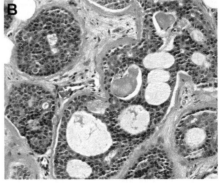

Fig. 10. Adenoid cystic (basal cell) carcinoma. Adenoid cystic (basal cell) carcinoma exhibits infiltrative features such as extraprostatic extension (*A. arrows*). The stroma surrounding glands demonstrates hyalinization (*B*).

DIFFERENTIAL DIAGNOSIS

Intraductal carcinoma: The term "ductal" in ductal adenocarcinoma refers to a specific ductal morphologic feature (pseudostratified tall columnar cells) in contrast to the acinar cytology such as simple/low cuboid epithelial cells with round nuclei and lack of papillary morphology in IDC-P. Ductal adenocarcinoma commonly spreads into preexisting prostatic ducts and therefore basal cells are focally preserved, mechanistically similar to IDC-P and may be diagnosed as ductal adenocarcinoma with intraductal spread.

Urothelial carcinoma: Centrally located ductal adenocarcinoma often presents with papillary or solid morphology and may be confused with high-grade, poorly differentiated urothelial carcinoma, which often has prominent cytological pleomorphism, nested morphology, and lacks acinar differentiation. A panel of PSA, PSMA, NKX3.1, CK903, p63, and GATA3 is helpful and typically is required for this differential diagnosis.

HGPIN: In needle biopsies, the PIN-like morphology of ductal carcinoma may be confused for HGPIN. The presence of numerous crowded glands is helpful to separate from HGPIN. Basal cell markers also may help in this differentiation, but the lack of basal cell staining in small focus does not rule out an HGPIN diagnosis. A definitive distinction may not be feasible in small needle biopsy samples, and the possibility of PIN-like ductal carcinoma should be raised.

ATYPICAL INTRADUCTAL PROLIFERATION

DEFINITION

An intraductal proliferation of prostatic secretory cells may occasionally show a greater degree of architectural complexity and/or cytologic atypia than a typical HGPIN, yet falls short of the strict diagnostic threshold for IDC-P. The terms "atypical cribriform lesion," "atypical intraductal cribriform proliferation," "low-grade intraductal carcinoma," and more recently "atypical proliferation suspicious for intraductal carcinoma" have all been proposed to designate this lesion. The term "AIP" is preferred as it generally includes all morphologic patterns that have been described in this lesion.

CLINICAL SIGNIFICANCE

Only limited data are available regarding the significance of AIP. In one study, AIP-associated carcinoma had similar clinicopathologic features as IDC-P-associated carcinoma showing higher grade and higher stage compared to acinar carcinoma without AIP/IDC-P.[48] Shah and colleagues[49] found that AIP identified in biopsy without concomitant IDC-P was associated with one or more features of adverse pathology, defined as $\geq$ GG3, IDC-P, CrP4, and pT3a/pT3b, in subsequent biopsy or radical prostatectomy. The study included 62 patients who had AIP without associated IDC-P in the initial biopsy. Thirteen patients who had concomitant GG1 or GG2 cancer (without cribriform architecture) underwent radical prostatectomy, 93% of which were found to have adverse pathology. In addition, 6 of 12 patients with AIP only in initial biopsy had a subsequent biopsy, three (50%) of which were found to harbor adverse pathology including one with IDC-P and two with GG3 cancer. In addition, AIP also shares molecular characteristics of IDC-P.[48,50,51] Comparing ERG and PTEN status between AIP and IDC-P, there was a similar frequency of ERG overexpression and PTEN loss among AIP, IDC-P, and invasive carcinoma.

In summary, AIP is a clinically significant lesion that needs to be recognized and reported. If only AIP is identified, further workup such as repeat biopsy and prostate mpMRI is warranted to rule out unsampled clinically significant cancer.

MORPHOLOGICAL FEATURES

Morphologically, like IDC-P, AIP is characterized by the involvement of several glands which exhibit frequent right-angle branching. AIP is typically characterized by loose cribriform proliferation that lacks intraluminal necrosis and/or severe nuclear atypia required for the diagnosis of IDC-P.[51] The most common morphological features include (1) intraductal proliferation with loose cribriform architecture (more luminal spaces relative to epithelium), but without significant nuclear pleomorphism or necrosis; (2) solid or dense cribriform structure incompletely spanning the glandular lumen; or (3) any lesion, regardless of the architecture, with significant nuclear atypia or pleomorphism beyond high-grade PIN, but falling short of the current diagnostic criteria for IDC-P. The great majority (>90%) of AIP cases demonstrate loose cribriform architecture.[51] PTEN and ERG biomarkers can be helpful in cases which are difficult, however, normal staining patterns (retained PTEN and negative ERG) would not rule out the diagnosis.[48] PTEN loss and ERG overexpression support the diagnosis of AIP over HGPIN. A representative example of AIP and the utility of PTEN and ERG biomarkers is shown in **Fig. 11**. A summary of the diagnostic approach to AIP is illustrated in **Fig. 12**.

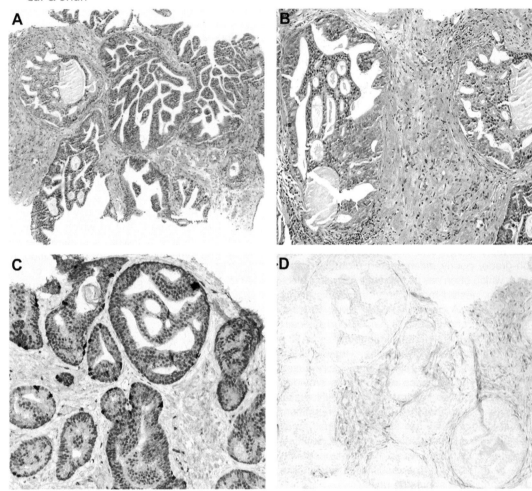

Fig. 11. Atypical intraductal proliferation, suspicious for intraductal carcinoma. Several glands present with lumen-spanning proliferation exhibiting loose cribriform architecture with morphological features worse than HGPIN but falling short of IDC-P (*A* and *B*). PIN4-ERG multiplex stains demonstrate the preservation of basal cells and nuclear ERG overexpression (*C*). PTEN is lost in epithelial cells of atypical cribriform glands with positive internal control (stromal cells), supporting the diagnosis of AIP over HGPIN (*D*).

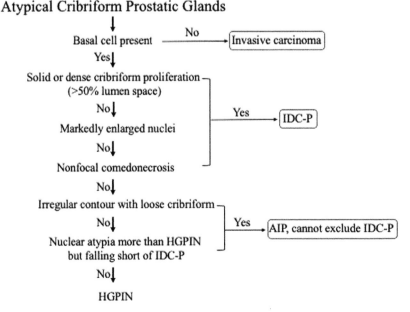

Fig. 12. Diagnostic algorithm of atypical prostatic cribriform lesions. (*Adapted from* Shah RB, Zhou M. Prostate Biopsy Interpretation: An Illustrated Guide. Second ed. Springer.)

Fig. 13. Central zone glands. In a prostate needle biopsy, the presence of isolated glands with loose cribriform proliferation may raise concern for AIP. The glands however have distinct cytoplasmic eosinophilia, a helpful clue to the diagnosis. Nuclei are bland and stream parallel to bridges.

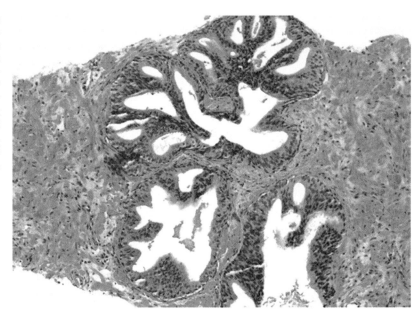

DIFFERENTIAL DIAGNOSIS

Central zone glands: Central zone gland histology is typically a mimicker of HGPIN; however prominent loose cribriform architecture in some cases may mimic AIP (**Fig. 13**). This histology is typically seen in biopsies from the base of the prostate. In the central zone, glands are complex with frequent papillary and undulating architecture with pseudostratified lining epithelium. At low magnification, glands demonstrate distinct cytoplasmic eosinophilia, a useful clue to the diagnosis. Roman bridges and loose cribriform architecture are common. Nuclei stream parallel to bridges in comparison to perpendicular orientation in AIP. Nuclear atypia is absent.

Cribriform HGPIN: AIP often exhibits loose cribriform architecture with "low-grade" morphology that overlaps with what in the past was referred to as "cribriform HGPIN," and falls short of the diagnostic criteria for IDC-P. The distinction between AIP and cribriform HGPIN is particularly problematic as there are no objective, reproducible morphologic criteria to distinguish between them. It is recommended to not diagnose cribriform HGPIN on biopsy, but rather use AIP in this setting especially due to management implications. The diagnosis of AIP warrants immediate repeat biopsy to rule out unsampled clinically significant PCa. In contrast, the patient with HGPIN diagnosis may not receive further follow-up biopsy.

SUMMARY

Cribriform lesions of the prostate gland are of wide-ranging significance from normal anatomical variation, benign proliferative lesions, premalignant, suspicious to frankly malignant and biologically aggressive. A systemic approach with careful assessment of several architectural and cytological features is crucially important to arrive at the correct diagnosis.

CLINICS CARE POINTS

- Reporting of CrP4 and IDC-P in both biopsy and RP settings is recommended due to their independent association with various adverse clinical outcomes

- The distinction between CrP4 and IDC-P is important specifically in two situations: when there is a lack of definitive infiltrative carcinoma and suspicion for IDC-P, and in the setting of GG1 infiltrative carcinoma where documentation of IDC-P is necessary to correctly assign GS to the case. In the setting of high-grade PCa, the distinction between the two is of little clinical significance

- Ductal adenocarcinoma commonly spreads into preexisting prostatic ducts and therefore basal cells are focally preserved. This phenomenon should not be confused with IDC-P or HGPIN. The diagnosis of ductal adenocarcinoma is based on cytological features

- The diagnosis of cribriform HGPIN in a biopsy setting is not recommended; such lesions should be reported as AIP, suspicious for IDC-P

DISCLOSURE

The authors have nothing to disclose.

REFERENCES

1. Epstein JI, Egevad L, Amin MB, et al. The 2014 international society of urological pathology (ISUP) consensus conference on gleason grading of prostatic carcinoma: definition of grading patterns and proposal for a new grading system. Am J Surg Pathol 2016;40(2):244–52.

2. Chen Z, Pham H, Abreu A, et al. Prognostic value of cribriform size, percentage, and intraductal carcinoma in Gleason Score 7 prostate cancer with Cribriform Gleason Pattern 4. Hum Pathol 2021. https://doi.org/10.1016/j.humpath.2021.09.005.

3. Hollemans E, Verhoef EI, Bangma CH, et al. Large cribriform growth pattern identifies ISUP grade 2 prostate cancer at high risk for recurrence and metastasis. Mod Pathol 2019;32(1):139–46.

4. Keefe DT, Schieda N, El Hallani S, et al. Cribriform morphology predicts upstaging after radical prostatectomy in patients with Gleason score 3 + 4 = 7 prostate cancer at transrectal ultrasound (TRUS)-guided needle biopsy. Virchows Arch 2015;467(4):437–42.

5. Kweldam CF, Kummerlin IP, Nieboer D, et al. Disease-specific survival of patients with invasive cribriform and intraductal prostate cancer at diagnostic biopsy. Mod Pathol 2016;29(6):630–6.

6. Kweldam CF, Wildhagen MF, Steyerberg EW, et al. Cribriform growth is highly predictive for postoperative metastasis and disease-specific death in Gleason score 7 prostate cancer. Mod Pathol 2015;28(3):457–64.

7. Kweldam CF, Kummerlin IP, Nieboer D, et al. Prostate cancer outcomes of men with biopsy Gleason score 6 and 7 without cribriform or intraductal carcinoma. Eur J Cancer 2016;66:26–33.

8. Hollemans E, Verhoef EI, Bangma CH, et al. Cribriform architecture in radical prostatectomies predicts oncological outcome in Gleason score 8 prostate cancer patients. Mod Pathol 2021;34(1):184–93.

9. van Leenders G, Kweldam CF, Hollemans E, et al. Improved prostate cancer biopsy grading by incorporation of invasive cribriform and intraductal carcinoma in the 2014 grade groups. Eur Urol 2020;77(2):191–8.

10. Epstein JI, Amin MB, Fine SW, et al. The 2019 genitourinary pathology society (GUPS) white paper on contemporary grading of prostate cancer. Arch Pathol Lab Med 2021;145(4):461–93.

11. van Leenders G, van der Kwast TH, Grignon DJ, et al. The 2019 international society of urological pathology (ISUP) consensus conference on grading of prostatic carcinoma. Am J Surg Pathol 2020;44(8):e87–99.

12. Flood TA, Schieda N, Keefe DT, et al. Utility of Gleason pattern 4 morphologies detected on transrectal ultrasound (TRUS)-guided biopsies for prediction of upgrading or upstaging in Gleason score 3 + 4 = 7 prostate cancer. Virchows Arch 2016;469(3):313–9.

13. Kweldam CF, Nieboer D, Algaba F, et al. Gleason grade 4 prostate adenocarcinoma patterns: an interobserver agreement study among genitourinary pathologists. Histopathology 2016;69(3):441–9.

14. Shah RB, Cai Q, Aron M, et al. Diagnosis of "cribriform" prostatic adenocarcinoma: an interobserver reproducibility study among urologic pathologists with recommendations. Am J Cancer Res 2021;11(8):3990–4001.

15. van der Slot MA, Hollemans E, den Bakker MA, et al. Inter-observer variability of cribriform architecture and percent Gleason pattern 4 in prostate cancer: relation to clinical outcome. Virchows Arch 2021;478(2):249–56.

16. Iczkowski KA, van Leenders G, Tarima S, et al. Cribriform prostate cancer: Morphologic criteria enabling a diagnosis, based on survey of experts. Ann Diagn Pathol 2021;52:151733.

17. van der Kwast TH, van Leenders GJ, Berney DM, et al. ISUP consensus definition of cribriform pattern prostate cancer. Am J Surg Pathol 2021;45(8):1118–26.

18. Iczkowski KA, Torkko KC, Kotnis GR, et al. Digital quantification of five high-grade prostate cancer patterns, including the cribriform pattern, and their association with adverse outcome. Am J Clin Pathol 2011;136(1):98–107.

19. Kovi J, Jackson MA, Heshmat MY. Ductal spread in prostatic carcinoma. Cancer 1985;56(7):1566–73.

20. Moch H, Humphrey PA, Ulbright TM, et al. WHO classification of tumours of the urinary system and male genital organs. 4th ed. Lyon CEDEX, France: International Agency for Research on Cancer; 2016.

21. Khani F, Epstein JI. Prostate biopsy specimens with Gleason 3+3=6 and intraductal carcinoma: radical prostatectomy findings and clinical outcomes. Am J Surg Pathol 2015;39(10):1383–9.

22. Miyai K, Divatia MK, Shen SS, et al. Heterogeneous clinicopathological features of intraductal carcinoma of the prostate: a comparison between "precursor-like" and "regular type" lesions. Int J Clin Exp Pathol 2014;7(5):2518–26.

23. Robinson BD, Epstein JI. Intraductal carcinoma of the prostate without invasive carcinoma on needle biopsy: emphasis on radical prostatectomy findings. J Urol 2010;184(4):1328–33.

24. Khani F, Wobker SE, Hicks JL, et al. Intraductal carcinoma of the prostate in the absence of high-grade invasive carcinoma represents a molecularly distinct

type of in situ carcinoma enriched with oncogenic driver mutations. J Pathol 2019;249(1):79–89.

25. Varma M. Intraductal carcinoma of the prostate: a guide for the practicing pathologist. Adv Anat Pathol 2021;28(4):276–87.

26. Varma M, Epstein JI. Head to head: should the intraductal component of invasive prostate cancer be graded? Histopathology 2021;78(2):231–9.

27. Kato M, Tsuzuki T, Kimura K, et al. The presence of intraductal carcinoma of the prostate in needle biopsy is a significant prognostic factor for prostate cancer patients with distant metastasis at initial presentation. Mod Pathol 2016;29(2):166–73.

28. Kimura K, Tsuzuki T, Kato M, et al. Prognostic value of intraductal carcinoma of the prostate in radical prostatectomy specimens. Prostate 2014;74(6):680–7.

29. Cohen RJ, Wheeler TM, Bonkhoff H, et al. A proposal on the identification, histologic reporting, and implications of intraductal prostatic carcinoma. Arch Pathol Lab Med 2007;131(7):1103–9.

30. Guo CC, Epstein JI. Intraductal carcinoma of the prostate on needle biopsy: histologic features and clinical significance. Mod Pathol 2006;19(12):1528–35.

31. Shah RB, Magi-Galluzzi C, Han B, et al. Atypical cribriform lesions of the prostate: relationship to prostatic carcinoma and implication for diagnosis in prostate biopsies. Am J Surg Pathol 2010;34(4):470–7.

32. Samaratunga H, Delahunt B, Egevad L, et al. Intraductal carcinoma of the prostate is an aggressive form of invasive carcinoma and should be graded. Pathology 2020;52(2):192–6.

33. Varma M, Egevad L, Delahunt B, et al. Reporting intraductal carcinoma of the prostate: a plea for greater standardization. Histopathology 2017;70(3):504–7.

34. Fine SW, Al-Ahmadie HA, Chen YB, et al. Comedonecrosis revisited: strong association with intraductal carcinoma of the prostate. Am J Surg Pathol 2018;42(8):1036–41.

35. Madan R, Deebajah M, Alanee S, et al. Prostate cancer with comedonecrosis is frequently, but not exclusively, intraductal carcinoma: a need for reappraisal of grading criteria. Histopathology 2019;74(7):1081–7.

36. Magers M, Kunju LP, Wu A. Intraductal carcinoma of the prostate: morphologic features, differential diagnoses, significance, and reporting practices. Arch Pathol Lab Med 2015;139(10):1234–41.

37. Kato M, Hirakawa A, Kobayashi Y, et al. Integrating tertiary Gleason pattern 5 into the ISUP grading system improves prediction of biochemical recurrence in radical prostatectomy patients. Mod Pathol 2019;32(1):122–7.

38. Saeter T, Vlatkovic L, Waaler G, et al. Intraductal carcinoma of the prostate on diagnostic needle biopsy predicts prostate cancer mortality: a population-based study. Prostate 2017;77(8):859–65.

39. Miyai K, Divatia MK, Shen SS, et al. Clinicopathological analysis of intraductal proliferative lesions of prostate: intraductal carcinoma of prostate, high-grade prostatic intraepithelial neoplasia, and atypical cribriform lesion. Hum Pathol 2014;45(8):1572–81.

40. Rijstenberg LL, Hansum T, Hollemans E, et al. Intraductal carcinoma has a minimal impact on Grade Group assignment in prostate cancer biopsy and radical prostatectomy specimens. Histopathology 2020;77(5):742–8.

41. Chen-Maxwell D, Prendeville S. Grading of prostate cancer: the impact of including intraductal carcinoma on the overall Grade Group assigned in diagnostic biopsies. Histopathology 2020;77(3):503–7.

42. Truong M, Hollenberg G, Weinberg E, et al. Impact of gleason subtype on prostate cancer detection using multiparametric magnetic resonance imaging: correlation with final histopathology. J Urol 2017;198(2):316–21.

43. Harmon SA, Brown GT, Sanford T, et al. Spatial density and diversity of architectural histology in prostate cancer: influence on diffusion weighted magnetic resonance imaging. Quant Imaging Med Surg 2020;10(2):326–39.

44. Tonttila PP, Ahtikoski A, Kuisma M, et al. Multiparametric MRI prior to radical prostatectomy identifies intraductal and cribriform growth patterns in prostate cancer. BJU Int 2019;124(6):992–8.

45. Prendeville S, Gertner M, Maganti M, et al. Role of magnetic resonance imaging targeted biopsy in detection of prostate cancer harboring adverse pathological features of intraductal carcinoma and invasive cribriform carcinoma. J Urol 2018;200(1):104–13.

46. Currin S, Flood TA, Krishna S, et al. Intraductal carcinoma of the prostate (IDC-P) lowers apparent diffusion coefficient (ADC) values among intermediate risk prostate cancers. J Magn Reson Imaging 2019;50(1):279–87.

47. Amin A. Prostate Ductal Adenocarcinoma. Appl Immunohistochem Mol Morphol 2018;26(7):514–21.

48. Hickman RA, Yu H, Li J, et al. Atypical intraductal cribriform proliferations of the prostate exhibit similar molecular and clinicopathologic characteristics as intraductal carcinoma of the prostate. Am J Surg Pathol 2017;41(4):550–6.

49. Shah RB, Nguyen JK, Przybycin CG, et al. Atypical intraductal proliferation detected in prostate needle biopsy is a marker of unsampled intraductal carcinoma and other adverse pathological features: a prospective clinicopathological study of 62 cases

with emphasis on pathological outcomes. Histopathology 2019;75(3):346–53.

50. Han B, Suleman K, Wang L, et al. ETS gene aberrations in atypical cribriform lesions of the prostate: Implications for the distinction between intraductal carcinoma of the prostate and cribriform high-grade prostatic intraepithelial neoplasia. Am J Surg Pathol 2010;34(4):478–85.

51. Shah RB, Yoon J, Liu G, et al. Atypical intraductal proliferation and intraductal carcinoma of the prostate on core needle biopsy: a comparative clinicopathological and molecular study with a proposal to expand the morphological spectrum of intraductal carcinoma. Histopathology 2017;71(5):693–702. https://doi.org/10.1111/his.13273.

52. Bottcher R, Kweldam CF, Livingstone J, et al. Cribriform and intraductal prostate cancer are associated with increased genomic instability and distinct genomic alterations. BMC Cancer 2018;18(1):8.

53. Elfandy H, Armenia J, Pederzoli F, et al. Genetic and epigenetic determinants of aggressiveness in cribriform carcinoma of the prostate. Mol Cancer Res 2019;17(2):446–56.

54. Lozano R, Salles DC, Sandhu S, et al. Association between BRCA2 alterations and intraductal and cribriform histologies in prostate cancer. Eur J Cancer 2021;147:74–83.

55. Chua MLK, Lo W, Pintilie M, et al. A prostate cancer "nimbosus": genomic instability and SChLAP1 dysregulation underpin aggression of intraductal and cribriform subpathologies. Eur Urol 2017;72(5):665–74.

56. Shah RB, Shore KT, Yoon J, et al. PTEN loss in prostatic adenocarcinoma correlates with specific adverse histologic features (intraductal carcinoma, cribriform Gleason pattern 4 and stromogenic carcinoma). Prostate 2019;79(11):1267–73.

57. Lotan TL, Gumuskaya B, Rahimi H, et al. Cytoplasmic PTEN protein loss distinguishes intraductal carcinoma of the prostate from high-grade prostatic intraepithelial neoplasia. Mod Pathol 2013;26(4):587–603.

58. Dawkins HJ, Sellner LN, Turbett GR, et al. Distinction between intraductal carcinoma of the prostate (IDC-P), high-grade dysplasia (PIN), and invasive prostatic adenocarcinoma, using molecular markers of cancer progression. Prostate 2000;44(4):265–70.

59. Bettendorf O, Schmidt H, Staebler A, et al. Chromosomal imbalances, loss of heterozygosity, and immunohistochemical expression of TP53, RB1, and PTEN in intraductal cancer, intraepithelial neoplasia, and invasive adenocarcinoma of the prostate. Genes Chromosomes Cancer 2008;47(7):565–72.

Diagnosis and Pathologic Reporting of Prostate Cancer in the Era of MRI-Targeted Prostate Biopsy

Benjamin L. Coiner, MD[a], Soroush Rais-Bahrami, MD[b,c,d], Jennifer B. Gordetsky, MD[e,f,*]

KEYWORDS

- PI-RADS • Prostatic adenocarcinoma • Cancer imaging • Gleason score • Grade group
- Pathology reporting

Key points

- Multiparametric MRI-targeted biopsy of the prostate in combination with standard-of-care, systematic extended sextant prostate biopsy improves the overall detection of prostate cancer, including low-grade cases.
- MRI-targeted biopsies are more likely to detect higher-grade disease and high-risk pathologic features.
- Targeted biopsy pathology should be routinely reported separately from systematic biopsies.
- Reporting of prostate cancer grade and tumor extent on each distinct MRI-targeted biopsy site is best done utilizing an aggregate approach to tissue cores obtained from that site.
- Pertinent benign histologic findings are recommended to be reported for targeted lesions with prostate imaging reporting and data system scores of 4–5 and no cancer identified on targeted cores.

Historically, the detection of prostate cancer relied upon a systematic yet random sampling of the prostate by transrectal ultrasound guided biopsy. This approach was a nontargeted technique that led to the under detection of cancers at biopsy and the upgrading of cancers at radical prostatectomy. Multiparametric MRI-targeted prostate biopsy allows for an image-directed approach to the identification of prostate cancer. MRI-targeted biopsy of the prostate is superior for the detection of clinically significant prostate cancer. As this technique has become more prevalent among urologists, pathologists need to recognize how this development impacts cancer diagnosis and reporting.

OVERVIEW

Historically, the detection of prostate cancer relied upon a systematic yet random sampling of the

[a] Vanderbilt University School of Medicine, 2209 Garland Avenue, Nashville, TN 37232, USA; [b] Department of Urology, University of Alabama at Birmingham, Birmingham, AL, USA; [c] Department of Radiology, University of Alabama at Birmingham, Birmingham, AL, USA; [d] O'Neal Comprehensive Cancer Center, University of Alabama at Birmingham, Faculty Office Tower 1107, 510 20th Street South, Birmingham, AL 35294, USA; [e] Department of Urology, Vanderbilt University Medical Center, Nashville, TN, USA; [f] Department of Pathology, Microbiology and Immunology, Vanderbilt University Medical Center, C-3320 MCN, 1161 21st Avenue South, Nashville, TN 37232, USA
* Corresponding author. Department of Pathology, Vanderbilt University Medical Center, C-3320 MCN, 1161 21st Avenue South, Nashville, TN 37232.
E-mail address: Jennifer.b.gordetsky@vumc.org
Twitter: @bencoiner (B.L.C.); Twitter: @RaisBahrami (S.R.-B.); Twitter: @jgordetsky (J.B.G.)

Surgical Pathology 15 (2022) 609–616
https://doi.org/10.1016/j.path.2022.07.002

prostate gland by needle core biopsy when there was a clinical suspicion of prostate cancer. This random sampling of the prostate was limited by ultrasound imaging technology, which was useful for transrectal identification of the prostate gland but insufficient for identifying regions suspicious for cancer. As systematic sampling of the prostate is a nontargeted approach, this technique led to the under detection of cancers at biopsy and a significant degree of upgrading of cancers at radical prostatectomy.[1] In the era of active surveillance, appropriate characterization and risk stratification of prostate cancer on biopsy is of the utmost clinical importance.[2] Advances in multiparametric (MP)-MRI have revolutionized detection of prostate cancer on imaging. This technique allows for an image-directed approach to the identification of prostate cancer. It has been shown that MRI-targeted biopsy of the prostate, whether alone or in combination with the traditional systematic approach, is superior for the appropriate detection and characterization of prostate cancer.[3–6] As this technique has become more prevalent among urologists, pathologists need to recognize how this development impacts cancer diagnosis and our role in reporting prostate cancer findings.

DISCUSSION

MULTIPARAMETRIC MRI OF THE PROSTATE

MP-MRI offers high-resolution imaging of soft tissues, especially useful in the detection of prostatic lesions suspicious for cancer. This technology is now a widely accepted tool alongside systematic transrectal ultrasound (TRUS) biopsy in prostate cancer diagnosis and management.[4,7–11] By using different imaging sequences, MP-MRI provides information from prostate anatomy and volume to lesion characteristics, such as cellularity, tissue density, and vascularity, and is a sensitive imaging method for detecting prostate cancer.[8,12] Lesion characteristics found via MP-MRI can then be used to estimate malignancy and tumor aggressiveness.[12,13] MP-MRI has also been shown to accurately identify local extra-prostatic spread and detect regional and metastatic disease spread.[14] As a result, compared to systematic TRUS biopsy, MP-MRI with or without subsequent MRI-targeted biopsy detects more clinically significant prostate cancer and overlooks more clinically insignificant prostate cancer.[7–10,12–16] In cases where cancer is first detected on systematic TRUS biopsy, MP-MRI has been shown to upgrade the Gleason score in a proportion of patients.[12] Mounting evidence suggests MP-MRI may both help patients avoid unnecessary biopsies and overtreatment of clinically insignificant prostate cancers. In addition, MRI-targeted biopsies provide additional pathologic information, leading to improved cancer detection and reduced misclassification of clinically significant prostate cancer.[3,4,7,8,10,12,14,17] Recent randomized clinical trials offer evidence supporting the use of prebiopsy MP-MRI as a universally beneficial risk assessment tool in patients being considered for biopsy.[4,17,18] However, evidence supporting the use of both MRI-targeted and systematic TRUS biopsy together exists. Ahdoot and colleagues advocated for the use of combined MRI-targeted and systematic TRUS biopsy, citing their findings that this combined approach led to an increased number of overall prostate cancer diagnoses, including clinically significant prostate cancer. They argue that a combined approach better ensures the biopsy is representative of the patient's tumor, as MRI-targeted biopsy alone may underestimate the grade of some tumors.[3] Multiple groups have found that MRI-targeted plus systematic confirmatory biopsy improves risk stratification in patients at the time of active surveillance enrollment.[19,20]

METHODS FOR TARGETED BIOPSY OF THE PROSTATE

Once a lesion suspicious for prostate cancer has been identified by MP-MRI and biopsy is indicated, three methods exist for MRI-targeted biopsy: in-bore, cognitive fusion, and MRI/ultrasound (MRI/US) software-based fusion.[12,14,15,21] In-bore MRI-guided biopsy is performed with the patient in the bore of the MRI scanner. The biopsy is performed during a separate scan after a suspicious lesion has been identified. Serial MRI scans guide the biopsy needle using a transrectal or transperineal approach. This method is limited by space, patient comfort, sedation needs, and safety requirements of the MRI environment. Cognitive fusion requires an experienced operator to view the MRI images showing a suspicious lesion before the biopsy, which is then cognitively translated by the operator to the images viewed while performing a TRUS biopsy. MRI/US fusion uses software to translate the lesion identified by MRI to a real-time image used for TRUS biopsy. In their systematic review, Wegelin and colleagues[15] found that all three methods of MRI-targeted biopsies had similar overall prostate cancer detection rates compared with systematic TRUS biopsy, but increased detection of clinically significant cancer and decreased detection of insignificant cancer. Their results showed in-bore biopsy to be similar to MRI/US fusion and superior to the cognitive fusion method for detection of prostate cancer.

PROSTATE IMAGING REPORTING AND DATA SYSTEM SCORING OF PROSTATE LESIONS

The Prostate Imaging Reporting and Data System (PI-RADS) is a standardized, 5-category risk-stratification system for prostate lesions detected by MP-MRI.[11] First established in 2012, PI-RADS has been validated and improved upon. PI-RADS version 2.0, published in 2016, was designed by the joint steering committee of the American College of Radiology, the European Society of Urogenital Radiology, and the AdMeTech Foundation to better standardize image acquisition, interpretation, and reporting.[11,13,22] Most recently, PI-RADS version 2.1 was published in 2019 to offer technical revisions and address specific limitations of PI-RADS version 2.0 that had been identified, including issues of inter-reader variability, clarification, and simplification of interpretation criteria.[11,22] Since its development and now widespread implementation, PI-RADS, used to interpret prostate MP-MRI and inform MRI-targeted biopsy, has improved prostate cancer diagnostic pathways, including the detection of clinically significant prostate cancers.[13,22–24] Mazzone and colleagues[25] discovered positive predictive values (PPVs) for PI-RADS 3, 4, and 5 to be 13%, 40%, and 69%, respectively, in their systematic review and meta-analysis of the PPV of PI-RADS version 2.0 categories. PI-RADS has also recently been incorporated into various externally validated prostate cancer prediction models, which consider additional variables, such as Prostate specific antigen (PSA), Digital rectal exam (DRE), and previous biopsy.[24]

PI-RADS category 1 denotes a most likely benign lesion, category 3 an indeterminate lesion, and category 5 a most likely malignant lesion. In the first version of PI-RADS, an overall score was established after considering different imaging parameters—T2 weighted imaging, diffusion-weighted imaging, dynamic contrast-enhanced (DCE) T1-weighted imaging, and magnetic resonance spectroscopic imaging (MRSI).[11] PI-RADS versions 2.0 and 2.1 have since revised the emphasis on these imaging parameters, decreasing emphasis on DCE T1-weighted imaging and no longer including MRSI.[11,13,22]

CURRENT CLINICAL GUIDELINES

A 2016 consensus statement from the American Urological Association (AUA) and the Society of Abdominal Radiology (SAR) offered a series of recommendations for MP-MRI and MRI-targeted biopsy in patients with a prior negative biopsy.[26] Patients with PI-RADS 3–5 lesions warrant repeat biopsy with image-guided targeting. The statement acknowledges that MRI/US fusion or in-bore targeting may be more optimal choices, although cognitive fusion remains reasonable if a skilled operator is available. Two targeted cores must be obtained from each target lesion identified by MRI. Concurrent systematic TRUS biopsy may be chosen on a case-specific basis. Repeat biopsy may be deferred in men with PI-RADS 1 or 2 lesions and an otherwise low clinical suspicion of prostate cancer. In instances of negative MRI-targeted biopsy, continued clinical and laboratory follow-up and consideration of additional biopsies is recommended. A 2018 guideline from the AUA, the American Society for Radiation Oncology, and the Society of Urologic Oncology for patients with clinically localized prostate cancer stated that MP-MRI may be considered as part of active surveillance and that all patients with localized prostate cancer who elect active surveillance must have accurate staging that includes systematic TRUS biopsy or MRI-targeted biopsy.[27]

The European Association of Urology, the European Association of Nuclear Medicine, the European Society for Radiotherapy and Oncology, the European Association of Urology Section of Urological Research, and the International Society of Geriatric Oncology Prostate Cancer Guideline Panel offered consensus statements for deferred active treatment (DAT) for localized prostate cancer in 2019.[28] Their recommendations involving MP-MRI were as follows: A DAT program should be included in which MP-MRI should be performed at some point. Patients may be excluded from consideration for DAT if the extent and/or stage of disease is high as seen on MP-MRI. For inclusion, both MRI-targeted and systematic biopsies should be performed. If MP-MRI is followed by systematic and targeted biopsy, there is no need for confirmatory biopsy. The number of positive cores from MRI-targeted biopsies should not be used to estimate the extent of disease or tumor volume. Instead, the number of positive sextants from systemic biopsy and/or volume of the dominant lesion as seen on MP-MRI (if PI-RADS version $2 \geq 3$) should be considered as indicators of tumor volume. MP-MRI characteristics of lesions should not be used alone to exclude patients from DAT in patients with $\leq$T2 disease. Perform repeat MRI-targeted and systematic biopsies if any changes occur in MP-MRI findings for patients on active surveillance.

In 2020, the AUA and SAR published an update on the use of MP-MRI for diagnosis, staging, and management of prostate cancer[18]: PI-RADS version 2.1 is strongly encouraged when reporting MP-MRI findings. In biopsy naïve patients, prebiopsy MP-MRI is recommended. In patients with lesions suspicious of prostate cancer, MRI-targeted biopsy combined with systematic TRUS biopsy is advisable until sufficient evidence exists supporting a low risk of missing clinically significant cancers with MRI-targeted biopsy alone. When a biopsy is deferred, it is advised to further stratify risk via secondary biomarkers and maintain close follow-up. In patients with a previous negative biopsy, prebiopsy MP-MRI is also recommended to identify lesions that may have been missed with prior systematic biopsy. MP-MRI can be used for risk stratification and guiding surgical interventions, but its low sensitivity for local extraprostatic extension limits its use alone as a staging tool. MP-MRI and MRI-targeted biopsy is strongly recommended for patients considering active surveillance.

CONSIDERATIONS AT THE TIME OF THE BIOPSY

It is recommended that MRI-targeted lesions be labeled appropriately and given a distinction from standard systematic prostate biopsies.[16,29,30] Identification of the number of distinct regions of interest that are targeted, location of the area sampled, and PI-RADS score are useful pieces of information that should be provided by the clinician. It is also useful for the clinician to specify the patient's PSA and how many cores were obtained from each targeted lesion, as cores can often fracture upon collection. Information in this regard that is provided on the pathology requisition should be included in the pathology report.

The number of cores sampled at the time of MRI-targeted prostate biopsy has been shown by multiple studies to impact the overall detection of prostate cancer as well as the detection of the highest grade within a region of interest.[12,29,31–35] Studies have shown that obtaining only one biopsy core per targeted lesion can lead to decreased detection of cancer or missing a higher-grade component of a lesion.[12] One study showed that obtaining only one biopsy core underestimated the presence of cancer or the highest grade in up to 9% of lesions.[12] Another study showed a two-core approach missed 16% of clinically significant cancers in biopsy-naïve patients, 27% in men with a prior negative biopsy, and 32% in men on active surveillance.[31] Most cancers and clinically significant cancers will be detected using two-core sampling per targeted lesion, with studies showing a 72%–89% detection of the

highest Gleason grade or clinically significant Gleason grade.[31,32] Indeed, a 2016 consensus statement by the AUA and SAR recommended that at least two cores be obtained from each suspicious lesion found on MRI.[26] However, this still leaves a significant proportion of men who would be missed, which could have serious implications for men on active surveillance. More recent studies have demonstrated an improvement in cancer detection and highest/clinically significant grade detection using a three-core approach for both in-bore MRI-guided biopsy and MRI/US fusion-guided biopsy of the prostate.[33–35]

REPORTING OF PATHOLOGY

There have been relatively few studies that have investigated the best methods of reporting pathologic findings on MRI-targeted prostate biopsy. The first study to do so compared an aggregate tissue approach to an individual core approach for grading of cancer and determination of tumor extent.[36] The authors found that an aggregate method, which evaluates all tissue taken from a single MRI-targeted lesion, was superior to reporting each core individually. The percent of tumor extent within the entire sampled tissue was better correlated with lesion volume, lesion density, and prediction of extraprostatic extension after radical prostatectomy.[36] A more recent study validated these findings in terms of prostate cancer grading.[37] They showed that providing a global/aggregate grade using all positive cores from a single lesion performed better than either the highest single core score or the largest volume grade. This method rarely leads to downgrading at the time of radical prostatectomy. The authors also noted that grade concordance improved as the number of positive cores per lesion increased (≥3), which likely represents a better sampling of the index lesion. Aggregate grading of MRI-targeted biopsies may also offer better prediction of extraprostatic extension and lymph node involvement when using the Memorial Sloan Kettering Cancer Center pre-prostatectomy nomogram.[38] The aggregate reporting method for MRI-targeted biopsies was recommended recently in consensus statements by both the Genitourinary Pathology Society and the International Society of Urological Pathology (ISUP).[16,30]

The reporting of benign findings on MRI-targeted prostate biopsy has also been commented upon in the literature. It is well recognized that there are benign histologic findings that correlate with false-positive findings on MRI.[39] MRI technology depends on vascularity and tissue density to help identify areas suspicious for prostatic adenocarcinoma. Benign entities, such as increased stromal/gland ratio, benign prostatic hyperplasia, vascular lesions, or certain types of inflammation may cause a high PIRADS score.[39–42] Efforts are being made to improve the detection of these false positive lesions to avoid unnecessary biopsies in men.[43] Reporting of benign histologic findings known to mimic cancer on targeted biopsy cores may help to clinically correlate a highly suspicious MRI region of interest (PIRADS 4–5) with a benign pathologic diagnosis and thereby effect patient management. As such, the ISUP consensus statement recommended benign histology reporting in targeted biopsy cores with a PIRADS score of 4 or 5 and no finding of cancer.[30]

DETECTION OF POOR PROGNOSTIC PATHOLOGY FEATURES

MRI-targeted prostate biopsy has been shown to be superior to standard systematic biopsy in the detection of clinically significant cancer and high-risk features.[3,5,44–49] Of particular interest is the detection of cribriform morphology on prostate biopsy. The presence of cribriform morphology is known to be a poor prognostic marker associated with upgrading of cancer on radical prostatectomy, the presence of extraprostatic disease, increased risk of biochemical recurrence, and decreased disease-specific survival and, as such, is contraindicated for active surveillance.[16,30] Studies have shown that the incorporation of MRI-targeted biopsy improves the detection of cribriform morphology.[48,49] In addition, MRI-targeted biopsy has been shown to improve the detection of extraprostatic extension and perineural invasion, which can help in the selection of patients for active surveillance.[44–47] A recent study looking at transperineal MRI-ultrasound fusion-targeted prostate biopsy combined with a standard template detected perineural invasion in over 30% of patients.[45] Perineural invasion identified on MRI-targeted biopsy was shown in one study to predict extraprostatic extension and early biochemical recurrence.[50]

It has long been recognized that MRI-targeted biopsies are sensitive to areas with higher grade prostate cancer.[51] This allows for better detection of clinically significant prostate cancer but can also lead to oversampling of higher-grade areas.[46] Thus, it is recognized that MRI-targeted biopsy alone is more prone to downgrading at prostatectomy than systematic biopsies. This risk may be reduced by aggregate reporting of targeted biopsies.[36,37] Studies have recommended the combination of both systemic and MRI-targeted biopsies for the most accurate prediction of grade and adverse pathologic findings on radical prostatectomy.[3,5]

MISSING THE TARGET?

Clinically significant prostate cancer is rarely missed on MRI-targeted prostate biopsy but can occur for a variety of reasons. The most common scenario in MRI/US fusion-guided prostate biopsy is misregistrations by the software.[52,53] These cases are associated with smaller volume tumors on MRI, and often low-grade prostate cancers are detected in the sextants immediately adjacent to the targeted region of interest.[52] One study looked at false-negative cases in patients who had been previously diagnosed with prostate cancer and subsequently underwent in-bore MRI-guided biopsy.[54] Several of these patients had MRI-invisible lesions, and most of them had Grade Group 1 disease. Patients with prostate volumes greater than 40 mL were also at higher risk of having a missed lesion. Interestingly, the authors found that cancers in the anterior gland had a lower false-negative rate as MRI-targeted biopsy has been shown to optimize the detection of commonly occult anterior gland prostate cancer lesions.[54] Another study found similar findings in terms of errors in lesion targeting and MRI-invisible lesions being most common.[53] However, they also noted that 7% of cases were lesions missed by the radiologist. They found that a lower PIRADS score, despite a high PSA, was associated with missing a clinically significant prostate cancer on MRI-targeted biopsy.[53]

SUMMARY

MP-MRI-targeted biopsy of the prostate in combination with standard, systematic prostate biopsy improves the detection of clinically significant prostate cancer and high-risk pathologic features. Appropriate documentation of clinical and radiographic information, such as PIRADS score and PSA, is important and should be considered for inclusion in the pathology report. Targeted biopsy pathology should be reported separately from systematic biopsies. Reporting of prostate cancer grade and tumor extent on MRI-targeted biopsy is best done utilizing an aggregate/global tissue approach for each individual lesion targeted. Pertinent benign histology findings are recommended to be reported for targeted lesions with PI-RADS scores of 4–5 that do not harbor cancer.

CLINICS CARE POINTS

- An aggregate reporting method, which evaluates all tissue taken from a single MRI-targeted lesion, is superior to reporting each core individually in terms of correlation of tumor extent with lesion volume, lesion density, and prediction of extraprostatic extension and grade at radical prostatectomy.

- MP-MRI and MRI-targeted biopsy is strongly recommended for patients considering active surveillance.

- In biopsy naïve patients, prebiopsy MP-MRI is recommended.

- In patients with a previous negative biopsy, prebiopsy MP-MRI is recommended to identify lesions that may have been missed with prior systematic biopsy.

- MP-MRI-targeted biopsy of the prostate in combination with standard, systematic prostate biopsy improves the detection of clinically significant prostate cancer and high-risk pathologic features.

DISCLOSURE

The authors have nothing to disclose.

REFERENCES

1. George AK, Pinto PA, Rais-Bahrami S. Multiparametric MRI in the PSA screening era. Biomed Res Int 2014;2014:465816-6.
2. Glaser ZA, Porter KK, Thomas Jv, et al. MRI findings guiding selection of active surveillance for prostate cancer: a review of emerging evidence. Translational Androl Urol 2018;7(Suppl 4):S411–9.
3. Ahdoot M, Wilbur AR, Reese SE, et al. MRI-targeted, systematic, and combined biopsy for prostate cancer diagnosis. N Engl J Med 2020;382(10):917–28.
4. Kasivisvanathan V, Rannikko AS, Borghi M, et al. MRI-targeted or standard biopsy for prostate-cancer diagnosis. N Engl J Med 2018. https://doi.org/10.1056/nejmoa1801993.
5. Gandaglia G, Ploussard G, Valerio M, et al. The key combined value of multiparametric magnetic resonance imaging, and magnetic resonance imaging–targeted and concomitant systematic biopsies for the prediction of adverse pathological features in prostate cancer patients undergoing radical prostatectomy. Eur Urol 2020;77(6):733–41.
6. Patel HD, Koehne EL, Shea SM, et al. Systematic versus targeted magnetic resonance imaging/ultrasound fusion prostate biopsy among men with visible lesions. J Urol 2022;207(1):108–17.
7. Siddiqui MM, Rais-Bahrami S, Turkbey B, et al. Comparison of MR/ultrasound fusion-guided biopsy with ultrasound-guided biopsy for the diagnosis of prostate cancer. JAMA 2015;313(4):390–7.
8. Ahmed HU, El-Shater Bosaily A, Brown LC, et al. Diagnostic accuracy of multi-parametric MRI and TRUS biopsy in prostate cancer (PROMIS): a paired validating confirmatory study. Lancet 2017;389(10071):815–22.
9. Gordetsky JB, Saylor B, Bae S, et al. Prostate cancer management choices in patients undergoing multiparametric magnetic resonance imaging/ultrasound fusion biopsy compared to systematic biopsy. Urol Oncol 2018;36(5):241.e7-13.
10. Drost F-JH, Osses D, Nieboer D, et al. Prostate magnetic resonance imaging, with or without magnetic resonance imaging-targeted biopsy, and systematic biopsy for detecting prostate cancer: a cochrane systematic review and meta-analysis. Eur Urol 2020;77(1):78–94.
11. Dutruel SP, Jeph S, Margolis DJA, et al. PI-RADS: what is new and how to use it. Abdom Radiol 2020;45(12):3951–60.
12. Hong CW, Rais-Bahrami S, Walton-Diaz A, et al. Comparison of magnetic resonance imaging and ultrasound (MRI-US) fusion-guided prostate biopsies obtained from axial and sagittal approaches. BJU Int 2015;115(5):772–9.
13. Padhani AR, Weinreb J, Rosenkrantz AB, et al. Prostate imaging-reporting and data system steering committee: PI-RADS v2 status update and future directions. Eur Urol 2019;75(3):385–96.
14. Gennaro K, Porter K, Gordetsky J, et al. Imaging as a personalized biomarker for prostate cancer risk stratification. Diagnostics 2018;8(4):80.
15. Wegelin O, van Melick HHE, Hooft L, et al. Comparing three different techniques for magnetic resonance imaging-targeted prostate biopsies: a systematic review of in-bore versus magnetic resonance imaging-transrectal ultrasound fusion versus cognitive registration. is there a preferred technique? Eur Urol 2017;517–31. https://doi.org/10.1016/j.eururo.2016.07.041.
16. Epstein JI, Amin MB, Fine SW, et al. The 2019 genitourinary pathology society (GUPS) white paper on contemporary grading of prostate cancer. Arch Pathol Lab Med 2021;461–93. https://doi.org/10.5858/arpa.2020-0015-ra.
17. Klotz L, Chin J, Black PC, et al. Comparison of multiparametric magnetic resonance imaging-targeted biopsy with systematic transrectal ultrasonography biopsy for biopsy-naive men at risk for prostate

cancer: a phase 3 randomized clinical trial. JAMA Oncol 2021;7(4):534–42.

18. Bjurlin MA, Carroll PR, Eggener S, et al. Update of the standard operating procedure on the use of multiparametric magnetic resonance imaging for the diagnosis, staging and management of prostate cancer. J Urol 2020;203(4):706–12.

19. O'Connor LP, Wang AZ, Yerram NK, et al. Combined MRI-targeted plus systematic confirmatory biopsy improves risk stratification for patients enrolling on active surveillance for prostate cancer. Urology 2020;144:164–70.

20. Lai WS, Gordetsky JB, Thomas Jv, et al. Factors predicting prostate cancer upgrading on magnetic resonance imaging–targeted biopsy in an active surveillance population. Cancer 2017;123(11): 1941–8.

21. Logan JK, Rais-Bahrami S, Turkbey B, et al. Current status of magnetic resonance imaging (MRI) and ultrasonography fusion software platforms for guidance of prostate biopsies. BJU Int 2014;641–52. https://doi.org/10.1111/bju.12593.

22. Turkbey B, Rosenkrantz AB, Haider MA, et al. Prostate imaging reporting and data system version 2.1: 2019 update of prostate imaging reporting and data system version 2. Eur Urol 2019;340–51. https://doi.org/10.1016/j.eururo.2019.02.033.

23. Padhani AR, Barentsz J, Villeirs G, et al. PI-RADS Steering Committee: the PI-RADS Multiparametric MRI and MRI-directed Biopsy Pathway. Radiology 2019;292(2):464–74.

24. Fang AM, Rais-Bahrami S. Magnetic resonance imaging–based risk calculators optimize selection for prostate biopsy among biopsy-naive men. Cancer 2021. https://doi.org/10.1002/cncr.33872.

25. Mazzone E, Stabile A, Pellegrino F, et al. Positive predictive value of prostate imaging reporting and data system version 2 for the detection of clinically significant prostate cancer: a systematic review and meta-analysis. Eur Urol Oncol 2021;4(5): 697–713.

26. Rosenkrantz AB, Verma S, Choyke P, et al. Prostate magnetic resonance imaging and magnetic resonance imaging targeted biopsy in patients with a prior negative biopsy: a consensus statement by AUA and SAR. J Urol 2016;196(6):1613–8.

27. Sanda MG, Cadeddu JA, Kirkby E, et al. Clinically localized prostate cancer: AUA/ASTRO/SUO Guideline. Part II: recommended approaches and details of specific care options. J Urol 2018;199(4):990–7.

28. Lam TBL, MacLennan S, Willemse PPM, et al. EAU-EANM-ESTRO-ESUR-SIOG prostate cancer guideline panel consensus statements for deferred treatment with curative intent for localised prostate cancer from an international collaborative study (DETECTIVE Study). Eur Urol 2019;790–813. https://doi.org/10.1016/j.eururo.2019.09.020.

29. Gordetsky JB, Hirsch MS, Rais-Bahrami S. MRI-targeted prostate biopsy: key considerations for pathologists. Histopathology 2020;18–25. https://doi.org/10.1111/his.14113.

30. Leenders G, Kwast T, Grignon DJ, et al. The 2019 international society of urological pathology (ISUP) consensus conference on grading of prostatic carcinoma. Am J Surg Pathol 2020;44(8):e87–99.

31. Lu AJ, Syed JS, Ghabili K, et al. Role of core number and location in targeted magnetic resonance imaging-ultrasound fusion prostate biopsy. Eur Urol 2019;76(1):14–7.

32. Kenigsberg AP, Renson A, Rosenkrantz AB, et al. Optimizing the number of cores targeted during prostate magnetic resonance imaging fusion target biopsy. Eur Urol Oncol 2018;1(5):418–25.

33. Song G, Ruan M, Wang H, et al. How many targeted biopsy cores are needed for clinically significant prostate cancer detection during transperineal magnetic resonance imaging ultrasound fusion biopsy? J Urol 2020;204(6):1202–8.

34. Subramanian N, Recchimuzzi DZ, Xi Y, et al. Impact of the number of cores on the prostate cancer detection rate in men undergoing in-bore magnetic resonance imaging-guided targeted biopsies. J Comput Assist Tomogr 2021;45(2):203–9.

35. Seyfried N, Mahran A, Panda A, et al. Diagnostic yield of incremental biopsy cores and second lesion sampling for in-gantry mri-guided prostate biopsy. Am J Roentgenol 2020;217(4):908–18. https://doi.org/10.2214/AJR.20.24918.

36. Gordetsky JB, Schultz L, Porter KK, et al. Defining the optimal method for reporting prostate cancer grade and tumor extent on magnetic resonance/ultrasound fusion–targeted biopsies. Hum Pathol 2018;76:68–75.

37. Deng F-M, Isaila B, Jones D, et al. Optimal method for reporting prostate cancer grade in MRI-targeted biopsies. Am J Surg Pathol 2022;46(1): 44–50.

38. Glaser ZA, Gordetsky JB, Bae S, et al. Evaluation of MSKCC Preprostatectomy nomogram in men who undergo MRI-targeted prostate biopsy prior to radical prostatectomy. Urol Oncol 2019;37(12): 970–5.

39. Gordetsky JB, Ullman D, Schultz L, et al. Histologic findings associated with false-positive multiparametric magnetic resonance imaging performed for prostate cancer detection. Hum Pathol 2019;83:159–65.

40. Rais-Bahrami S, Nix JW, Turkbey B, et al. Clinical and multiparametric MRI signatures of granulomatous prostatitis. Abdom Radiol 2017;42(7):1956–62.

41. Sheridan AD, Nath SK, Aneja S, et al. MRI-ultrasound fusion targeted biopsy of prostate imaging reporting and data system version 2 category 5 lesions found false-positive at multiparametric prostate MRI. Am J Roentgenol 2018;210(5):W218–25.

42. Hupe MC, Offermann A, Tharun L, et al. Histomorphological analysis of false positive PI-RADS 4 and 5 lesions. Urol Oncol 2020;38(7):636.e7-12.

43. Stavrinides V, Syer T, Hu Y, et al. False positive multiparametric magnetic resonance imaging phenotypes in the biopsy-naïve prostate: are they distinct from significant cancer-associated lesions? lessons from PROMIS. Eur Urol 2021;79(1):20–9.

44. Gold SA, Shih JH, Rais-Bahrami S, et al. When to biopsy the seminal vesicles: a validated multiparametric magnetic resonance imaging and target driven model to detect seminal vesicle invasion of prostate cancer. J Urol 2019;201(5):943–9.

45. Wu CL, Kim M, Wu S, et al. Transperineal multiparametric magnetic resonance imaging-ultrasound fusion-targeted prostate biopsy combined with standard template improves perineural invasion detection. Hum Pathol 2021;117:101–7.

46. Gordetsky JB, Nix JW, Rais-Bahrami S. Perineural invasion in prostate cancer is more frequently detected by multiparametric MRI targeted biopsy compared with standard biopsy. Am J Surg Pathol 2016;40(4):490–4.

47. Baumgartner EM, Porter KK, Nix JW, et al. Detection of extraprostatic disease and seminal vesicle invasion in patients undergoing magnetic resonance imaging-targeted prostate biopsies. Translational Androl Urol 2018;7:S392–6.

48. Prendeville S, Gertner M, Maganti M, et al. Role of magnetic resonance imaging targeted biopsy in detection of prostate cancer harboring adverse pathological features of intraductal carcinoma and invasive cribriform carcinoma. J Urol 2018;200(1):104–13.

49. Gao J, Zhang Q, Fu Y, et al. Combined clinical characteristics and multiparametric MRI parameters for prediction of cribriform morphology in intermediate-risk prostate cancer patients. Urol Oncol 2020;38(4):216–24.

50. Truong M, Rais-Bahrami S, Nix JW, et al. Perineural invasion by prostate cancer on MR/US fusion targeted biopsy is associated with extraprostatic extension and early biochemical recurrence after radical prostatectomy. Hum Pathol 2017;66:206–11.

51. Gordetsky JB, Thomas JV, Nix JW, et al. Higher prostate cancer grade groups are detected in patients undergoing multiparametric MRI-targeted biopsy compared with standard biopsy. Am J Surg Pathol 2017;41(1):101–5.

52. Coker MA, Glaser ZA, Gordetsky JB, et al. Targets missed: predictors of MRI-targeted biopsy failing to accurately localize prostate cancer found on systematic biopsy. Prostate Cancer Prostatic Dis 2018;21(4):549–55.

53. Williams C, Ahdoot M, Daneshvar MA, et al. Why does magnetic resonance imaging-targeted biopsy miss clinically significant cancer? J Urol 2022;207(1):95–107.

54. Elfatairy KK, Filson CP, Sanda MG, et al. In-Bore MRI-guided prostate biopsies in patients with prior positive transrectal us-guided biopsy results: pathologic outcomes and predictors of missed cancers. Radiol Imaging Cancer 2020;2(5):e190078.

Molecular Genetics of Prostate Cancer and Role of Genomic Testing

Dilara Akhoundova, MD[a,b], Felix Y. Feng, MD[c],
Colin C. Pritchard, MD, PhD[d], Mark A. Rubin, MD[a,e],*

KEYWORDS

- Prostate cancer • Molecular profiling • Homologous recombination deficiency
- Microsatellite instability • Targeted treatment • PARP inhibitors • Genomic classifiers
- Germline testing

Key points

- PCa molecular landscape is profoundly heterogeneous and a classification into 7 molecular subgroups has been proposed based on molecular profiling of localized PCa (TCGA cohort).

- For localized PCa, several genomic classifiers are available to predict risk of distant metastasis, or/and PCa-related mortality. These assays can support clinical decision making regarding active surveillance or indication of adjuvant therapy following radical prostatectomy.

- In metastatic disease, main therapeutically actionable alterations are HRD, MSI-H, and CDK12 deficiency. Alterations in DNA damage response genes are present in 19% of localized and up to 31% of metastatic PCas. Genomic instability assays assessing HRD may predict sensitivity to PARP inhibitors.

- MSI-H (1–5%) sensitizes to immune checkpoint inhibitors (ICIs) and can be identified by immunohistochemistry (IHC), microsatellite PCR, or NGS, as well as sequencing of mismatch repair (MMR) genes. CDK12-deficient PCas (1%–5%) present variable degrees of sensitivities to ICIs.

- Germline testing is recommended in patients with personal history of high or very-high-risk localized PCa, regional or metastatic PCa, as well as family history of PCa.

ABSTRACT

Prostate cancer (PCa) is characterized by profound genomic heterogeneity. Recent advances in personalized treatment entail an increasing need of genomic profiling. For localized PCa, gene expression assays can support clinical decisions regarding active surveillance and adjuvant treatment. In metastatic PCa, homologous recombination deficiency, microsatellite instability-high (MSI-H), and CDK12 deficiency constitute main actionable alterations. Alterations in DNA repair genes confer variable sensitivities to poly(ADP-ribose)polymerase inhibitors, and the use of genomic instability assays as predictive biomarker is still incipient. MSI can be assessed by immunohistochemistry To date there is a lack of consensus as to testing standards.

Funded by: SWISS2021.

[a] Department for BioMedical Research, University of Bern, Murtenstrasse 24, Bern 3008, Switzerland; [b] Department of Medical Oncology, Inselspital, University Hospital of Bern, Bern 3010, Switzerland; [c] Department of Radiation Oncology, University of California, 1600 Divisadero Street, Suite H-1031, San Francisco, CA 94115, USA; [d] Department of Laboratory Medicine and Pathology, University of Washington, 1959 NE Pacific St Seattle, WA 98195-7110, USA; [e] Bern Center for Precision Medicine, Inselspital, University Hospital of Bern, Bern, 3008, Switzerland
* Corresponding author.
E-mail address: mark.rubin@dbmr.unibe.ch

surgpath.theclinics.com

OVERVIEW

Comprehensive molecular profiling of large cohorts of primary prostate cancer (PCa) and metastatic PCa (mPCa), using genome-wide next-generation sequencing (NGS) approaches, has significantly contributed to the characterization of the profoundly heterogeneous molecular landscape of PCa.[1–5] These studies have identified main therapeutically actionable molecular subtypes of PCa, such as homologous recombination-deficient (HRD), defined as harboring alterations in the homologous recombination repair pathway (HRR)[6] and more strictly an HRD mutational signature[7,8]; microsatellite instability-high (MSI-H); or CDK12-deficient tumors.[1–5] In localized disease, multiple studies have shown that gene expression assays performed on PCa biopsies or prostatectomy samples can predict risk of metastatic progression and PCa-specific mortality,[9–13] and current clinical guidelines integrate these assays as a useful tool to support clinical decision making regarding active surveillance and indication of intensification of therapy following radical prostatectomy (RP).[14]

In the metastatic disease scenario, recent clinical studies have demonstrated efficacy of targeted treatment of specific molecular subtypes of PCa, such as poly(ADP-ribose)polymerase (PARP) inhibitors for HRD PCas,[15–19] and immune checkpoint inhibitors (ICIs) for MSI-H[20,21] and a subset of CDK12-deficient[22] PCas. These advances in PCa precision oncology treatment have motivated an increasing demand on genomic testing for patients with mPCa, starting from early treatment lines.[23] In this article, the molecular alterations reported in localized and advanced PCa are summarized, and main molecular diagnostic assays are reviewed, with focus on gene expression assays for localized PCa and genomic instability and MSI assays for advanced disease.

MOLECULAR LANDSCAPE OF LOCALIZED AND METASTATIC PROSTATE CANCER

Most frequent genomic alterations in localized PCa and mPCa are fusions implicating members of the E26 transformation-specific (ETS) transcription factors family. Concretely, the TMPRSS2-ERG fusion is the overall most frequent molecular alteration, found in 40% to 50% of PCas.[1,2,4,24,25] Following the ETS fusions, most frequent genomic alterations in localized PCa are found in PTEN (17%), most frequently homozygous deletions; SPOP (11%); TP53 (8%); and FOXA1 (4%).[1] Based on whole exome sequencing (WES) data from 333

primary PCas, The Cancer Genome Atlas (TCGA) Research Network proposed PCa classification into the following 7 molecular subtypes: PCas with ERG (46%), ETV1 (8%), ETV4 (4%), and FLI1 (1%) fusions and SPOP- (11%), FOXA1-(3%), and IDH1-mutated (1%) PCas.[1] SPOP mutations are the most frequent mutations in localized PCa and are mutually exclusive with the ETS fusions.[1] This molecular classification could cluster 74% of the analyzed tumors. The remaining "not-clusterable" group of PCa tumors (26%) was enriched in mutations in TP53, KDM6A, and KMT2D; deletions in chromosomes 6 and 16; as well as MYC and CCND1 amplifications (**Fig. 1**).

In addition, molecular profiling data from several cohorts of mPCa are available. Whole genome sequencing (WGS) of the CPCT-02 cohort, consisting of 197 metastatic castration-resistant PCas (mCRPC), revealed that 68% of the cases could be clustered into the 7 subtypes proposed by the TCGA classification, and that the therapeutically actionable subtypes HRD, MSI-H, and CDK12[−/−] (tandem duplication genotype) did not show correlation with the TCGA subgroups.[4] Other studies have shown that CDK12 alterations are relatively mutually exclusive with SPOP, ETS fusions, TP53, and PTEN/PIK3CA alterations.[22,26] In the CPCT-02 cohort, mutations in AR, TP53, ZMYM3, APC, RB1, CDK12, ERF, and ZFP36L2 were significantly enriched in mCRPC when compared with the TCGA cohort.[4] WES and transcriptomics profiling of the SU2C-PCF cohort including 150 patients with mCRPC showed that most frequently altered genes in mCRPC are AR (62.7%), most frequently amplifications; ETS-family members (56.7%); TP53 (53.3%); and PTEN (40.7%). Also in this cohort, AR and TP53 alterations were enriched in mCRPC when compared with primary PCas, with AR and GNAS mutations being uniquely found in mCRPC.[2] In addition to the ETS fusions, other fusions uncovered involved BRAF, RAF1, PIK3CA/B, and RSPO2.[2] From a therapeutical point of view, whereas SPOP mutations are associated with longer response to androgen receptor signaling inhibitors (ARSI), shorter responses have been associated with alterations in RB1, TP53, and AR. Moreover, alterations in RB1 have been correlated with shorter overall survival (OS)[3] (see **Fig. 1**).

ALTERATIONS IN DNA REPAIR

Alterations in Homologous Recombination, Fanconi Anemia Pathway, and CDK12

Alterations in DNA damage response (DDR) genes have been reported in 19% of the 333 primary PCa tumors from the TCGA cohort, including alteration

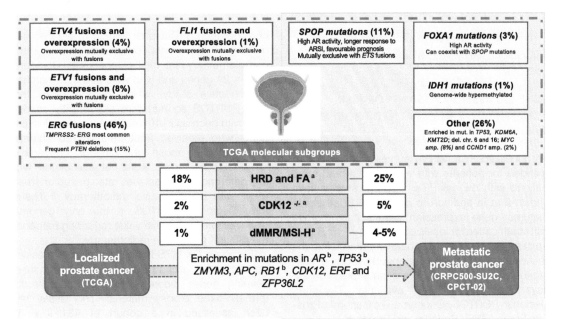

Fig. 1. Molecular landscape of localized and metastatic prostate cancer. Genomic alterations reported from the analysis of the TCGA, CRPC500-SU2C, and CPCT-02 cohorts are illustrated. amp., amplification; ARSI, androgen receptor signaling inhibitors; chr., chromosome; del., deletions; dMMR/MSI-H, mismatch repair deficient, microsatellite instable-high; FA, Fanconi anemia pathway; mut., mutations; OS, overall survival. [a]Actionable alterations; [b]Alterations in RB1, AR, and TP53 associated with shorter response to ARSI and RB1 additionally with shorter OS.

in the distinct genes involved in the HRR[6–8] and Fanconi anemia (FA) pathways, as well as CDK12.[1,27] Similarly, the SU2C-PCF cohort reported alterations in DDR genes in 23% of the cases.[2,3] A cohort of 3476 PCas (1660 samples from localized stage and 1816 mPCa samples) has been molecularly profiled using the FoundatioNOneCDx assay.[5] Alterations in the HRR and FA pathways have been uncovered in 24.4% of the cases, with most frequent alterations found in BRCA2 (9.8%) and ATM (5.2%).[5] In addition, 5.6% of the cases had alterations in CDK12.[5] In the TCGA cohort of localized PCas, the most frequent alterations were found in FANCD2 (7%), ATM (4%), BRCA2 (3%), and RAD51 C (3%),[1] and, in the mCRPC SU2C-PCF cohort, in BRCA2 (13%) and ATM (7.3%).[2,27]

Alterations in Mismatch Repair Genes

MSI-H or mismatch repair deficiency (dMMR) has been reported in 1% to 5% of PCas.[1,2,28,29] In the SU2C-PCF, 3 cases of MSH2 (2%) and 1 case of MLH1 (0.7%) mutations have been reported, corresponding to hypermutated tumors with high tumor mutational burden (TMB).[2] In the PCa cohort analyzed by FoundationOneCDx assay, 4% of the cases harbored alterations in MMR genes (most frequently in MSH2 and MSH6, followed by MLH1 und PMS2) and 0.1% in POLE (V411 E).[5] In a cohort of 433 patients

with mPCa, who underwent liquid biopsy with targeted cell-free DNA (cfDNA) sequencing, pathogenic mutations in MSH2 or MSH6 were uncovered in 2.3% of the cases.[28]

GERMLINE ALTERATIONS

Main germline alterations reported in PCa involve DDR and MMR genes. In the SU2C-PCF cohort, germline alterations in DDR genes were found in 8% of the patients, most frequently BRCA2 mutations (5.3%), followed by ATM (1.3%) and BRCA1 (0.7%).[2] In a study including 3607 men diagnosed with PCa and who received germline testing, germline variants associated with PCa were identified in 17.2% of patients,[30] with most frequent alterations found in BRCA2 (4.7%), CHEK2 (2.9%), MUTYH (2.4%), and ATM (2.0%). In this study distinct assays had been used, covering between 2 and 80 genes. Alterations in HOXB13 were reported in 1.1%, and in MMR genes (MLH1, MSH2, MSH6 and PMS2), in 1.7% of the patients. Screening for germline alterations across 20 DDR genes in a cohort of 692 unselected patients with mPCa uncovered pathogenic mutations involving 16 genes in 11.8% of the studied cohort, with most frequent alterations in BRCA2 (5.3%), ATM (1.6%), CHEK2 (1.9%), and BRCA1 (0.9%).[31] When compared with metastatic cohorts, the frequency of germline alterations in localized PCa (TCGA) was 4.6%.[1]

THE ROLE OF GENOMIC TESTING IN LOCALIZED AND ADVANCED PROSTATE CANCER

GENE EXPRESSION ASSAYS FOR RISK STRATIFICATION IN LOCALIZED PROSTATE CANCER

For localized PCa, active surveillance is recommended for patients with very-low-risk and most patients with low-risk PCa.[14] Several studies have shown that in addition to clinical and pathologic features, gene expression assays can improve risk stratification for localized PCa.[11–13,32,33] Based on this, these assays have been integrated into the routine assessment and therapeutic decision making for localized PCa.[34] Five gene expression assays are commercially available: Decipher, Decipher PORTOS, Oncotype Dx Genomic Prostate Score (GPS), Prolaris, and ProMark.[34]

Decipher is a 22 gene-expression assay suitable for formalin-fixed paraffin-embedded (FFPE), both PCa biopsy and prostatectomy material,[9] which was developed based on an originally whole-transcriptome panel.[35] In a prospective registry of 855 patients receiving PCa biopsy, high-risk scores on the Decipher Biopsy test predicted shorter time to treatment in patients undergoing active surveillance and shorter time to treatment failure in patients receiving local treatment.[36] In the post-RP setting, the prognostic value of Decipher has been assessed within the NRG/RTOG 9601 trial, which randomized patients with PCa with biochemical recurrence and pT3N0 or pT2N0 disease with positive margins, to receive salvage radiotherapy with placebo versus salvage radiotherapy with antiandrogen therapy (bicalutamide for 2 years).[9,37] The analysis of 352 RP samples from this study using the Decipher classifier showed that the test was independently prognostic for distant metastasis, PCa-specific mortality, and OS, when used as a continuous score (0 to 1.0), or following a risk category classification.[9] In addition, this study suggested that patients with lower Decipher scores derived little or no benefit from the addition of antiandrogen therapy to salvage radiotherapy, whereas those patients with higher Decipher scores obtained much more benefit from the antiandrogen therapy. Moreover, a meta-analysis including 5 retrospective studies and a total of 855 patients evaluated the prognostic role of Decipher post-RP, and confirmed that the test can successfully predict the 10-year metastasis risk.[10] As a consequence of these studies, the National Comprehensive Cancer Network (NCCN) guidelines now recommend consideration of Decipher testing to aid decision making in the postoperative setting.[14] Another complementary test, the Decipher PORTOS score, covers 24 genes and was validated in a matched retrospective study, which demonstrated that high PORTOS scores were significantly associated with decreased 10-year metastasis risk in patients who received postoperative radiotherapy compared with those who did not; conversely, low PORTOS scores were not associated with any difference in metastases rates based on treatment with postoperative radiotherapy.[38] Therefore, Decipher PORTOS is the only genomic classifier with predictive value regarding response to adjuvant or salvage radiotherapy.[34]

Oncotype DX GPS is another gene-expression panel consisting of 12 PCa-related and 5 housekeeping genes (score 0 to 100), suitable for formalin-fixed biopsy material. This assay has been assessed in a cohort of 431 low- to intermediate-risk PCa biopsies, showing correlation with adverse pathologic features (Grade Group $\geq$ 3 or extraprostatic extension), biochemical recurrence, and risk of metastasis.[11] However, a more recent study in a large prospective cohort of 432 patients treated with active surveillance failed to validate the GPS test, and suggested that adding GPS to a model containing Prostate-specific antigen (PSA) kinetics and diagnostic Gleason grading did not significantly improve stratification of risk for adverse pathology over the clinical variables alone.[39]

Prolaris is a broader gene-expression panel including 31 cell cycle-related and 5 housekeeping genes, which can be performed on FFPE material and has shown prognostic value when applied to biopsies and RP samples, being able to predict 10-year metastatic risk after RP and PCa-specific mortality after conservative treatment.[12,13,34] The NCCN guidelines propose the use of Decipher or Prolaris to support risk assessment in patients with unfavorable intermediate- to high-risk localized PCa and a life expectancy of at least 10 years, and allow the use of any of the 3 tests (Decipher, Prolaris, or Oncotype DX Prostate) for patients with low to favorable intermediate risk.[14] ProMark is an 8 protein-based assay, which showed ability to predict adverse pathologic features (Grade Group $\geq$ 2 or T $\geq$ 3b) when applied to PCa biopsies.[40]

GENOMIC INSTABILITY ASSAYS TO ASSESS HOMOLOGOUS RECOMBINATION DEFICIENCY

To date a limited number of studies have evaluated the role of HRD scores in PCa as a predictive biomarker of response to PARP inhibitors or platin-based chemotherapy. For ovarian cancer, Myriad Genetics MyChoice CDx is the only US Food and Drug Administration (FDA)-approved test developed to assess HRD. This assay calculates a genomic instability score (GIS) taking into account genomewide loss of heterozygosity (LOH), telomeric allelic imbalance, and large-scale state transitions, with a score greater than or equal to 42 classified as high. In addition, the assay detects variants and large rearrangements in BRCA1 and BRCA2.[41] GIS analysis has been performed in a cohort of 557 localized PCas, and showed that patients with BRCA2 alterations and higher HRD scores had longer progression-free survival (PFS) on olaparib.[42] Interestingly, tumors with alterations in ATM and CHEK2 had lower scores when compared with BRCA2-altered samples.[42]

TruSight Oncology 500 HRD test is a recently developed assay, combining targeted NGS (Illumina TruSight Oncology 500) with Myriad HRD assay. Illumina TruSight Oncology 500 interrogates for single nucleotide variants, deletions, insertions, and copy number variants in a total of 523 genes, as well as for fusions in 55 genes, providing also information on MSI status and TMB. The combined assay showed high agreement with the results of Myriad MyChoice CDx Plus regarding presence of BRCA mutations and GIS in ovarian cancer.[43]

FoundationOneCDx assay provides information on genomic LOH (gLOH) score. This score is calculated as percentage of LOH genome, with gLOH of 16 or higher considered as "LOH high." FoundationOneCDx assay has been used for tumor tissue testing in the PROFound phase 3 trial, which compared the efficacy of treatment with olaparib versus physician's choice in patients with mCRPC with alterations in HRD-related genes who progressed to a previous treatment with ARSI, showing prolonged PFS and OS for patients with BRCA1, BRCA2, and ATM alterations.[15,44] In a cohort of 3476 PCas molecularly characterized using the FoundationOneCDx assay,[5] gLOH scores were high in tumors harboring BRCA1, BRCA2, ATR, and FANCA alterations, whereas only a minority of CDK12-altered tumors presented a high score.[5]

Classifier of Homologous Recombination Deficiency (CHORD) is a genome-wide random forest-based approach, developed to detect tumor chromosomal instability.[45] In a cohort of 3504 solid tumors, analyzed by WGS, the CHORD was able to distinguish between "BRCA1-like" (BRCA1 alterations) and "BRCA2-like" (BRCA2, PALB2, and RAD51 C alterations) phenotypes.[45] Another supervised learning algorithm, HRDetect, is a lasso logistic regression model developed to identify BRCA1 and BRCA2 mutational signatures in breast cancer tumors.[46,47] This algorithm, applied to a cohort of 311 PCa samples analyzed by WGS, correctly discriminated samples with biallelic BRCA1/2 mutations, as well as identified further BRCA1/2 nonmutant cases with a high HRDetect scores (>0.7). HRDetect showed lower specificity when applied to WES data from the same cohort.[47]

MICROSATELLITE INSTABILITY TESTING

Alterations in MMR genes have been reported in 4% to 5% of mCRPC.[2,3,5] MSI status has been classically assessed by IHC for MLH1, MSH2, MSH6, and PMS2 proteins.[48–50] For IHC scoring, a product of intensity of the staining (0–3) and percentage of positive cells (0–3, 0 [0%], 1 [1%–33%], 2 [34%–66%], and 3 [67%–100%]) is calculated, with a product score of 3 or less classified as "loss of protein expression."[51] An alternative strategy is to assess MSI status by sequencing of specific microsatellite (or tandem repeats) loci using polymerase chain reaction (PCR). With this approach, panels of 5 (Bethesda,[52] OncoMate MSI Dx Analysis System[53]) to 8 (LMR MSI Analysis System[54]) microsatellite loci have been developed. In colorectal cancer (CRC), MSI-H detection by IHC has shown a 91.9% agreement with the detection by PCR, with high negative predictive and low positive predictive values, when compared with PCR.[55] Over the past years, NGS approach has enabled parallel assessment of multiple microsatellite loci.[56] Most of these NGS panels have been optimized for CRC (MSIPlus,[57] ColoSeq[58]). In a cohort of 91 PCas, with MSI status additionally tested by deep targeted sequencing of the MMR genes, 5-marker PCR panel had a sensitivity of 72.4% and a specificity of 100%, and larger NGS panels (>60 markers) showed a sensitivity of 93.1% and a specificity of 98.4%.[56] MSIsensor is an algorithm developed to detect somatic microsatellite alterations from paired normal-tumor-targeted NGS data.[59,60] A cohort of 1033 localized PCas and mPCas with available normal tumor NGS data (MSK-Impact)[61] has been analyzed with this algorithm, uncovering MSI-H or dMMR tumors in 3.1% of the cases, with 29.1% of these samples harboring pathogenic germline alterations in Lynch syndrome-related genes.[29] Half of these patients with MSI-H/dMMR showed more than 50% PSA declines under anti-PD1/PD-L1 ICIs.[29] MSI status in PCa can be also evaluated by liquid biopsy and cfDNA analysis (Guardant360 CDx,[62] FoundationOne Liquid CDx[63]) (Table 1).

Table 1
Summary of available homologous recombination deficiency and microsatellite instability tissue-based assays

Method	Assay/Analysis Method	Score and Threshold	Interpretation
HRD tumor testing			
Targeted NGS	Myriad Genetics MyChoice CDx	• LOH + LST + TAI (threshold ≥ 42) • Variants and large rearrangements in 15 genes (*ATM, BARD1, BRCA1, BRCA2, BRIP1, CDK12, CHEK1, CHEK2, FANCL, PALB2, PPP2R2A, RAD51 B, RAD51 C, RAD51D,* and *RAD54 L*).	• GIS • Pathogenicity of variants
	Myriad Genetics MyChoice CDx Plus	• LOH + LST + TAI (threshold ≥ 42) • Variants and large rearrangements in *BRCA1* and *BRCA2*	• GIS • Pathogenicity of variants
	TruSight Oncology 500 HRD	• SNV, indels, CNV in 523 genes, rearrangements in 55 genes • MSI and TMB • LOH + LST + TAI (threshold ≥ 42)	• Genomic alterations • MSI and TMB • GIS
	FoundationOneCDx	• SNV, indels, CNV in 324 genes, rearrangements in selected genes • MSI and TMB • gLOH ≥ 16	• Genomic alterations • MSI and TMB • gLOH low/high
Genome-wide NGS (WGS, WES)	CHORD	• Biallelic loss (deep deletion), presence of LOH, pathogenicity of variants • Threshold ≥ 0.5	• Probability of *BRCA1/2* deficiency • HRD
	HRDetect	• Mutational signatures analysis, HRD index score, analysis of variants in *BRCA1/2* and other HRR-related genes • Threshold > 0.7	• Probability of *BRCA1/2* deficiency • HRD
MSI testing			
IHC of MMR proteins	MLH1, MSH2, MSH6, and PMS2	• Intensity of staining: 0–3 • Percentage of positivity: 0–3 • Product score (threshold ≤ 3)	• Loss of MMR protein expression (dMMR)

PCR of microsatellites	Bethesda panel	• 5 microsatellite markers: 2 mononucleotide (Bat25, Bat26) and 3 dinucleotide (D2S123, D5S346, and D17S250) • Threshold: ≥ 2 markers positive for shifts in the allelic bands	• MSS • MSI-L (1 marker) • MSI-H (≥ 2 markers)
	MSI Analysis System Version 1.2/OncoMate MSI Dx Analysis System	• 5 SMR markers (BAT-25, BAT-26, NR-21, NR-24, and MONO-27) and 2 pentanucleotide repeat markers (Penta C and Penta D) • Threshold: ≥ 2 markers positive for shifts in the allelic bands	• MSS • MSI-L (1 marker) • MSI-H (≥ 2 markers)
	LMR MSI Analysis System	• 4 SMR markers (BAT-25, BAT-26, NR-21, and MONO-27), 4 LMR markers (BAT-52, BAT-56, BAT-59, and BAT-60), and 2 pentanucleotide repeat markers (Penta C and Penta D) • Threshold: ≥ 3 markers positive for shifts in the allelic bands	• MSS • MSI-L (1–2 markers) • MSI-H (≥ 3 markers)
NGS	MSIPlus	• Optimized for CRC • 16 microsatellite markers and hotspots in KRAS, NRAS, and BRAF	• MSI-H (following mSINGS score)
	ColoSeq	• Optimized for CRC • SNV, deletions or rearrangements in MMR-related genes (MLH1, MSH2, MSH6, PMS2, EPCAM, APC, MUTYH) and 24 additional genes	• Variant interpretation
	NGS-targeted panels including MMR genes (eg, MSK-Impact)	• MSISensor score ≥ 10	• MSI-H
Targeted sequencing of MMR genes	Any NGS-targeted panel covering MMR genes	• SNV, indels, CNV in MMR genes	• Variant interpretation

Abbreviations: CNV, copy number variations; LMR, long mononucleotide repeats; LST, large-scale transitions; MSI-L, MSI-low; MSS, microsatellite stable; SMR, single mononucleotide repeats; SNV, single nucleotide variants; TAI, telomeric allelic imbalance; TMB, tumor mutational burden.

GERMLINE HOMOLOGOUS RECOMBINATION DEFICIENCY TESTING

In the PROfound phase 3 study,[15] BRCAanalysis CDx identified germline *BRCA1/2* alterations in blood samples of the 16% of the included patients. This HRD germline population constituted 53.5% of all patients with tumor *BRCA1/2* alterations in the study. When considering the 62 evaluable patients with a positive BRCAanalysis CDx test for germline *BRCA1/2* alterations, their PFS was 10.12 versus 1.87 months for olaparib versus physician's choice (hazard ratio, 0.08, $P < 0.0001$).[64,65] For tumor tissue testing, FoundationOneCDx assay was used in the study.[15] Myriad's BRACAnalysis CDx is currently FDA approved for patients with ovarian, breast, and pancreatic cancers and PCa who meet criteria for germline testing to identify pathogenic *BRCA1* and *BRCA2* mutations. For PCa, the NCCN guidelines recommend germline testing for patients with personal history of PCa, diagnosed at any age and starting from high-risk localized stage, as well as for patients with familiar history of PCa (Table 2). It is recommended that germline panels include the Lynch syndrome-related genes *MLH1*, *MSH2*, *MSH6,* and *PMS2*, and the HRD genes *BRCA1*, *BRCA2*, *ATM*, *PALB2,* and *CHEK2*.[14] Other genes, such as *HOXB13*, should also be considered.[14,66]

DISCUSSION

Over the past years, tumor molecular characterization has been progressively integrated into the clinical management of patients with localized PCa and mPCa.[14] For localized PCa, multiple pretreatment risk stratification algorithms are available based on clinical and pathologic features (eg, GS, PSA level, clinical T stage).[67] For patients with biopsied PCas and NCCN low to favorable intermediate risk, genomic classifiers, independently or in combination with multiparametric MRI,[68] can help identify better candidates for active surveillance, although further validation is needed for some of these classifiers.[14,34] For patients who have biochemical recurrence after RP, the NCCN guidelines recommend that physicians consider adding androgen deprivation therapy (ADT) to salvage radiotherapy for patients; the use of genomic classifiers such as Decipher may help identify patients most likely to benefit from the addition of ADT to salvage radiotherapy in this setting. Across the spectrum of localized PCa, several gene expression classifiers are

Table 2
National Comprehensive Cancer Network guidelines recommendation for germline testing in patients with diagnosis of prostate cancer

Family history			Personal history	
Family members*	**Tumor type**	**Age at diagnosis**	**Tumor type**	**Age at diagnosis**
Germline testing is recommended			**Germline testing is recommended**	
At least 1 (1st degree)	PCa**	</=60	PCa (from high risk localized to metastatic)	Any
	Breast, CRC or endometrial	</=50	Breast	Any
			Germline testing may be considered	
At least 1 (1st, 2nd or 3rd degree)	Male breast, ovarian, exocrin pancreatic	Any	PCa (intermediate risk and intraductal/cribriform histology)	Any
	PCa (from high risk localized to metastatic)	Any	PCa and previous other cancer ***	Any
At least 2 (1st, 2nd or 3rd degree)	PCa** or Breast	Any		
At least 3 (1st or 2nd degree)	Lynch-related cancers	Especially if <50		
Mutation (pathogenic/likely pathogenic) in *BRCA1, BRCA2, ATM, PALB2, CHEK2, MLH1, MSH2, MSH6, PMS2, EPCAM*				
Ashkenazi Jewish ancestry				

available as prognostic tools to aid in risk stratification for clinical decision making.

For advanced PCa, recent advances in targeted therapeutic approaches have increased the clinical need to screen mPCa tumors for targetable molecular alterations. Most relevant therapeutic advances have been made for DDR[15–17] and MSI-H tumors,[20,21] as well as CDK12-altered PCas.[22] However, despite these relevant advances, targeted treatment with PARP inhibitors and immunotherapy is successful only in a subset of DDR,[17] MSI-H,[29] and CDK12-altered PCas,[22,69] and further development and validation of solid predictive biomarkers is needed. For instance, distinct HRD genotypes harbor different degrees of sensitivities to PARP inhibitors.[15,17] Beyond germline alterations in BRCA1 and BRCA2, biomarker analysis from the TOPAR-B phase 2 trial showed that PCas with homozygous BRCA2 and PALB2 deficiency, as well as tumors with loss of ATM protein expression, had most benefit from treatment with olaparib.[17] In ovarian cancer, first-line maintenance treatment with olaparib in combination with bevacizumab is indicated for patients with HRD tumors assessed by Myriad Genetics MyChoice CDx, based on the results of the PAOLA-1 phase 3 trial.[70] In PCa, still limited studies are available correlating GIS score with efficacy of PARP inhibitors.[15,42]

For MSI-H/dMMR tumors, the KEYNOTE-158 phase 2 study assessed the efficacy of pembrolizumab in distinct MSI-H/dMMR tumor entities, including 6 patients with mPCa, showing an overall response rate of 34.3% and a median OS of 23.5 months (95% confidence interval, 13.5–not reached) for the entire study cohort.[71] MSI status was assessed either by IHC or 5 microsatellite loci PCR panel.[71] Based on this and other studies, pembrolizumab is currently approved for MSI-H/dMMR mPCas, which progressed after at least 1 prior systemic treatment line.[72] Moreover, for patients with uncovered pathogenic or likely pathogenic mutations in Lynch syndrome-associated genes, germline counseling and/or testing is recommended, as well as for patients with personal or familiar history of PCa (see **Table 2**). Clinical and molecular features of CDK12-altered mPCas have been analyzed in a retrospective study, which included 60 patients, 51.7% of them harboring a biallelic alteration in CDK12.[22] The study showed that CDK12-altered tumors had poor responses to ARSI and taxane-based chemotherapy, lack of response to PARP inhibitors, and variable responses to PD-1 inhibitors (pembrolizumab and nivolumab).[22] Mechanistically, the lack of response to PARP inhibitors of this molecular subtype of PCa has been correlated with a genomic instability phenotype distinct from HRD, characterized by tandem duplications and gene fusions.[22] Finally, recent studies have been assessing the role of liquid biopsy for molecular subtyping and identification of predictive biomarkers in advanced PCa.[62,63,73]

Surgical pathologists play a critical role in triaging tissue for molecular biomarker testing in PCa. It is important for pathologists to understand when biomarker testing may be appropriate, and how these tests are performed. Pathologists should be aware that preanalytic and histopathologic factors may affect these tests. Because these assays are validated only on FFPE specimens containing untreated PCa, specimens that were previously frozen or fixed in nonformalin fixatives should not be used for these tests. In addition, tumors that have been treated with radiation or ADT are not eligible for these assays. When choosing tissue for these tests, pathologists should pick the most representative tissue blocks with the highest Gleason grade and largest tumor volume. Pathologists should also make sure there is sufficient tumor in the tissue submitted for testing.

SUMMARY

Molecular tumor profiling has gained relevance in personalized clinical management and precision oncology treatment of localized PCa and mPCa. Use of gene expression assays for genomic risk stratification can support decision algorithm regarding active surveillance or indication of intensification of therapy in localized PCa. For mPCa, tumor molecular characterization by NGS, as well as by assays assessing HRD and MSI status, are essential to predict benefit form molecularly targeted therapies, such as PARP inhibitors and immunotherapy. Moreover, because PCa tumor responses to targeted treatment are still highly heterogeneous, further development and validation of robust predictive biomarkers is required.

CLINICS CARE POINTS

- Molecular tumor testing is essential in metastatic PCa, in order to identify patients with targetable alterations, such as HRD and dMMR/MSI-H tumors.

- Genomic classifiers may help identify patients most likely to benefit from the addition of ADT to radiotherapy in the biochemical recurrence setting.

> • Germline testing should be offered to patients with metastatic or nodal positive PCa, as well as to a subset of patients with high risk localized PCa.

ACKNOWLEDGMENTS

The authors thank Dr Mariana Ricca at the University of Bern for editorial support. This work has been supported by funding from the following research foundations: SPHN SOCIBP, Krebsliga Schweiz (Swiss Cancer League), Nuovo-Soldati Foundation for Cancer Research, ISREC Fondation Recherche Cancer, and Werner and Hedy Berger-Janser Foundation. The figure 1 has been created using images from BioRender.com.

DISCLOSURE

D. Akhoundova and. C.C. Pritchard declare no conflicts of interests. F.Y. Feng serves on the Scientific Advisory Board of Artera, BlueStar Genomics, SerImmune, and the Immuno-Oncology Program for Bristol Myers Squibb, and has consulted for Foundation Medicine, Tempus, Janssen, Astellas, Bayer, Myovant, Roivant, and Novartis. M.A. Rubin is a coinventor on patents in the area for diagnosis and therapy in prostate cancer for ETS fusions (University of Michigan and the Brigham and Women's Hospital), SPOP mutations (Cornell University), and EZH2 (University of Michgian).

REFERENCES

1. The molecular taxonomy of primary prostate cancer. Cell 2015;163(4):1011–25.
2. Robinson D, Van Allen EM, Wu YM, et al. Integrative clinical genomics of advanced prostate cancer. Cell 2015;161(5):1215–28.
3. Abida W, Cyrta J, Heller G, et al. Genomic correlates of clinical outcome in advanced prostate cancer. Proc Natl Acad Sci 2019;116(23):11428–36.
4. van Dessel LF, van Riet J, Smits M, et al. The genomic landscape of metastatic castration-resistant prostate cancers reveals multiple distinct genotypes with potential clinical impact. Nat Commun 2019;10(1):5251.
5. Chung JH, Dewal N, Sokol E, et al. Prospective comprehensive genomic profiling of primary and metastatic prostate tumors. JCO Precis Oncol 2019;3. https://doi.org/10.1200/po.18.00283.
6. Li X, Heyer W-D. Homologous recombination in DNA repair and DNA damage tolerance. Cell Res 2008; 18(1):99–113. https://doi.org/10.1038/cr.2008.1.
7. Gulhan DC, Lee JJ-K, Melloni GEM, et al. Detecting the mutational signature of homologous recombination deficiency in clinical samples. Nat Genet 2019;51(5):912–9.
8. Rosenthal R, McGranahan N, Herrero J, et al. deconstructSigs: delineating mutational processes in single tumors distinguishes DNA repair deficiencies and patterns of carcinoma evolution. Genome Biol 2016;17(1):31.
9. Feng FY, Huang HC, Spratt DE, et al. Validation of a 22-gene genomic classifier in patients with recurrent prostate cancer: an ancillary study of the NRG/RTOG 9601 randomized clinical trial. JAMA Oncol 2021;7(4):544–52.
10. Spratt DE, Yousefi K, Deheshi S, et al. Individual Patient-level meta-analysis of the performance of the decipher genomic classifier in high-risk men after prostatectomy to predict development of metastatic disease. J Clin Oncol 2017;35(18):1991–8.
11. Cullen J, Rosner IL, Brand TC, et al. A biopsy-based 17-gene genomic prostate score predicts recurrence after radical prostatectomy and adverse surgical pathology in a racially diverse population of men with clinically low- and intermediate-risk prostate cancer. Eur Urol 2015;68(1):123–31.
12. Cooperberg MR, Simko JP, Cowan JE, et al. Validation of a Cell-cycle progression gene panel to improve risk stratification in a contemporary prostatectomy cohort. J Clin Oncol 2013;31(11):1428–34.
13. Cuzick J, Stone S, Fisher G, et al. Validation of an RNA cell cycle progression score for predicting death from prostate cancer in a conservatively managed needle biopsy cohort. Br J Cancer 2015;113(3):382–9.
14. Schaeffer E, Srinivas S, Antonarakis ES, et al. NCCN guidelines insights: prostate cancer, version 1.2021. J Natl Compr Canc Netw 2021;19(2):134–43.
15. de Bono J, Mateo J, Fizazi K, et al. Olaparib for metastatic castration-resistant prostate cancer. N Engl J Med 2020;382(22):2091–102.
16. Mateo J, Porta N, Bianchini D, et al. Olaparib in patients with metastatic castration-resistant prostate cancer with DNA repair gene aberrations (TOPARP-B): a multicentre, open-label, randomised, phase 2 trial. Lancet Oncol 2020;21(1):162–74.
17. Carreira S, Porta N, Arce-Gallego S, et al. Biomarkers associating with PARP inhibitor benefit in prostate cancer in the TOPARP-B trial. Cancer Discov 2021;11(11):2812–27.
18. Chi KN, Rathkopf DE, Smith MR, et al. Phase 3 MAGNITUDE study: First results of niraparib (NIRA) with abiraterone acetate and prednisone (AAP) as first-line therapy in patients (pts) with metastatic castration-resistant prostate cancer (mCRPC) with and without homologous recombination repair (HRR) gene alterations. J Clin Oncol 2022;40(6_suppl):12.
19. Saad F, Armstrong AJ, Thiery-Vuillemin A, et al. PROpel: Phase III trial of olaparib (ola) and abiraterone (abi) versus placebo (pbo) and abi as first-line

20. Le DT, Uram JN, Wang H, et al. PD-1 blockade in tumors with mismatch-repair deficiency. N Engl J Med 2015;372(26):2509–20.

21. Le DT, Durham JN, Smith KN, et al. Mismatch repair deficiency predicts response of solid tumors to PD-1 blockade. Science 2017;357(6349):409–13.

22. Antonarakis ES, Velho PI, Fu W, et al. CDK12-altered prostate cancer: clinical features and therapeutic outcomes to standard systemic therapies, poly (ADP-Ribose) polymerase inhibitors, and PD-1 inhibitors. JCO Precision Oncol 2020;(4):370–81.

23. Merseburger AS, Waldron N, Ribal MJ, et al. Genomic testing in patients with metastatic castration-resistant prostate cancer: a pragmatic guide for clinicians. Eur Urol 2021;79(4):519–29.

24. Tomlins SA, Rhodes DR, Perner S, et al. Recurrent fusion of TMPRSS2 and ETS transcription factor genes in prostate cancer. Science 2005;310(5748):644–8.

25. Tomlins SA, Bjartell A, Chinnaiyan AM, et al. ETS gene fusions in prostate cancer: from discovery to daily clinical practice. Eur Urol 2009;56(2):275–86.

26. Wu YM, Cieślik M, Lonigro RJ, et al. Inactivation of CDK12 delineates a distinct immunogenic class of advanced prostate cancer. Cell 2018;173(7):1770–82.e14.

27. Lozano R, Castro E, Aragón IM, et al. Genetic aberrations in DNA repair pathways: a cornerstone of precision oncology in prostate cancer. Br J Cancer 2021;124(3):552–63.

28. Ritch E, Fu SYF, Herberts C, et al. Identification of hypermutation and defective mismatch repair in ctDNA from metastatic prostate cancer. Clin Cancer Res 2020;26(5):1114–25.

29. Abida W, Cheng ML, Armenia J, et al. Analysis of the prevalence of microsatellite instability in prostate cancer and response to immune checkpoint blockade. JAMA Oncol 2019;5(4):471–8.

30. Nicolosi P, Ledet E, Yang S, et al. Prevalence of germline variants in prostate cancer and implications for current genetic testing guidelines. JAMA Oncol 2019;5(4):523–8.

31. Pritchard CC, Mateo J, Walsh MF, et al. Inherited DNA-repair gene mutations in men with metastatic prostate cancer. N Engl J Med 2016;375(5):443–53.

32. Kim HL, Li P, Huang H-C, et al. Validation of the Decipher Test for predicting adverse pathology in candidates for prostate cancer active surveillance. Prostate Cancer Prostatic Dis 2019;22(3):399–405.

33. Klein EA, Haddad Z, Yousefi K, et al. Decipher genomic classifier measured on prostate biopsy predicts metastasis risk. Urology 2016;90:148–52.

34. Eggener SE, Rumble RB, Armstrong AJ, et al. Molecular biomarkers in localized prostate cancer: ASCO guideline. J Clin Oncol 2020;38(13):1474–94.

35. Erho N, Crisan A, Vergara IA, et al. Discovery and validation of a prostate cancer genomic classifier that predicts early metastasis following radical prostatectomy. PLoS One 2013;8(6):e66855.

36. Vince RA, Jiang R, Qi J, et al. Impact of Decipher Biopsy testing on clinical outcomes in localized prostate cancer in a prospective statewide collaborative. Prostate Cancer Prostatic Dis 2021. https://doi.org/10.1038/s41391-021-00428-y.

37. WU Shipley, Seiferheld W, Lukka HR, et al. Radiation with or without antiandrogen therapy in recurrent prostate cancer. N Engl J Med 2017;376(5):417–28.

38. Zhao SG, Chang SL, Spratt DE, et al. Development and validation of a 24-gene predictor of response to postoperative radiotherapy in prostate cancer: a matched, retrospective analysis. Lancet Oncol 2016;17(11):1612–20.

39. Lin DW, Zheng Y, McKenney JK, et al. 17-gene genomic prostate score test results in the canary prostate active surveillance study (PASS) cohort. J Clin Oncol 2020;38(14):1549–57.

40. Blume-Jensen P, Berman DM, Rimm DL, et al. Development and clinical validation of an in situ biopsy-based multimarker assay for risk stratification in prostate cancer. Clin Cancer Res 2015;21(11):2591–600.

41. Patel JN, Braicu I, Timms KM, et al. Characterisation of homologous recombination deficiency in paired primary and recurrent high-grade serous ovarian cancer. Br J Cancer 2018;119(9):1060–6.

42. Lotan TL, Kaur HB, Salles DC, et al. Homologous recombination deficiency (HRD) score in germline BRCA2- versus ATM-altered prostate cancer. Mod Pathol 2021;34(6):1185–93.

43. Weichert W, Qiu P, Lunceford J, et al. Assessing homologous recombination deficiency (HRD) in ovarian cancer: Optimizing concordance of the regulatory-approved companion diagnostic and a next-generation sequencing (NGS) assay kit. J Clin Oncol 2022;40(16_suppl):e17571.

44. Hussain M, Mateo J, Fizazi K, et al. Survival with olaparib in metastatic castration-resistant prostate cancer. N Engl J Med 2020;383(24):2345–57.

45. Nguyen L, Martens J WM, Van Hoeck A, et al. Pan-cancer landscape of homologous recombination deficiency. Nat Commun 2020;11(1):5584.

46. Davies H, Glodzik D, Morganella S, et al. HRDetect is a predictor of BRCA1 and BRCA2 deficiency based on mutational signatures. Nat Med 2017;23(4):517–25.

47. Sztupinszki Z, Diossy M, Krzystanek M, et al. Detection of molecular signatures of homologous recombination deficiency in prostate cancer with or without BRCA1/2 mutations. Clin Cancer Res 2020;26(11):2673–80.

48. Lynch HT, Snyder CL, Shaw TG, et al. Milestones of Lynch syndrome: 1895–2015. Nat Rev Cancer 2015;15(3):181–94.

49. Hampel H, Frankel WL, Martin E, et al. Screening for the lynch syndrome (hereditary nonpolyposis colorectal cancer). N Engl J Med 2005;352(18):1851–60.

50. Lindor NM, Burgart LJ, Leontovich O, et al. Immunohistochemistry versus microsatellite instability testing in phenotyping colorectal tumors. J Clin Oncol 2002;20(4):1043–8.

51. Lee JH, Cragun D, Thompson Z, et al. Association between IHC and MSI testing to identify mismatch repair-deficient patients with ovarian cancer. Genet Test Mol Biomarkers 2014;18(4):229–35.

52. Boland CR, Thibodeau SN, Hamilton SR, et al. A National Cancer Institute Workshop on Microsatellite Instability for cancer detection and familial predisposition: development of international criteria for the determination of microsatellite instability in colorectal cancer. Cancer Res 1998;58(22):5248–57.

53. Bacher JW, Flanagan LA, Smalley RL, et al. Development of a fluorescent multiplex assay for detection of MSI-high tumors. Dis Markers 2004;20:136734.

54. Lin JH, Chen S, Pallavajjala A, et al. Validation of long mononucleotide repeat markers for detection of microsatellite instability. J Mol Diagn 2022;24(2):144–57.

55. Chen ML, Chen JY, Hu J, et al. Comparison of microsatellite status detection methods in colorectal carcinoma. Int J Clin Exp Pathol 2018;11(3):1431–8.

56. Hempelmann JA, Lockwood CM, Konnick EQ, et al. Microsatellite instability in prostate cancer by PCR or next-generation sequencing. J Immunother Cancer 2018;6(1):29.

57. Hempelmann JA, Scroggins SM, Pritchard CC, et al. MSIplus for integrated colorectal cancer molecular testing by next-generation sequencing. J Mol Diagn 2015;17(6):705–14.

58. Pritchard CC, Smith C, Salipante SJ, et al. ColoSeq provides comprehensive lynch and polyposis syndrome mutational analysis using massively parallel sequencing. J Mol Diagn 2012;14(4):357–66.

59. Middha S, Zhang L, Nafa K, et al. Reliable pancancer microsatellite instability assessment by using targeted next-generation sequencing data. JCO Precis Oncol 2017;2017. https://doi.org/10.1200/po.17.00084.

60. Niu B, Ye K, Zhang Q, et al. MSIsensor: microsatellite instability detection using paired tumor-normal sequence data. Bioinformatics 2014;30(7):1015–6.

61. Abida W, Armenia J, Gopalan A, et al. Prospective genomic profiling of prostate cancer across disease states reveals germline and somatic alterations that may affect clinical decision making. JCO Precis Oncol 2017;2017. https://doi.org/10.1200/po.17.00029.

62. Barata P, Agarwal N, Nussenzveig R, et al. Clinical activity of pembrolizumab in metastatic prostate cancer with microsatellite instability high (MSI-H) detected by circulating tumor DNA. J Immunother Cancer 2020;8(2). https://doi.org/10.1136/jitc-2020-001065.

63. Trujillo B, Wu A, Wetterskog D, et al. Blood-based liquid biopsies for prostate cancer: clinical opportunities and challenges. Br J Cancer 2022. https://doi.org/10.1038/s41416-022-01881-9.

64. Available at: https://s3.amazonaws.com/myriad-library/technical-specifications/BRCATechSpecs_Integrated.pdf.

65. Available at: https://www.accessdata.fda.gov/cdrh_docs/pdf14/p140020c.pdf.

66. Giri VN, Knudsen KE, Kelly WK, et al. Implementation of germline testing for prostate cancer: philadelphia prostate cancer consensus conference 2019. J Clin Oncol 2020;38(24):2798–811.

67. Zelic R, Garmo H, Zugna D, et al. Predicting prostate cancer death with different pretreatment risk stratification tools: a head-to-head comparison in a nationwide cohort study. Eur Urol 2020;77(2):180–8.

68. Salmasi A, Said J, Shindel AW, et al. A 17-gene genomic prostate score assay provides independent information on adverse pathology in the setting of combined multiparametric magnetic resonance imaging fusion targeted and systematic prostate biopsy. J Urol 2018;200(3):564–72.

69. Rescigno P, Gurel B, Pereira R, et al. Characterizing CDK12-mutated prostate cancers. Clin Cancer Res 2021;27(2):566–74.

70. Ray-Coquard I, Pautier P, Pignata S, et al. Olaparib plus bevacizumab as first-line maintenance in ovarian cancer. N Engl J Med 2019;381(25):2416–28.

71. Marabelle A, Le DT, Ascierto PA, et al. Efficacy of pembrolizumab in patients with noncolorectal high microsatellite instability/mismatch repair–deficient cancer: results from the phase II KEYNOTE-158 study. J Clin Oncol 2020;38(1):1–10.

72. Available at: https://www.accessdata.fda.gov/drugsatfda_docs/label/2021/125514s096lbl.pdf.

73. Herberts C, Annala M, Sipola J, et al. Deep whole-genome ctDNA chronology of treatment-resistant prostate cancer. Nature 2022. https://doi.org/10.1038/s41586-022-04975-9.

Update on Flat and Papillary Urothelial Lesions
Genitourinary Pathology Society Consensus Recommendations

Eva Compérat, MD[a,b],*, André Oszwald, MD[a],
Gabriel Wasinger, MD[a], Shahrokh Shariat, MD[c],
Mahul Amin, MD[d,e]

KEYWORDS

- Flat lesion • Papillary lesion • Urothelial neoplasia • GUPS

Key points

- Genitourinary Pathology Society recommends "flat urothelial hyperplasia" be called "atypical urothelial proliferation-flat."
- Urothelial dysplasia is a rare diagnosis with significant interobserver variability. The diagnosis should be made with extreme caution, especially if the patient already has a clinical history of carcinoma in situ (CIS) or if there has been no previous history of bladder cancer.
- The diagnosis of CIS is primarily based on morphology, with only a supportive role of immunohistochemistry.

ABSTRACT

The reporting recommendations on "flat and papillary urothelial neoplasia," published in 2 position articles by the Genitourinary Pathology Society in July 2021, was a collective contribution of 38 multidisciplinary experts aiming to clarify nomenclature, classification of flat and papillary urothelial neoplasia and controversial issues. In this review, we discuss some of these recommendations including nomenclature, practical approaches, and their importance for clinical practice.

INTRODUCTION

In July 2021, the Genitourinary Pathology Society (GUPS) published reporting recommendations on "flat and papillary urothelial neoplasia," included in 2 articles and authored by a panel of 38 invited multidisciplinary experts, including urologic pathologists, urologists, and oncologists. This update includes a new approach to lesions with "mixed morphologic features,"[1] and early patterns of urothelial neoplasia, which were not addressed in the World Health Organisation (WHO) GU bluebook 2022, such as "hyperplasia,"[2] "urothelial

---

[a] Department of Pathology, General Hospital of Vienna, Medical University of Vienna, Vienna, Austria; [b] Department of Pathology, Sorbonne University, Assistance Publique-Hôpitaux de Paris, Hôpital Tenon, Paris, France; [c] Department of Urology, Comprehensive Cancer Center, Medical University of Vienna, Vienna, Austria; [d] Department of Pathology and Laboratory Medicine, University of Tennessee Health Science, Memphis, TN, USA; [e] Department of Urology, USC, Keck School of Medicine, Los Angeles, CA, USA
* Corresponding author. Department of Pathology, General Hospital of Vienna, Medical University of Vienna, Vienna, Austria.
E-mail address: eva.comperat@meduniwien.ac.at

Surgical Pathology 15 (2022) 629–640
https://doi.org/10.1016/j.path.2022.07.009

proliferation of uncertain malignant potential (UPUMP),"[3] and inverted lesions. Other important settings, such as heterogeneous noninvasive papillary tumors with a high-grade focus, will also be discussed briefly in this article according to the GUPS recommendations (Boxes 1 and 2).

FLAT UROTHELIAL LESIONS

In the WHO 2004 classification, urothelial hyperplasia was defined as a markedly thickened mucosa without cytologic atypia, and that these features are often seen as a "shoulder" lesion adjacent to low-grade papillary urothelial lesions. Clonal analysis showed that these lesions are related to concomitant papillary tumors.[4] In the WHO 2016 classification, the lesion was renamed to "UPUMP." The definition retained the description of a marked thickening of the urothelium without true papillary formation, showing no or minimal cytologic atypia, and included lesions previously designated as flat and papillary hyperplasia.

The use of UPUMP and papillary hyperplasia is still lacking consensus, although they are encountered both clinically and histologically in daily practice. The GUPS authors suggest calling "flat urothelial hyperplasia" as "atypical proliferative urothelial lesions (AUP)." This denomination can also describe mixed patterns, which means that some parts are flat, others have a more papillary aspect, but no fibro-vascular cores. With regards to "flat urothelial hyperplasia," the authors underline the evolution of the concept as described above.[5] They reiterate the importance of morphologic criteria, such as notably thickened urothelium (typically >9 layers), increased cell density, and minimal to absent cytologic atypia. Furthermore, slight and moderate undulations without true papillary cores are acceptable. GUPS recommends using the term "AUP-flat" for lesions previously called flat hyperplasia and recommends

including a comment that this lesion might be reactive, a shoulder lesion of a low-grade urothelial neoplasia or a precursor of early noninvasive low-grade neoplasia. AUP-flat does not seem to be closely associated with subsequent urothelial neoplasia but the data are sparse.[6] One study showed the development of subsequent neoplasia in 15% of patients with de novo hyperplasia and in 40% of patients with hyperplasia in the context of prior neoplasia. The authors reported that the greatest risk of progression is associated with early papillary formation.[7] Some authors claimed that these atypical urothelial proliferations can also be found in patients with chronic cystitis but once again data are sparse.[8]

Underlying molecular alterations have shown to involve alterations in chromosome 9, 11 and 17, as well as FGFR3 mutations.[9] In addition, mouse models showed that the maintenance of urothelial hyperplasia in transgenic mice depends on continuous expression of FOXA1 and activated HRAS, and that mutated receptor tyrosine kinases FOXA1 and/or other downstream effectors may mediate oncogene addiction in urothelial hyperplasia.[10] So far, these results have not yet been confirmed in humans.

To be distinguished from flat hyperplasia (AUP-F; Fig. 1) are lesions displaying both increased numbers of urothelial layers and more than a slight undulation of the surface contour but again without cytologic atypia or true papillae (Fig. 2). These were formerly termed papillary hyperplasia and included in UPUMP, and are now designated "AUP-tented" per GUPS recommendations (see Fig. 2). These lesions may clinically present as a dome-shaped or ill-defined papillary lesion. In summary, both AUP-flat and AUP-tented remain in the spectrum of benign or perhaps precursor lesions.

In contrast, it is important to mention that the terminology of dysplasia and carcinoma in situ (CIS), which are also flat lesions, is still being

---

Box 1
Key updates and recommendations on flat urothelial lesions

"Flat Urothelial Hyperplasia" is Recommended be Called "Atypical Urothelial Proliferation-Flat"

Urothelial dysplasia is a rare diagnosis with significant interobserver variability. The diagnosis should be made with extreme caution, especially if the patient already has a clinical history of CIS or if there has been no previous history of bladder cancer

The diagnosis of CIS is primarily based on morphology, with only a supportive role of IHC, if needed

Keratinizing squamous metaplasia must be reported, with a comment on its extent (focal vs extensive)

CIS with glandular features represents a divergent differentiation of urothelial carcinoma

When CIS with glandular differentiation is excluded, many nonpapillary glandular precursors have low-grade or high-grade features, mostly arising in the background of cystitis glandularis with extensive intestinal metaplasia

Box 2
Recommendations for nomenclature of flat and papillary noninvasive urothelial lesions

Recommendations for nomenclature of flat and papillary noninvasive urothelial lesions (excluding endophytic aspects)

Flat lesions

Atypical urothelial proliferation-flat

Dysplasia

Urothelial carcinoma in situ

Papillary lesions

Atypical urothelial proliferation-tented urothelial papilloma

Papillary urothelial neoplasm of low malignant potential noninvasive papillary urothelial carcinoma low grade

Noninvasive papillary urothelial carcinoma high grade

Papillary urothelial lesions

discussed in the WHO 2022 classification. Dysplasia is defined as a lesion encompassing changes that are thought to be preneoplastic in nature, but cytologically fall short of the diagnosis of CIS. It is important to note that dysplasia is not a synonym of intraepithelial neoplasia. Moreover, dysplasia should not be diagnosed based on immunohistochemistry results falling short of CIS. Because data on dysplasia are limited and largely historic, the term should only be used in cases unequivocally not representing reactive changes but falling short of the morphologic threshold for CIS. Due to poor interobserver reproducibility and poor understanding of the biological behavior and respective management criteria, many experts reserve this term only for cases with a history of bladder cancer. In de novo settings, it is recommended to use descriptive nomenclature such as "urothelial atypia, see comment" and suggest close clinical follow-up and rebiopsy, particularly if symptoms or clinical lesions are present or persist.[1]

CIS is a high-grade intraepithelial lesion with significant cytologic atypia. Lesions may be unifocal or multifocal, small or extensive, cystoscopically invisible or recognizable. In case of extensive and/or multifocal CIS, it must be emphasized that CIS can even involve the urinary tract outside

Fig. 1. AUP-flat with no cytologic atypia.

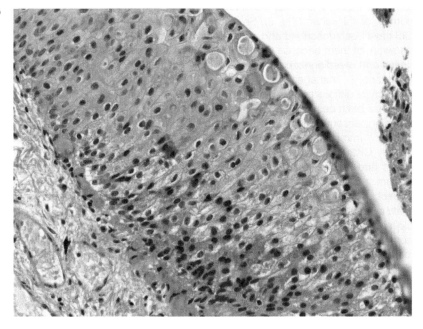

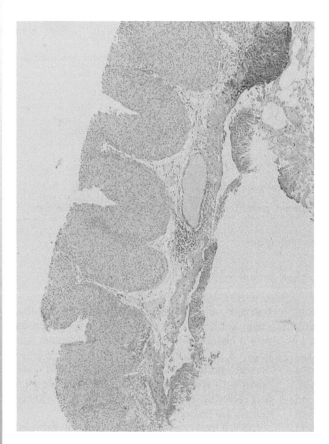

Fig. 2. AUP-tented. The thickened urothelium is arranged into narrow papillary folds. However, there are no discrete detached papillary fronds.

the bladder, therefore positive cytology can be seen even in the absence of visible bladder lesions.[11]

CIS is diagnosed based on the cytonuclear features in a mucosa that may be denuded, thinned, normal, or thickened (**Fig. 3**). Several patterns of CIS have been described and pathologists should be aware of them because CIS is both underdiagnosed and overdiagnosed in clinical practice with important management consequences.[12] Recently, a difficult pattern with plasmacytoid features has been described, recognizable by cellular rounding, eccentric nuclei, and eosinophilic cytoplasm.[13] Immunohistochemistry can be helpful (mostly CK20+/CD44− immune phenotype), with MIB-1 and racemase overexpression in the urothelium. p53 IHC has been advocated, although correct interpretation is key due to scattered positivity in reactive conditions (wild type pattern). Nuclear p53 must be strong and diffuse, or entirely absent (null phenotype)[14] in all/most lesional (atypical) cells, and the findings should be interpreted strictly in the context of morphology. Sometimes, CIS may not involve the full thickness, such patterns as "undermining," "overriding," or "pagetoid"[12] (**Fig. 4**) are diagnostically challenging and

may be seen at frozen sections because the patterns most likely represent intraurothelial spread of CIS away from the main lesion.

With regards to flat lesions, pathologists may also encounter other flat lesions such as flat squamous or glandular lesions. In case of flat squamous lesions, the squamous metaplasia without keratinization is the most frequent and is commonly seen in women. Caution is warranted when there is keratinization; these patients have a higher risk to develop squamous CIS and invasive squamous cell carcinoma when keratinizing metaplasia is extensive (>50% of the bladder mucosal surface),[15] often with coexistent squamous dysplasia.[16]

Urothelial CIS may have glandular features, and this pattern is usually associated with invasive urothelial carcinoma with or without glandular differentiation (**Fig. 5**). In contrast, primary noninvasive glandular lesions are extremely rare and follow patterns in the gastrointestinal tract of low-grade and high-grade dysplasia. They occur in the setting of chronic irritation and intestinal metaplasia. These lesions may be precursor lesions or may be seen as shoulder or surface lesions with adenocarcinomas in the bladder. Intestinal

Fig. 3. Urothelial carcinoma in situ in its denuded form.

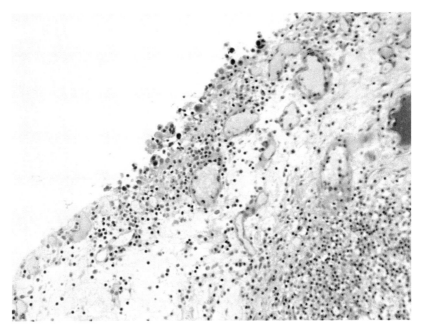

metaplasia and dysplasia display several molecular mutations (*APC, ROS, ATM*), which are different from the classic urothelial CIS.[17] Although diagnostically not discriminatory, the most common genetic alterations shared between different glandular neoplasms in the bladder include *TP53, APC* (in the Wnt pathway), and *KRAS* (in the MAPK pathway) mutations.[17] Pathologists should also pay attention whether the sampled lesion is from a neobladder with mucosa from the intestinal tract because malignancy can also develop in this type of mucosa.[18,19]

One of the areas of significant disagreement pertains to the grading of noninvasive papillary urothelial neoplasms between pathologists in the United States and in some parts of Europe. Urologists in the United States consistently use the ISUP 1998 system, adopted by WHO 2004 and WHO 2016 and recommended by the College of American Pathologists reporting of bladder cancer guidelines, as well as the eighth edition of the AJCC staging manual. The noninvasive papillary urothelial neoplasms are classified as papilloma, papillary urothelial neoplasm of low malignant

Fig. 4. Urothelial carcinoma in situ with "pagetoid" spread. The surface is replaced by atypical cells.

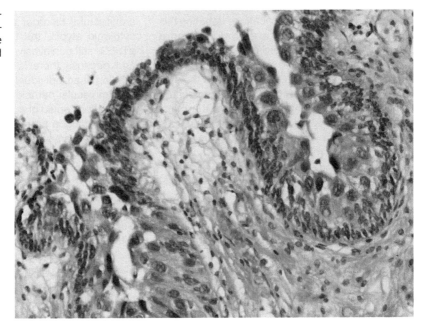

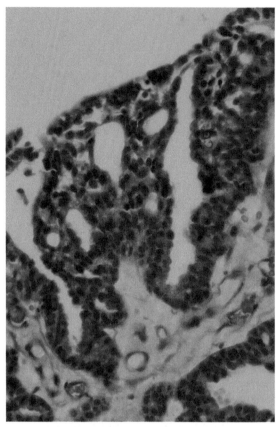

Fig. 5. Urothelial carcinoma in situ with pseudoglandular differentiation.

potential (PUNLMP), low-grade and high-grade urothelial carcinoma. In contrast, some European pathologists and urologists use a 4-tiered system, which means LG/G1, LG/G2, HG/G2, and HG/G3. There have been several publications debating this issue for which references are provided, and a detailed discussion of the pros and cons of using a 2-tiered versus a 4-tier system is beyond the scope of this article. The GUPS endorses the system that is promulgated since 1998 and advocated in the WHO 2016 version.[20–22] One of the many reasons to adopt a 2-tiered system in 1998 was that in case of a 3-tiered system, many cases ended up in the middle group, which could be very heterogeneous. A 2-tiered system for carcinomas allows a lower interobserver variability and a better treatment decision.[23]

This system for all noninvasive urothelial tumors is still a 3-tiered system because it includes PUNLMP low-grade (pTaLG) and high-grade tumors. PUNLMP is chosen for a group of papillary neoplasms with thickened urothelial lining with minimal cytologic and architectural atypia; these tumors are never invasive at the time of initial diagnosis, and only progress to invasive disease through subsequent progression to low-grade and then high-grade tumors. Most commonly, they remain the same stage or progress toward pTaLG lesions.[24] In case of a greater degree of architectural disorder accompanied with distinct cytologic atypia, the tumor would be classified pTaLG, still noninvasive. Grading is a "hot" topic, and because there is opportunity for improving grading at an individual patient level, contributions from molecular pathology and artificial intelligence applications could greatly enhance the clinical utility of grading in future. Furthermore, we must be aware that any refinement of the classification should be reproducible worldwide by any pathologist and not only by specialist genitourinary pathologists. For the LG-HG classification for noninvasive carcinoma, in use for more than 2-decades, there are several detailed descriptions. Besides relevance to clinical management, the 2-tiered system for noninvasive carcinomas reflects the underlying molecular pathways of bladder carcinogenesis.[25]

One of the topics where the GUPS article adds a new perspective to practicing pathologists is the grading in heterogeneous tumors based on the features seen in the "worst areas." In cases of noninvasive low-grade papillary tumors, it is important for pathologists not to overlook small areas of the high-grade component and to standardize how to factor in a high-grade area into the final grade assignment for a particular case. According to several studies, grade heterogeneity exists in between 5% and 32% of tumors.[26,27] Unfortunately, differences in criteria and design do not allow to directly compare studies to determine the optimal cutoff threshold. Cheng and colleagues suggested to consider all tumors with more than 5% of a high-grade component as high-grade lesions.[27] Stage progression and disease-specific survival of tumors with less than 5% were similar to those of pure pTaLG tumors. Gofrit and colleagues suggested in a study of 642 cases that a cutoff of 10% could be used to define these mixed-grade carcinomas.[26] Clinical outcome was similar to LG tumors and significantly better than HG tumors. The 5-year progression-free survival was 99%, 97%, and 74%, respectively, for LG, mixed grade, and HG tumors. The 5-year disease-specific survival (DSS) was 100%, 99.5%, and 88%, respectively, for LG, mixed grade, and noninvasive HG carcinomas.[26] Therefore, DSS was significantly worse in patients with high-grade tumors ($P < .0001$) but similar between those with high-grade and mixed-grade lesions ($P = .679$).

A recent article by Downes and colleagues suggested that fibroblast growth factor receptor 3 (FGFR3) mutations are a hallmark of the low-grade pathway, with subsequent progression to muscle invasion when a homozygous CDKN2A deletion occurs in FGFR3 mutant tumors.[28] The authors hypothesized that the grade heterogeneity represents the morphologic manifestation of molecular changes associated with disease progression. They examined a small number of patients with nonmuscle invasive bladder cancer (n = 29). The grade heterogeneity in urothelial carcinoma was characterized by increased MIB-1 expression, and particularly in the FGFR3 mutant pathway, with homozygous deletions of CDKN2A in low-grade and high-grade areas. These findings suggest that CDKN2A deletion occurs before grade progression. Therefore, the authors suggested to assign the highest grade to urothelial carcinomas with grade heterogeneity.[28] GUPS suggests that 10% may be used as a cutoff in a low-grade papillary urothelial carcinoma, using terminology such as "noninvasive low-grade papillary urothelial carcinoma with a focal (<10%) noninvasive high-grade component." However, 2022 WHO classification uses 5% as the cutoff threshold. As discussed above, the support for use both 5% and 10% as the cutoff points exists in the literature. Use of such diagnostic nomenclature may be accompanied by a comment "There is limited data on the prognostic significance of a minor component of high-grade tumor in an otherwise low-grade carcinoma, and the studies suggest that they generally behave more like low-grade tumors." This cutoff would also allow to minimize the exposure to adjuvant therapies for these patients. The problem at the moment is the lack of meaningful large prospective studies allowing to compare different cutoff thresholds.

Urologists use several clinical and pathologic factors to classify bladder cancers into low-risk, intermediate-risk, and high-risk, which is important for follow-up and treatment (Tables 1 and 2).

The intravesical treatment with Bacillus Calmette–Guérin is the treatment of choice for all high-grade lesions but can have many side effects. Mixed tumors (<10%) according to the few existing data seem to behave more like low-grade tumors. Other factors, such as the presence of CIS and size of tumor and prior treatment, must also be considered. In the future, molecular data as given in the Downes study might also be helpful to decide how to report and treat these carcinomas.[28] GUPS expects in the upcoming years to have more data to validate a cutoff of high grade component because this is also a question of medical utility and cost efficacy.

Another issue discussed in the GUPS article is how to report LG papillary urothelial carcinomas in which both the papillary and the invasive components are LG. LG T1 carcinomas are rare. This is also applicable for such carcinoma subtypes with deceptively bland histology as nested and microcystic subtypes. For such tumors, GUPS recommends using these types of comments: "invasive urothelial carcinomas that are morphologically low grade are uncommon and have a similar prognosis stage for stage compared with invasive urothelial carcinoma that are morphologically high grade; there are no data to suggest there should be differences in therapy based on the histologic grade of the invasive component."[29] The prognosis of T1LG tumors has not been explored in large studies. In the article of Toll and colleagues, 41 patients were examined but follow-up data were poor and no definitive conclusion could be drawn. Four patients developed recurrence, nevertheless all were alive without disease after 49 months of follow-up.[29]

For T1 tumors, only a few other studies have been undertaken to investigate the extent and location of the invasive component (papillary stalk vs base). In the article of Lawless and colleagues,

Table 1
Risk groups for bladder cancer classification, according to European Association of Urology (EAU) guidelines for nonmuscle invasive bladder cancer[22]

Risk Group	Clinicopathological Factors	Management[a]
Low	A primary, single, Ta/T1 LG/G1 tumor <3 cm in diameter without CIS in a patient <70 y A primary Ta LG/G1 tumor without CIS with at most one of the additional clinical risk factors (see below*)	Surveillance
Intermediate	Patients without CIS who are not included in either the low-risk, high-risk, or very high-risk group	Mostly surveillance
High	All T1 HG/G3 without CIS, except those included in the very high-risk group All CIS patients, except those included in the very high-risk group stage, grade with additional clinical risk factors: • Ta LG/G2 or T1G1, no CIS with all 3 risk factors • Ta HG/G3 or T1 LG, no CIS with at least 2 risk factors T1G2 no CIS with at least 1 risk factor	+/− second look Bacillus Calmette–Guérin (BCG) instillations
Very high	Stage, grade with additional clinical risk factors*: • Ta HG/G3 and CIS with all 3 risk factors • T1G2 and CIS with at least 2 risk factors • T1 HG/G3 and CIS with at least 1 risk factor T1 HG/G3 no CIS with all 3 risk factors	+/− second look BCG instillations

Very complex, please go to the EAU guidelines 2022.[11]
  [a] Additional clinical risk factors are the following: age greater than 70 y, multiple papillary tumors, tumor diameter of 3 cm or greater.

T1 papillary urothelial carcinomas were retrospectively reviewed and characterized as focal invasion confined to the papillary stalk, focal invasion of the tumor base, or extensive invasion of the tumor base. The data showed clearly that patients with tumors with extensive invasion at the base of the stalk (where invasion typically occurs) had a higher risk of progression and death resulting from bladder cancer than patients with only focal invasion at the base or invasion within the stalk of the tumor ($P < .0001$). Interestingly, the presence of unconventional carcinoma subtypes was not significantly associated with the risk of recurrence ($P = .21$). Such data suggest that reporting the site and extent of lamina propria invasion in patients with T1 papillary urothelial carcinomas will allow better risk stratification for progression than grade.[30,31] These data have not been confirmed in large-scale studies.

The GUPS article also suggests that tissue immunomarkers are not routinely recommended in clinical practice for grading urothelial carcinomas. Some studies showed that an overexpression of Aurora-A, MIB-1, loss of CD44, and increased CK20 (especially in CIS) correlated with the tumor grade[32] and, although pathologists variably (and infrequently) use immunohistochemical markers to grade bladder cancer, the opinion

Table 2
Correlations and findings in endophytic urothelial neoplasia

Inverted Papilloma	No Atypia
Inverted PUNLMP	No to minimal atypia
Inverted papillary urothelial carcinoma, noninvasive low-grade	Moderate to severe atypia
Inverted papillary urothelial carcinoma, noninvasive high-grade	Moderate to severe atypia

of pathology societies has always been consistent to not use immunohistochemistry in grading of noninvasive bladder cancer.

Another pertinent question based on emerging data is whether molecular grading should be done with the help of immunohistochemistry in muscle invasive bladder cancers. Several panels have been suggested. The aim is to select between basal (CD44, CK5/6, CK 14, p63) and luminal (CK20, GATA3, FOXA1, Uroplakin II) markers to refine the diagnosis on a molecular level. Simple phenotypes, only tested with 2 cytokeratins might already be interesting (eg, CK20 and CK5/6).[33] Bontoux and colleagues recently tested a 4-antibody panel to detect luminal and basal markers (CK5/6, CK14, GATA3, FOXA1) and demonstrated that CK14 was a better marker than CK5/6 for basal/squamous cell carcinomas. They also found that higher stages (pT3-4) more often displayed the basal markers.[34] Nevertheless, GUPS does not currently recommend the use of antibodies for molecular classification. Aided by prospective studies, these markers might in the long-term gain increased value in routine practice, especially as the literature has demonstrated different behaviors of luminal and basal bladder cancers and different responses to chemotherapies.[35] Thus, we have currently not reached the threshold for consistent application in routine pathology practice or for patient management.

Another important topic in the GUPS article is urothelial neoplasms with exclusive or predominant inverted growth. These lesions are relatively uncommon and mostly occur in the bladder,

followed by the upper urinary tract. The most common are inverted papillomas, which by definition are benign lesions and well-known to urologic pathologists (Fig. 6).[36] From a diagnostic perspective, these endophytic lesions may be challenging in that they may be difficult to distinguish from an invasive lesion. Similar to their exophytic counterpart, these lesions display a wide range of morphologic and cytologic features, from inverted papilloma, inverted PUNLMP, to inverted noninvasive low-grade and high-grade papillary urothelial carcinomas. It is much more common to see urothelial tumors that show both mixed exophytic and endophytic growth; in such cases, it is not necessary to mention the inverted growth pattern in pathology reports. From a histologic point of view, the tumors show branching and anastomosing cords in conjunction with smooth, pushing, and expansile borders. Grading of these lesions should be based on criteria applicable to their better-known exophytic counterparts. Thus, if an inverted proliferation has increased cell density and thickness, it is considered as inverted PUNLMP. If there is cytologic atypia, it should be graded low-grade or high-grade based on extent of architectural disarray and cytologic atypia. As a matter of practical application, a lesion may be designated "inverted" when it is either pure or at least displays greater than 80% of inverted histology. Depending on whether the tumor is predominantly or exclusively endophytic, terminology such as "papillary urothelial carcinoma, low grade with predominant greater than 80% inverted growth pattern, no evidence of invasion" or

Fig. 6. Inverted papilloma, the most frequent and benign inverted lesion.

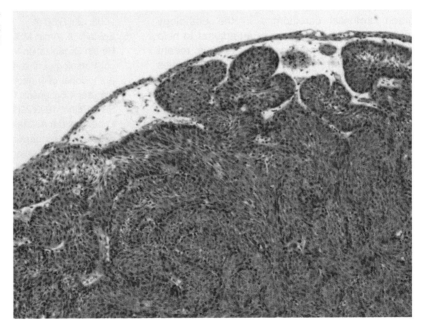

"papillary urothelial carcinoma, low grade with exclusive inverted growth, no evidence of invasion" is adequate.

From a differential diagnostic perspective, one of the most critical areas for the surgical pathologist is to accurately recognize destructive invasion into the lamina propria and distinguish it from tumors with inverted growth patterns. This observation has ramifications for stage assignment as well as for management. With respect to endophytic tumors, one of the major hurdles is the current lack of data regarding the biological potential and outcome of these lesions. From the limited literature that is available, it seems that inverted tumors have lower progression rates. In an article from Maxwell and colleagues, the authors evaluated 189 primary PUNLMP (177 exophytic, 12 inverted). No recurrence or progression was documented on follow-up for PUNLMPs that demonstrated exclusively inverted growth.[37] Another article from Arslankoz and colleagues aimed to evaluate the impact of the inverted pattern on recurrence in patients with newly diagnosed noninvasive, low-grade papillary urothelial carcinoma of the urinary bladder. Tumors with inverted pattern showed a lower recurrence rate than pure exophytic tumors (37.5% vs 52.1%), a longer time to first recurrence (mean 34 vs 21.5 months) and fewer recurrence episodes ($P = .482, .564,$ and 0.051, respectively). All recurring inverted cases recurred only once during follow-up. No tumor with greater than 80% inverted architecture recurred. The results demonstrate that inverted lesions seem to have a better outcome in terms of disease recurrence. To indicate the presence and percentage of the inverted pattern in low-grade urothelial carcinomas in the pathology report might be considered as an adjunct to help long-term patient management.[38] Some recent studies demonstrated chromosomal abnormalities by UroVysion fluorescence testing. Inverted lesions often displayed FGFR3, TERT promoter, TP53, CDKN1A, and PIK3CA mutations.[39]

SUMMARY

The GUPS articles were a collective contribution from 32 urologic pathologists and 6 urologists and oncologists from 10 countries around the world. The purpose was to clarify nomenclature and classification and to propose practice approach and/or nomenclature in areas that have not received formal recognition by the WHO and other subspecialty textbooks. Most importantly, it identifies areas where there is a gap in knowledge and need for further collaborative, multi-institutional, or prospective studies. Although the rapid advances have been made in the molecular underpinnings of urothelial carcinoma, and some promising developments have occurred in artificial intelligence applications in pathology, these are yet to create an impact in current clinical application. It is anticipated that, in the future, they will make substantial improvements to our efforts in grading bladder cancer particularly at individual patient level.

DISCLOSURE

The authors have nothing to disclose.

REFERENCES

1. Amin MB, Comperat E, Epstein JI, et al. The Genitourinary Pathology Society Update on Classification and Grading of Flat and Papillary Urothelial Neoplasia With New Reporting Recommendations and Approach to Lesions With Mixed and Early Patterns of Neoplasia. Adv Anat Pathol 2021;28(4): 179–95.
2. JN E, G S, JI E, et al. World Health Organization Classification fo Tumour. Pathology and Genetics of Tumours of the Urinary System and Male Genital Organs. Bd 2004;1.
3. Humphrey PA, Moch H, Cubilla AL, et al. The 2016 WHO Classification of Tumours of the Urinary System and Male Genital Organs-Part B: Prostate and Bladder Tumours. Eur Urol 2016;70(1):106–19.
4. Obermann EC, Junker K, Stoehr R, et al. Frequent genetic alterations in flat urothelial hyperplasias and concomitant papillary bladder cancer as detected by CGH, LOH, and FISH analyses. J Pathol 2003;199(1):50–7.
5. Epstein JI, Amin MB, Reuter VR, et al. The World Health Organization/International Society of Urological Pathology consensus classification of urothelial (transitional cell) neoplasms of the urinary bladder. Bladder Consensus Conference Committee. Am J Surg Pathol 1998;22(12):1435–48.
6. Lopez-Beltran A, Cheng L, Andersson L, et al. Preneoplastic non-papillary lesions and conditions of the urinary bladder: an update based on the Ancona International Consultation. Virchows Arch 2002; 440(1):3–11.
7. Lowenthal BM, Sahoo D, Amin MB, et al. Urothelial Proliferation of Unknown Malignant Potential Involving the Bladder: Histopathologic Features and Risk of Progression in De Novo Cases and Cases With Prior Neoplasia. Arch Pathol Lab Med 2020;144(7):853–62.
8. Knüchel-Clarke R, Gaisa NT. [Preneoplastic lesions and precursors of urothelial cancer]. Pathologe 2016;37(1):33–9.

9. van Oers JMM, Adam C, Denzinger S, et al. Chromosome 9 deletions are more frequent than FGFR3 mutations in flat urothelial hyperplasias of the bladder. Int J Cancer 2006;119(5):1212–5.

10. Yee CH, Zheng Z, Shuman L, et al. Maintenance of the bladder cancer precursor urothelial hyperplasia requires FOXA1 and persistent expression of oncogenic HRAS. Sci Rep 2019;9(1):270.

11. Babjuk M, Burger M, Capoun O, et al. European Association of Urology Guidelines on Non-muscle-invasive Bladder Cancer (Ta, T1, and Carcinoma in Situ). Eur Urol 2022;81(1):75–94.

12. McKenney JK, Gomez JA, Desai S, et al. Morphologic expressions of urothelial carcinoma in situ: a detailed evaluation of its histologic patterns with emphasis on carcinoma in situ with microinvasion. Am J Surg Pathol 2001;25(3):356–62.

13. Sangoi AR, Falzarano SM, Nicolas M, et al. Carcinoma In Situ With Plasmacytoid Features: A Clinicopathologic Study of 23 Cases. Am J Surg Pathol 2019;43(12):1638–43.

14. Neal DJ, Amin MB, Smith SC. CK20 versus AMACR and p53 immunostains in evaluation of Urothelial Carcinoma in Situ and Reactive Atypia. Diagn Pathol 2020;15(1):61.

15. Khan MS, Thornhill JA, Gaffney E, et al. Keratinising squamous metaplasia of the bladder: natural history and rationalization of management based on review of 54 years experience. Eur Urol 2002;42(5):469–74.

16. McKenney JK. Precursor lesions of the urinary bladder. Histopathology 2019;74(1):68–76.

17. Pires-Luis AS, Martinek P, Alaghehbandan R, et al. Molecular Genetic Features of Primary Nonurachal Enteric-type Adenocarcinoma, Urachal Adenocarcinoma, Mucinous Adenocarcinoma, and Intestinal Metaplasia/Adenoma: Review of the Literature and Next-generation Sequencing Study. Adv Anat Pathol 2020;27(5):303–10.

18. Ozkaptan O, Cubuk A, Dincer E, et al. Adenocarcinoma in Orthotopic Neobladder 19 Years After Radical Cystoprostatectomy. J Coll Physicians Surg Pak 2021;30(5):588–90.

19. Armah HB, Krasinskas AM, Parwani AV. Tubular adenoma with high-grade dysplasia in the ileal segment 34 years after augmentation ileocystoplasty: report of a first case. Diagn Pathol 2007;2:29.

20. Varma M, Delahunt B, van der Kwast T. Grading Noninvasive Bladder Cancer: World Health Organisation 1973 or 2004 May Be the Wrong Question. Eur Urol 2019;76(4):413–5.

21. van der Kwast T, Liedberg F, Black PC, et al. a. International Society of Urological Pathology Expert Opinion on Grading of Urothelial Carcinoma. Eur Urol Focus 2021. S2405-4569(21)00096-101.

22. Sylvester RJ, Rodríguez O, Hernández V, et al. a. European Association of Urology (EAU) Prognostic Factor Risk Groups for Non-muscle-invasive Bladder Cancer (NMIBC) Incorporating the WHO 2004/2016 and WHO 1973 Classification Systems for Grade: An Update from the EAU NMIBC Guidelines Panel. Eur Urol 2021;79(4):480–8.

23. Soukup V, Čapoun O, Cohen D, et al. Prognostic Performance and Reproducibility of the 1973 and 2004/2016 World Health Organization Grading Classification Systems in Non-muscle-invasive Bladder Cancer: A European Association of Urology Non-muscle Invasive Bladder Cancer Guidelines Panel Systematic Review. Eur Urol 2017;72(5):801–13.

24. Compérat E, Larré S, Roupret M, et al. Clinicopathological characteristics of urothelial bladder cancer in patients less than 40 years old. Virchows Arch 2015;466(5):589–94.

25. Compérat E, Amin M, Reuter V. Reply re: Murali Varma, Brett Delahunt, Theodorus van der Kwast. Grading Noninvasive Bladder Cancer: World Health Organisation 1973 or 2004 May Be the Wrong Question. Eur Urol 2019;76:413-5: Two Decades of World Health Organisation/International Society of Urological Pathology Bladder Cancer Grading: Time to Reflect on Accomplishments and Plan Refinement in the Molecular Era, Not Regress to Readoption of a 45-year-old Classification. Eur Urol 2019;76(4):416–7.

26. Gofrit ON, Pizov G, Shapiro A, et al. Mixed high and low grade bladder tumors–are they clinically high or low grade? J Urol 2014;191(6):1693–6.

27. Cheng L, Weaver AL, Leibovich BC, et al. Predicting the survival of bladder carcinoma patients treated with radical cystectomy. Cancer 2000;88(10):2326–32.

28. Downes MR, Weening B, van Rhijn BWG, et al. Analysis of papillary urothelial carcinomas of the bladder with grade heterogeneity: supportive evidence for an early role of CDKN2A deletions in the FGFR3 pathway. Histopathology 2017;70(2):281–9.

29. Toll AD, Epstein JI. Invasive low-grade papillary urothelial carcinoma: a clinicopathologic analysis of 41 cases. Am J Surg Pathol 2012;36(7):1081–6.

30. Lawless M, Gulati R, Tretiakova M. Stalk versus base invasion in pT1 papillary cancers of the bladder: improved substaging system predicting the risk of progression. Histopathology 2017;71(3):406–14.

31. Pan CC, Chang YH, Chen KK, et al. Constructing prognostic model incorporating the 2004 WHO/ISUP classification for patients with non-muscle-invasive urothelial tumours of the urinary bladder. J Clin Pathol 2010;63(10):910–5.

32. Compérat E, Camparo P, Haus R, et al. Aurora-A/STK-15 is a predictive factor for recurrent behaviour in non-invasive bladder carcinoma: a study of 128 cases of non-invasive neoplasms. Virchows Arch 2007;450(4):419–24.

33. Rebola J, Aguiar P, Blanca A, et al. Predicting outcomes in non-muscle invasive (Ta/T1) bladder cancer: the role of molecular grade based on luminal/

basal phenotype. Virchows Arch 2019;475(4): 445–55.

34. Bontoux C, Rialland T, Cussenot O, et al. A four-antibody immunohistochemical panel can distinguish clinico-pathological clusters of urothelial carcinoma and reveals high concordance between primary tumor and lymph node metastases. Virchows Arch 2021;478(4):637–45.

35. Witjes JA, Bruins HM, Cathomas R, et al. a. European Association of Urology Guidelines on Muscle-invasive and Metastatic Bladder Cancer: Summary of the 2020 Guidelines. Eur Urol 2020;79(1):82–104.

36. Amin MB, Smith SC, Reuter VE, et al. Update for the practicing pathologist: The International Consultation On Urologic Disease-European association of urology consultation on bladder cancer. Mod Pathol 2015;28(5):612–30.

37. Maxwell JP, Wang C, Wiebe N, et al. Long-term outcome of primary Papillary Urothelial Neoplasm of Low Malignant Potential (PUNLMP) including PUNLMP with inverted growth. Diagn Pathol 2015;10:3.

38. Arslankoz S, Kulaç İ, Ertoy Baydar D. The Influence of Inverted Growth Pattern on Recurrence for Patients with Non-Invasive Low Grade Papillary Urothelial Carcinoma of Bladder. Balkan Med J 2017;34(5): 464–8.

39. Almassi N, Pietzak EJ, Sarungbam J, et al. Inverted urothelial papilloma and urothelial carcinoma with inverted growth are histologically and molecularly distinct entities. J Pathol 2020;250(4):464–5.

Urothelial Carcinoma
Divergent Differentiation and Morphologic Subtypes

Jatin Gandhi, MD[a,1], Jie-Fu Chen, MD[b,1],
Hikmat Al-Ahmadie, MD[b,*]

KEYWORDS

• Urothelial carcinoma • Divergent differentiation • Subtype

Key points

- Bladder cancers are morphologically heterogeneous and molecularly unique.
- Clinical uncertainty as to the prognostic implications of some of the subtypes.
- Some subtypes of urothelial carcinoma (UC) have phenotype–genotype signatures.
- Most histologic subtypes are genomically similar to classic UC.

ABSTRACT

Urothelial carcinoma (UC) is known to encompass a wide spectrum of morphologic features and molecular alterations. Approximately 15% to 25% of invasive UC exhibits histomorphologic features in the form of "divergent differentiation" along other epithelial lineages, or different "subtypes" of urothelial or sarcomatoid differentiation. It is recommended that the percentage of divergent differentiation and or subtype(s) be reported whenever possible. Recent advances in molecular biology have led to a better understanding of the molecular underpinning of these morphologic variations. In this review, we highlight histologic characteristics of the divergent differentiation and subtypes recognized by the latest version of WHO classification, with updates on their molecular and clinical features.

OVERVIEW

Bladder cancer is the sixth most common cancer in the US, with an estimated 83,730 (4.4% of all cancer cases) new cases and 17,200 deaths in 2021 (2.8% of all cancers).[1–3] Cancers arising in the urinary bladder demonstrate a wide spectrum of histopathologic features which can be focal or extensive. It is estimated that approximately 15% to 25% of invasive urothelial carcinoma (UC) exhibit morphologic variations,[4,5] which can occur in the form of "divergent differentiation" along other epithelial lineages such as squamous, glandular, trophoblastic, or small cell/high-grade neuroendocrine differentiation, singly or in combination.[6–8] Additionally, several "subtypes" (formerly known as "variants") of UC have been described with distinctive histologic, and to some extent, immunohistochemical (IHC) features, with evidence suggesting derivation from a urothelial origin. The histologic complexity is supported by the distinct molecular alterations in at least a subset of these subtypes, which further substantiates the biology of intratumoral and intertumoral heterogeneity in UC and its potential clinical applications. Similar to the previous editions, the 5th edition of the WHO classification recognizes the morphologic

This article was supported in part by Sloan Kettering Institute for Cancer Research Cancer Center Support Grant (P30CA008748), SPORE in Bladder Cancer (P50CA221745), NCI (P01CA221757), and NCI (R01CA233899).
[a] Department of Pathology and Laboratory Medicine, Emory University School of Medicine, 1364 Clifton Rd, Atlanta, GA 30322, USA; [b] Department of Pathology and Laboratory Medicine, Memorial Sloan Kettering Cancer Center, 1275 York Avenue, New York, NY 10065, USA
[1] Two authors contributed equally.
* Corresponding author. Department of Pathology and Laboratory Medicine, Memorial Sloan Kettering Cancer Center, 1275 York Avenue, New York, NY 10065
E-mail address: alahmadh@mskcc.org

Surgical Pathology 15 (2022) 641–659
https://doi.org/10.1016/j.path.2022.07.003

surgpath.theclinics.com

Table 1
Summary of subtypes and divergent differentiation of urothelial carcinoma (UC)

Category	Figure	Reference#
Divergent differentiation of urothelial carcinoma (UC)		
Squamous cell neoplasms/UC with squamous differentiation (SQD)		10,11,16,17
(Pure) Squamous cell carcinoma (SCC)	Fig. 1	18–20
Verrucous carcinoma		18,21–24
Glandular neoplasms/UC with glandular differentiation		11,12,17,25,26
(Pure) Adenocarcinoma	Fig. 2	12,25–30
Tumors of mullerian type/UC with mullerian differentiation		
Clear cell adenocarcinoma (CCA)	Fig. 3	31–39
Endometrioid carcinoma (EDCA)		18,31,32,36
High-grade neuroendocrine carcinoma		
Small cell carcinoma (SMCC)	Fig. 4	8,40–49
Large cell neuroendocrine carcinoma (LCNEC)	Fig. 4	41,50
UC with trophoblastic differentiation	Fig. 5	10,51–53
Histologic subtypes of UC		
Micropapillary urothelial carcinoma (MPUC)	Fig. 6	10,54–63
Plasmacytoid urothelial carcinoma (PUC)	Fig. 7	8,15,64–69
Nested urothelial carcinoma (NVUC) and large nested UC	Fig. 8	70–81
Tubular/microcystic UC		10,82,83
Lymphoepithelioma-like urothelial carcinoma (LELC)	Fig. 8	84–87
Lipid-rich UC	Fig. 8	88–90
Clear cell (glycogen-rich) UC		91
Giant cell UC	Fig. 8	92–95
Sarcomatoid UC	Fig. 8	8,96–102
Poorly differentiated UC	Fig. 8	103
Urachal and diverticular neoplasms		
Urachal carcinoma		26,104–116

Adapted from WHO Classification of Urinary and Male Genital Tumours, 5th ed. 2022; Ref. 9

diversity of UC with 10 subtypes (**Table 1**), and the guidelines recommend reporting the percentage of divergent differentiation and or subtype(s) whenever possible.[9] This review will highlight the various morphologic criteria for the diagnosis of subtypes of UC and their clinical relevance. Updates on the molecular characteristics of these subtypes will also be discussed.

UROTHELIAL CARCINOMA WITH DIVERGENT DIFFERENTIATION

UC with squamous differentiation (SqD): SqD is one of the most frequent forms of divergent differentiation, observed in up to ~40% of high-grade and/or high-stage disease.[4,6,10,11] It is important to note that conventional urothelial carcinoma (UC-NOS) not uncommonly exhibits many morphologic features also seen with squamous cell carcinoma (SCC), including polygonal cell shape, abundant light eosinophilic cytoplasm,

distinct cell border, and peritumoral lymphocytic aggregates. Therefore, it is recommended that the term squamous differentiation in UC is used only when more specific features of squamous morphology are seen, such as intercellular bridges or keratinization (**Fig.** 1A, B). Tumors with SqD characteristically cluster with the basal/squamous subtypes on gene expression profiling, characterized by overexpression of basal and stem-like markers (CD44, CK5, CK6, and CK14), epidermal growth factor receptor (EGFR) and desmocollins (DSC1-3) and desmogleins (DSG1–4), TGM1 (transglutaminase 1), and PI3 (elafin); and low expression of markers associated with urothelial phenotype and histogenesis (uroplakins, GATA3, FOXA1, PPARG, and thrombomodulin).[12–15] In the series of radical cystectomy (RC), UC with SqD is associated with higher stage at presentation; however, the recurrent-free survival (RFS) and cancer-specific survival (CSS) in cases with SqD was similar to UC-NOS in stage-matched

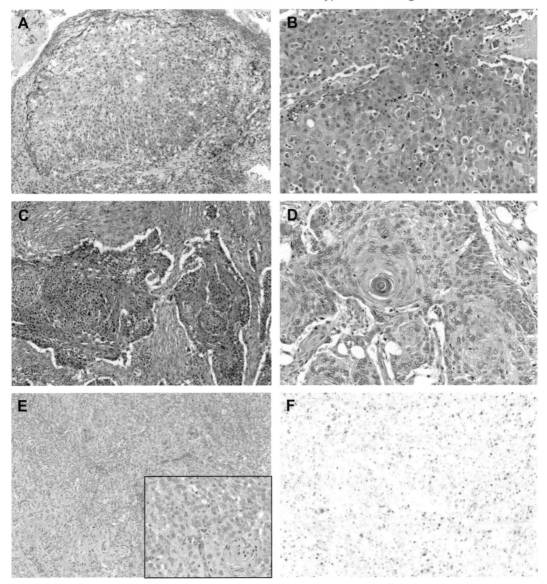

Fig. 1. Squamous differentiation of urothelial carcinoma (UC) and squamous cell carcinoma of the bladder. (*A–B*) Examples of squamous differentiation with transition from adjacent conventional urothelial carcinoma in the bladder. (*C–D*) Pure squamous cell carcinoma can also occur in the bladder. (*E*) In rare cases, the carcinoma is associated with high-risk human papillomavirus (HPV), with basaloid morphology (high-power view in inset) and positive RNA in situ hybridization for high-risk HPV (*F*).

analysis.[16,17] In addition, the clinical outcome seemed more favorable compared with the other subtypes of UC.[17]

Squamous cell carcinoma: Primary SCC of the urinary bladder (**Fig.** 1C, D) is extremely rare in the Western world with an overall worldwide incidence of 3.4% in women and 1.3% in men. SCC is the most frequent type of bladder cancer following UC, comprising 2.1 to 6.7% of all bladder malignancies.[18] In addition to the usual risk factors such as smoking, arsenic, and aromatic amines exposure, important predisposing risk factors include chronic irritation associated with chronic urinary tract infection, calculi, prolonged catheterization (such as in patients with spinal cord injury or neurogenic bladder) and Schistosomiasis.[18] Rarely, human papillomavirus (HPV) has been associated with bladder SCC, with similar morphology to those seen in cervical or oropharyngeal counterparts with basaloid, poorly differentiated appearance and little to no keratin formation (**Fig.** 1E, F).[19] Given the rarity of these cases, diagnostic consideration should also include HPV-related carcinoma arising from

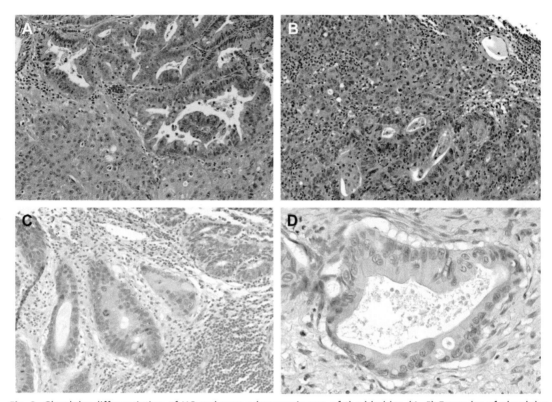

Fig. 2. Glandular differentiation of UC and pure adenocarcinoma of the bladder. (*A, B*) Examples of glandular differentiation with transition from adjacent conventional urothelial carcinoma in the bladder. (*C, D*) Rarely, pure adenocarcinoma can also occur in the bladder. The example in these figures shows resemblance to adenocarcinoma of gastrointestinal origin with acinar and cribriform architecture which is lined by pseudostratified epithelium.

cervical, anal, urethral, or penile origin. The diagnosis of pure SCC is generally reserved for keratin-forming squamous neoplasm, lacking any identifiable conventional UC component (invasive or noninvasive). Areas of keratinization and glassy pink cytoplasm are recognizable within the carcinoma in many cases. Grading pure SCC of the bladder is generally dependent on the amount of keratinization.[6] The histologic spectrum can be variable and may include large nest formation, clear cell change, pseudocystic changes, bizarre atypia and spindle cell morphology, and sarcomatoid transformation. The precursor surface lesions, ie, keratinizing squamous metaplasia/dysplasia or extensive condyloma acuminata may be observed in the vicinity with characteristic cystoscopy findings. Oncologic outcomes remain unclear when compared with UC with SqD, as some studies found no survival differences between pure SCC and UC with SqD if treated with RC and pelvic lymph node dissection,[16] whereas other studies reported bladder SCC to be more aggressive than UC-NOS after adjusting for stage and other prognostic parameters.[18,20]

Verrucous carcinoma of the urinary bladder is an extremely rare and clinically indolent tumor in the urinary tract with an exophytic filiform growth pattern. It is commonly observed in males in their 5th decade with higher incidences in areas endemic to Schistosomiasis.[18,21,22] The relationship with HPV is uncertain although progression from condyloma acuminatum has been documented in anecdotal case reports.[23,24] Grossly, these tumors are solitary, exophytic, fungating, and filiform. Microscopically, the tumor is frequently characterized by papillomatosis, acanthosis, and hyperkeratosis with pushing borders. The cytologic atypia is minimal. High-grade areas or frank stromal infiltration makes the diagnosis of verrucous carcinoma unsuitable. Overall prognosis is highly favorable although the data are very limited.[21]

Urothelial carcinoma with glandular differentiation: Glandular differentiation is common in UC and can be seen in up to 18% of cases.[4] True glandular differentiation is defined by the presence of glandular spaces resembling tubular or enteric glands (**Fig. 2**A, B) with occasional tumors exhibiting abundant extracellular mucin and mimicking colloid carcinoma. Intracytoplasmic mucin can be observed in 14% to 63% of cases.[6] The expression of MUC5AC and CDX2 by immunohistochemistry might be useful in highlighting glandular differentiation. Recent studies suggested that UC with glandular differentiation is genomically related to UC-NOS with a similar frequency of alterations in TERT promoter (~76%), chromatin-modifying genes (eg, KDM6A, KMT2D, and ARID1A), and DNA damage response (DDR) genes. These findings can help to distinguish UC with glandular differentiation from pure adenocarcinomas of the urinary bladder, which typically have molecular profiles similar to colorectal adenocarcinomas (see additional discussion of adenocarcinoma later in discussion).[12,25,26] Similar to SqD, UC with glandular differentiation had a higher stage at presentation; however, it is not associated with adverse survival outcome compared with conventional UC after adjusting for stage.[11,17,26]

Adenocarcinoma: Primary adenocarcinoma of the bladder is rare accounting for 0.5–2% of all bladder cancers in the US. Implicated predisposing factors include long-standing intestinal metaplasia, bladder exstrophy, chronic irritation, and obstruction due to nonfunctioning bladder or endemic schistosomiasis. Grossly, the tumors are frequently solid or sessile. Microscopically, primary bladder adenocarcinoma can be of enteric, mucinous, mixed, and not otherwise specified (NOS) types. The enteric type is identical to its gastrointestinal counterpart, exhibiting acinar, cribriform, villous, or solid architectural patterns, lined by pseudostratified epithelium and luminal necrosis (**Fig. 2**C, D). The mucinous type is composed of abundant extracellular mucin with floating tumor cells that may seem signet-ring, gland-forming, or sheet-like. The mixed type includes an admixture of enteric and mucinous types. Adenocarcinoma NOS is applicable to tumors not fulfilling any of the above features. There is not a uniformly accepted grading system for bladder adenocarcinoma. Surface glandular changes may coexist and include villous adenoma and high-grade dysplasia. By immunohistochemistry, bladder adenocarcinoma is usually positive for CK20 and CDX2 which cannot distinguish between primary adenocarcinoma from metastasis or direct extension from a colorectal primary.[27,28] Knowledge of precedent clinical history of primary gastrointestinal malignancy and radiologic and/or endoscopic evaluation is generally helpful in establishing a site of origin of bladder adenocarcinomas. Recent genomic studies on adenocarcinomas of the bladder demonstrated a high incidence of oncogenic alterations in TP53, KRAS, and PIK3CA, similar to frequencies observed in colorectal adenocarcinoma, and significantly lower incidence of APC alterations compared with colorectal adenocarcinoma. They typically don't harbor alterations commonly seen in UC such as mutations in TERT promoter, FGFR3, or chromatin-modifying genes.[12,25,26,29] When matched for stage, primary bladder adenocarcinoma has a similar outcome to UC.[30] Primary treatment modalities include surgery followed by adjuvant chemotherapy to control distant metastasis and/or adjuvant radiotherapy for better local control.

Adenocarcinomas of Müllerian type: Müllerian-type adenocarcinoma may rarely develop in the bladder and is thought to either arise from a pre-existing Müllerian precursor within deeper layers of the bladder wall such as endometriosis and Mullerianosis or be of urothelial derivation.[31,32] These carcinomas resemble their Mullerian-type counterparts in the female genital tract, such as clear cell adenocarcinoma (CCA) and endometrioid adenocarcinoma (EdCA). They are most commonly pure but may rarely be mixed with a urothelial component. CCA is the more common form of these 2 entities and, in contrast to other bladder carcinomas, these tumors have a female predominance.[33–35] Macroscopically, CCA occurs most commonly in the bladder neck and seems as a papillary or sessile, large solitary mass.[33] Microscopically, it resembles the female ovarian counterpart exhibiting tubulocystic pattern with basophilic secretions, hyalinized papillary cores or solid sheet-like growth patterns. Hobnail nuclei with appreciable cytologic atypia mitotic activity are frequently seen with accompanying hemorrhage and necrosis (**Fig. 3**). The histopathological appearance of EdCA is similar to its counterparts in the ovary and endometrium, often containing back-to-back endometrioid-type glands with squamous metaplasia or other metaplastic changes.[18,36] Useful IHC markers for CCA include PAX8, keratin 7, EMA, HNF1ß, and CA125.[6,34] IHC for (loss of) ARID1A expression has been proposed as multiple recent genomic studies have found CCA to have frequent ARID1A mutations, although the clinical utility in bladder tumors remains to be evaluated.[37] Other genomic characteristics of CCA include PIK3CA alterations, single-nucleotide alterations (SNVs), copy number alterations (CNVs) with the absence of TERT alterations (when exclusively pure CCA), hence supporting a nonurothelial differentiation.[34,38,39] The main differential diagnosis of CCA includes nephrogenic adenoma. Due to the shared PAX8 immunoreactivity, the distinction is often entirely morphologic based on significant cytologic atypia, high mitotic rate, necrosis, and deeply invasive

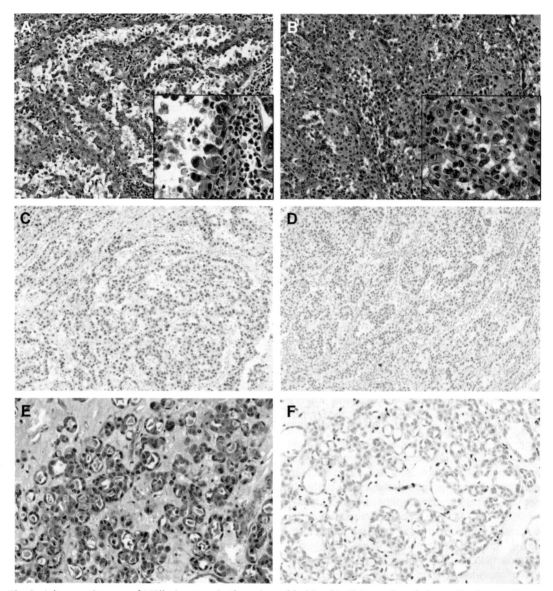

Fig. 3. Adenocarcinomas of Müllerian type in the urinary bladder. (*A, B*) Examples of clear cell adenocarcinoma (CCA) that shows tubulocystic pattern (*A*) with hyalinized papillary cores or solid sheet-like growth patterns (*B*). Nuclear hobnailing and prominent cytologic atypia are shown in the high-power view (insets). The tumor cells are typically positive for PAX8 (*C*) and may be positive for HNF1ß (*D*). (*E*) Another example of CCA demonstrates microcystic/glandular growth pattern and absence of ARID1A expression by immunohistochemistry (*F*), which corresponds to *ARID1A* mutation.

glands with stromal changes in CCA. The immunoprofile for EdCA is similar to the female genital counterparts, including ER and PR expression. Prognosis and management of these tumors are currently uncertain due to the scarcity of cases.

Neuroendocrine carcinoma of the urinary bladder: Small cell carcinoma (SmCC) of the urinary bladder is rare and associated with an aggressive course.[40,41] Morphologically, it is indistinguishable from its pulmonary counterpart and exhibits small cells with high nuclear to cytoplasmic ratio, nuclear molding, abundant mitotic figures and necrosis (Fig. 4A–C). Although most of the SmCC is associated with UC-NOS suggesting its urothelial origin, pure SmCC in the urinary bladder also exists. By IHC, the tumor often expresses neuroendocrine markers CD56, synaptophysin, chromogranin, and INSM1.[8,42,43] Various keratins are also expressed, mostly as focal and perinuclear dot-like patterns, reflective of the limited amount of cytoplasm in

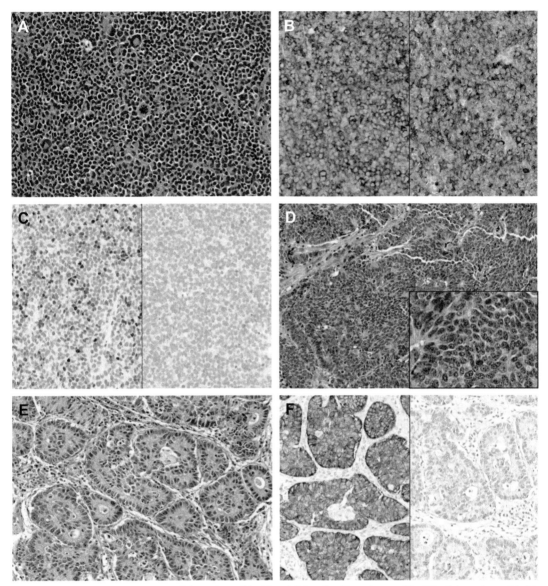

Fig. 4. Neuroendocrine carcinoma of the urinary bladder. (*A*) Small cell carcinoma (SmCC) of the urinary bladder exhibits characteristic small cells with high nuclear to cytoplasmic ratio, nuclear molding, abundant mitotic figures, and necrosis that are virtually identical SmCC in the lung. The tumor cells are classically positive for neuroendocrine markers including synaptophysin (*B left*), chromogranin (*B right*), and INSM1 (*C left*), and exhibit loss of RB expression *(C right)*. (*D, E*) Large cell neuroendocrine carcinoma (LCNEC) exhibits variable architectural patterns; the example in (*D*) shows a solid and vaguely rosette-like growth pattern, while the example in (*E*) exhibits prominent glandular architecture. LCNEC usually contains large high-grade polygonal tumor cells with variable amounts of cytoplasm and prominent nucleoli (*D inset*). The tumor cells are positive for neuroendocrine markers such as synaptophysin (*F left*) and chromogranin (*F right*) in more variable degrees.

tumor cells. Recently, novel neuroendocrine markers NEUROD1, ASCL1, POU2F3, YAP1, and DLL3 identified subgroups of bladder SmCC similar to those recently reported in lung SmCC.[44,45] ASCL1 and NEUROD1 expression was generally associated with higher expression of traditional neuroendocrine markers synaptophysin, chromogranin and

INSM1, and was mutually exclusive with POU2F3 expression. In contrast, POU2F3+ tumors were associated with lower expression of the same traditional neuroendocrine markers. The clinical significance of this classification is yet to be determined. By expression profiling, SmCC is characterized by a urothelial-to-neural phenotypic switch associated

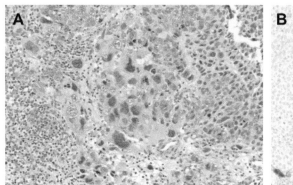
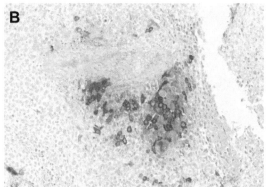

Fig. 5. UC with trophoblastic differentiation. (*A*) Example of clusters of syncytiotrophoblasts in the background of conventional UC, with IHC evidence of β-HCG expression in (*B*).

with the downregulation of both luminal and basal markers and dysregulation of the epithelial-to-mesenchymal transition network.[46,47] The genomic profile of SmCC is generally similar to that of UC with high levels of APOBEC mutation signature, high level of chromosomal instability and genomic doubling, and higher rates of *TP53*, *RB1*, and *TERT* promoter mutations.[40,46–48] The preferred treatment modality for SmCC consists of a combination of neoadjuvant chemotherapy and further consolidation by RC.[41,49]

Large cell neuroendocrine carcinoma (LCNEC) is a rare and still poorly characterized tumor of the bladder that is traditionally included in small-cell/high-grade neuroendocrine carcinoma category.[6] These tumors are high-grade, exhibiting neuroendocrine features and high mitotic activity by light microscopy, and showing evidence of neuroendocrine differentiation by immunohistochemistry. In contrast to SmCC, LCNEC consist of large high-grade polygonal tumor cells with variable amounts of cytoplasm and prominent nucleoli. They have variable architectural patterns such as nests, trabeculae, organoid, and palisaded (**Fig.** 4D–F). They may be pure or, more often, admixed with components of urothelial, glandular, squamous, or SmCC. Many of the tumors may be misclassified as poorly differentiated or glandular when associated with UC-NOS due to their growth patterns. By immunostains, LCNEC tumors express pancytokeratin and neuroendocrine markers. There are limited data on the molecular features of LCNEC, but early evidence suggests a similar genomic profile to SmCC, characterized by high tumor mutational burden and consistently harboring *TP53*, *RB1*, and *TERT* promoter mutations.[50] The currently preferred treatment modality is similar to SmCC whenever possible (neoadjuvant chemotherapy followed by cystectomy) with immunotherapy as an alternative option in the metastatic setting.[41,50]

UC with trophoblastic differentiation: Trophoblastic differentiation can occur in up to 5.5% of UC in the urinary bladder and 10.2% in the upper urinary tract.[51] UC with trophoblastic differentiation can be subdivided into (a) UC with scattered syncytiotrophoblasts (**Fig.** 5A), (b) UC with choriocarcinomatous differentiation and (c) UC with expression of β-HCG but no recognizable trophoblasts.[10] IHC stain for β-HCG can be positive in most of the cases (**Fig.** 5B), although the expression can frequently be seen in adjacent UC-NOS.[51,52] Some studies have suggested that urine or serum β-HCG levels may serve as a biomarker in assessing the response to therapy.[53] Positivity of other germ cell markers such as hydroxyl-δ-5-steroid dehydrogenase (HSD3B1) or Sal-like protein 4 (SALL4) have also been demonstrated, but the clinical utility remains to be further investigated.[52] Due to the limited case number in the literature, the molecular pathogenesis of trophoblastic differentiation in UC has not been well-defined. Trophoblastic differentiation seems to be associated with higher stage at presentation, but the presence of trophoblastic differentiation did not seem to predict adverse outcomes in multivariate analysis.[51,52]

HISTOLOGIC SUBTYPES OF UROTHELIAL CARCINOMA

Micropapillary urothelial carcinoma: Micropapillary urothelial carcinoma (MPUC) is a rare and aggressive form of UC, reported in 0.6 to 2.2% of cases, and is commonly seen in men with a mean age of 66 years. This subtype frequently presents as a high-stage disease and has a natural tendency for lymphatic vascular invasion and nodal metastasis.[6,10] Morphologically the reproducible features include the presence of multiple small clusters of tumor cells with reversal of polarity, embedded in a back-to-back lacunar/retraction

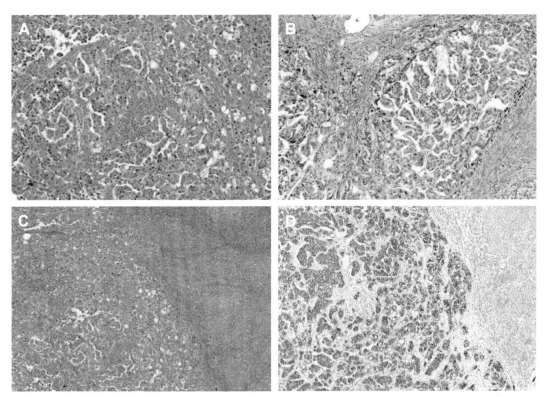

Fig. 6. Micropapillary urothelial carcinoma (MPUC). (*A, B*) Examples of classic MPUC exhibit multiple small clusters of tumor cells with reversal of polarity, embedded in a back-to-back lacunar/retraction space and lacking true fibrovascular cores. (*C*) MPUC (left) may exist with conventional UC (right). (*D*) IHC for HER2neu demonstrates overexpression of HER2, which corresponds to the amplification of the *ERBB2* gene in the MPUC area; note that the adjacent UC-NOS only shows weak membranous expression.

space and lacking a true fibrovascular core (**Fig. 6**A, B). Retraction spaces associated with MPUC can often mimic vascular invasion while lacking definitive endothelial lining. It is also not to be confused with the retraction artifacts that are frequently present in bladder tumors as a result of tissue processing. It has been shown that multiple nests within the same lacunar space had the highest association with a diagnosis of MPUC among the morphologic features.[54] Noninvasive UC with micropapillary architecture should not be regarded as MPUC. Although these unrelated features may be associated, they should not be considered as precursors for MPUC.[55] MPUC has consistently been reported to harbor higher rates of *ERBB2* gene alterations (including amplification and mutation) than UC-NOS and other UC subtypes (**Fig. 6**C, D). By expression profiling, these tumors are typical of luminal subtype and characterized by the enrichment of *PPARG* and suppression of p63 target genes.[56–60] The aggressive nature of MPUC has been recognized from the time this entity was coined as this tumor is generally associated with a higher rate of locally

advanced disease. However, more studies are showing that when compared with pure UC, MPUC was not associated with increased recurrence or mortality following RC.[61–63]

Plasmacytoid urothelial carcinoma: Plasmacytoid urothelial carcinoma (PUC) is a rare variant (<1%) of UC, histologically exhibiting discohesive single or small clusters of cells that resemble plasma cells or monocytes with a minimal stromal response (**Fig. 7**).[6,64] The invasive tumor cells typically infiltrate the bladder wall as single cells, linear cords, solid expansile or loose alveolar nests, or diffuse sheets.[8] These tumors invariably contain signet ring cells with intracytoplasmic vacuoles, but characteristically lack extracellular mucin. Patients with PUC frequently have local recurrences and peritoneal carcinomatosis, with an increased incidence of cancer-specific mortality. Extravesical spread of the disease can be as high as 28% for patients who undergo preoperative chemotherapy, despite the absence of radiographic progression after systemic therapy, rendering them unresectable at the time of surgery.[65] PUC is associated with higher rates of positive surgical

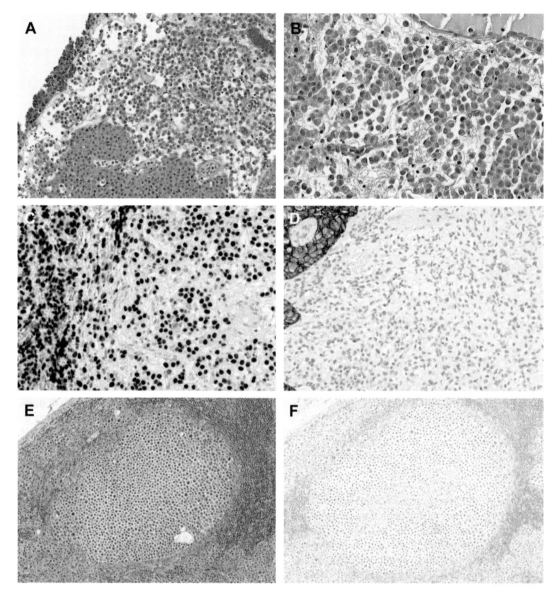

Fig. 7. Plasmacytoid urothelial carcinoma (PUC). (*A*, *B*) Examples of PUC that show the infiltrative growth of discohesive single or small clusters of cells that resemble plasma cells. The tumor cells are typically positive for GATA-3 (*C*) but show abnormal expression of E-cadherin (*D*), which corresponds to the alteration of the *CDH1* gene. (*E*) PUC has a high rate of lymph node metastasis. (*F*) IHC for E-cadherin demonstrates the absence of expression in PUC involving a lymph node.

margins and lymph node involvement and can be upstaged in up to 73% cases following RC.[66] Overall survival is still significantly lower following adjuvant or neoadjuvant chemotherapy for PUC compared with UC-NOS, with an overall downstaging rate of ~21%, pathologic complete response of ~12% and response rates ranging from 38% to 53%.[65,66] Genomically, PUC harbors a relatively high mutation rate with a median tumor mutation burden (TMB) of 14.9 mutations/Mb in one study.[65] Notably, these tumors harbor *CDH1* truncating mutations, and less frequently *CDH1*

promoter hypermethylation, which is pathognomonic to this histologic type. Therefore, the loss of E-cadherin expression (or less frequent presence of cytoplasmic labeling only; Fig. 7D), and abnormal expression of p120 (cytoplasmic expression and loss of membranous staining) is a characteristic immunoprofile.[67,68] Aside from *CDH1* alterations, the overall genomic landscape of PUC is similar to that of UC-NOS, with frequent mutations in chromatin modifiers, cell cycle regulators, and *TERT* promoter which may be useful to distinguish from other tumors with similar

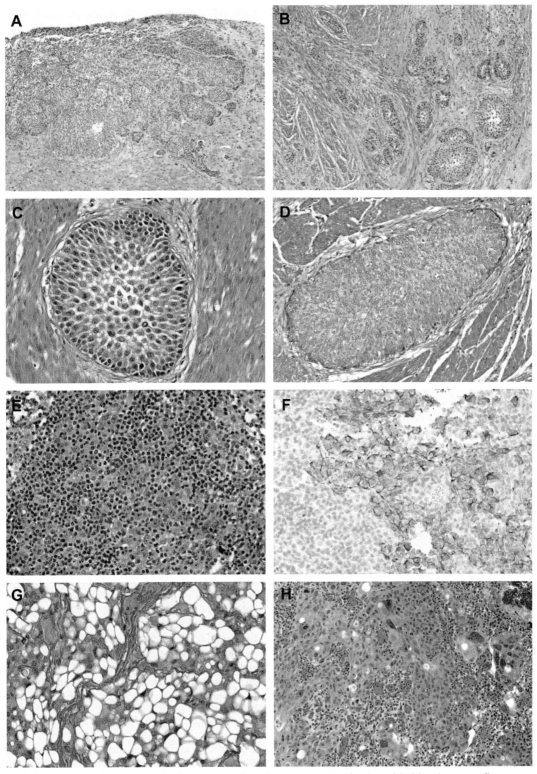

Fig. 8. (*A*) Nested subtype of UC (NVUC) in superficial lamina propria of urinary bladder shows confluent nests and cord-like growth with florid von Brunn nests-like areas. Note the morphologic resemblance to benign or non-neoplastic entities such as proliferative cystitis and von Brunn nest hyperplasia. (*B, C*) NVUC characteristically exhibits deceptively bland cytology, jagged tumor–stroma interface, and minimal desmoplastic response.

morphology such as lobular mammary carcinoma and diffuse-type gastric adenocarcinoma, particularly in metastatic setting.[69] So far, no germline CDH1 mutations have been identified in patients with PUC.[15,67]

Nested subtype (including large nested) of urothelial carcinoma: Nested subtype (including large nested) of urothelial carcinoma (NVUC) is a rare variant of UC that despite the characteristic deceptively bland morphologic features, can be associated with aggressive clinical course.[6,70–72] Histologically, NVUC has a characteristic growth pattern composed of the proliferation of small round to ovoid irregular nests of urothelial cells with banal cytology, jagged tumor-stroma interface and minimal desmoplastic response in the superficial compartment making its diagnosis challenging on initial biopsy or transurethral resection (Fig. 8A–C). The architectural pattern of the nested component can also be variably admixed with confluent nests, cord-like growth, cystitis cystica-like areas, and tubular growth pattern.[73] The large nested subtype of UC, as the name suggests, consists of large irregular and infiltrating nests, associated with stromal reaction and has an overall bland histologic feature (Fig. 8D).[71,72] Diagnostically, this subtype may be difficult to identify as it invariably shares overlapping morphologic features with a number of benign or nonneoplastic entities such as proliferative cystitis, von Brunn nest hyperplasia, nephrogenic adenoma, or inverted papilloma.[71,74,75] However, many cases can present with scattered but deeply invasive tumor foci of similar morphologic features, supporting its aggressive nature. By immunohistochemistry, NVUC typically have a luminal phenotype with frequent expression of FOXA1, GATA3, and CK20.[76–78] Interestingly, despite the overall luminal expression pattern, some NVUC tumors can exhibit CK5/6 expression with distinct localization at the basal layers of tumor nests.[78] Moreover, more than half of NVUC show nuclear PAX8 expression.[79,80] Relevant genomic findings in NVUC include the high rate of TERT promoter mutations, which is typically not detected in benign mimickers.[76,79,81] Additionally, occasional mutations in TP53, JAK3, and CTNNB1 have been reported in a study on large nested UC, while FGFR3 mutations were identified in the vast majority of cases.[77]

Tubular and Microcystic urothelial carcinomas: UC exhibiting tubular and microcystic features with overall bland cytologic features have been rarely reported.[82] These 2 entities are closely related to NVUC due to the bland appearing cells lining the tubules or microcystic structures making their recognition and distinction from NVUC challenging. In fact, microcystic and tubular morphology is present in a significant number of NVUC. The lining cells may exhibit mucinous contents.[6] Similar to nested subtypes, the tumor–stroma interface is jagged and irregular including the involvement of muscularis propria, which is an indication of its malignant behavior.[9] The differential diagnosis includes cystitis cystica *et* glandularis, and sometimes CCA.[10,83]

Lymphoepithelioma-like urothelial carcinoma: Lymphoepithelioma-like urothelial carcinoma (LELC) of the bladder is rare and exhibits similar morphologic features to its namesake in the nasopharynx and stomach characterized by a syncytial growth of high-grade epithelial cells with large pleomorphic nuclei, vesicular chromatin, prominent nucleoli, and ill-defined cytoplasmic borders, and are associated dense lymphoplasmacytic infiltrate (Fig. 8E, F).[84,85] It is, however, not associated with Epstein–Barr virus (EBV).[84,86,87] These tumors are male predominant, commonly seen between 5th and 7th decade, and associated with a component of UC in most of cases.[86,87] RNA expression and IHC profiling of LELC revealed that these tumors are enriched for basal-squamous molecular subtype markers (express KRT5, KRT6, and KRT14), are microsatellite stable and overexpress PD-L1 (∼93%).[85]

Lipid-rich urothelial carcinoma: These rare urothelial tumors have large neoplastic cells with optically clear empty multivacuolated cells resembling lipoblasts (Fig. 8G). They are typically admixed with UC-NOS, with variable amounts of the lipid-rich areas within the tumor.[6,88] The lipid-rich contents within the neoplastic cells have been verified by electron microscopy, Sudan Black B, and Oil Red stains.[89,90] The background UC is invariably high grade and invasive. The common differential diagnosis includes the signet ring component

---

(D) Large nested subtype consists of large irregular and infiltrating nests, and may associate with stromal reaction and has an overall bland histologic feature. (E) Lymphoepithelioma-like urothelial carcinoma (LELC) consists of syncytial growth of high-grade epithelial cells in the background of dense lymphoplasmacytic infiltrate. The tumor cells harbor large pleomorphic nuclei, vesicular chromatin, prominent nucleoli, and ill-defined cytoplasmic borders, and are evident by pan-cytokeratin staining (F). (G) Lipid-rich urothelial carcinoma demonstrates large neoplastic cells with optically clear empty multivacuolated cells resembling lipoblasts. (H) Example of giant cell urothelial carcinoma with loosely cohesive nests or single cells of anaplastic giant cells.

(glandular differentiation) of UC, heterologous lipo-sarcomatous elements of a sarcomatoid carcinoma or a liposarcoma itself. Due to the limited number of reported cases of lipid-rich UC, the associated clinical outcome is difficult to determine.

Clear cell (glycogen-rich) urothelial carcinoma: Clear cell (glycogen-rich) UC is a rare manifestation of UC that is characterized by solid and nested architecture and composed of cells with prominent cytoplasmic membranes with voluminous clear cytoplasm.[6,91] Diagnostic considerations may include involvement by clear cell renal cell carcinoma or CCA of Mullerian origin. However, clear cell UC lacks the characteristic vascular pattern typically seen in clear cell RCC and the tubulocystic architecture, hobnailed nuclei, and hyalinized stroma that are typically seen in Mullerian type CCA. Periodic acid–Schiff (PAS) and PAS-diastase (PAS-D) stains highlight the presence of glycogen within clear cells. By immunohistochemistry, clear cell UC typically expresses CK7, GATA3, CK5, and CD44, consistent with its urothelial phenotype.

Giant cell urothelial carcinoma: Giant cell UC is a very rare subtype of UC with only a handful of cases reported in the literature and is often accompanied by UC-NOS.[92–95] Morphologically, the tumor consists of loosely cohesive expansile and infiltrating nests or single cells of anaplastic giant cells (Fig. 8H). Tumor cells have abundant eosinophilic cytoplasm and may contain intracytoplasmic vacuoles. Necrosis and atypical mitotic forms are readily seen. Identifying a classic UC component or carcinoma in situ may be the key to diagnosis in challenging cases. The giant cells typically express keratins and other markers associated with urothelial phenotype, which helps distinguish them from histologic mimickers such as osteoclastic or trophoblastic cells.[92,94]

Sarcomatoid urothelial carcinoma: This is a rare form of biphasic bladder cancer, in which a component of the tumor exhibits mesenchymal differentiation, commonly nondescript spindled appearance, which may or may not be associated with heterologous differentiation (osseous, cartilaginous, myogenic, angiogenic, and so forth) and myxoid change in the stroma (Fig. 9A–E).[6,96,97] Sarcomatoid UC may be associated with prior radiation therapy and/or cyclophosphamide treatment.[97] Morphologically, the epithelial component may contain UC-NOS, squamous, glandular, or high-grade neuroendocrine carcinoma elements, and may imperceptibly merge with sarcomatoid histology.[98,99] To establish a diagnosis of sarcomatoid UC, one of the following must be identified: (1) epithelial differentiation on H&E examination; (2) variable keratin expression in the sarcomatous areas, often high molecular keratins CK 34ßE12 or CK5/6; and or (3) GATA3 expression in the sarcomatous areas.[8] The genomic landscape of sarcomatoid UC is overall similar to that of UC-NOS with the enrichment of *TP53, RB1, and PIK3CA* mutations.[100,101] By expression profiling, sarcomatoid UC is linked to the basal/squamous subtype with downregulated of luminal markers, dysregulation of epithelial–mesenchymal transition (EMT) network and overexpression of EMT markers, and overexpression of programmed death-ligand 1 (PD-L1).[101] Sarcomatoid UC is associated with higher stage at presentation and independently associated with worse survival compared with UC-NOS. Despite the worse outcome, sarcomatoid UC has similar pathologic response rates to neoadjuvant chemotherapy to those of UC-NOS.[102]

Poorly differentiated urothelial carcinoma: In the current WHO 2022, this tumor encompasses tumors such as the undifferentiated carcinoma with osteoclastic giant cells and any other tumors in which a substantial component of the neoplasm does not show a definitive line of differentiation (Fig. 9F).[9] These tumors often lose lineage-specific markers (GATA3, uroplakin 2); however, variably express markers of epithelial differentiation (cytokeratins AE1/AE3, Cam 5.2, CK7 and/or EMA). The multinucleated osteoclast-like giant cells in this tumor often express CD68.[103] The presence of conventional UC components or carcinoma in situ is usually diagnostic of poorly differentiated UC.

URACHAL CARCINOMA

Urachal carcinomas are extremely rare bladder cancers arising from urachal remnants with an incidence ranging from 0.01% to 0.7% in Western and European countries.[6,104–106] Mucosuria is present in up to one-fourth of the patients. Urachal carcinomas are usually located in the bladder dome or anterior bladder wall, and often are deeply invasive into perivesical soft tissue.[107] Urachal remnants may be identified adjacent to the neoplasms after adequate sampling, and are usually lined by cuboidal or urothelial lining and may exhibit enteric metaplasia or adenomatous changes. These tumors are generally cystic and attempts are being made to subdivide them, based on the cellularity and atypia, into mucinous cystadenoma, mucinous cystic tumors of low malignant potential, and mucinous cystadenocarcinoma.[6,108,109] Although adenocarcinoma is the most common urachal carcinoma, other tumor types have been also reported including urothelial,

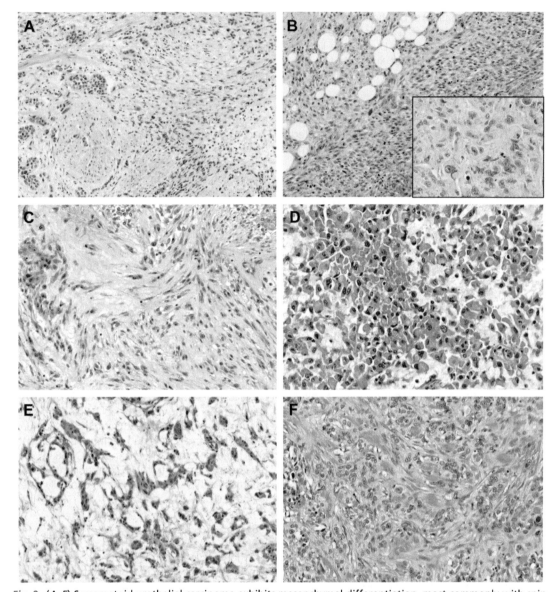

Fig. 9. (A–E) Sarcomatoid urothelial carcinoma exhibits mesenchymal differentiation, most commonly with spindled appearance (A, B). Myxoid stromal change may be observed in various degrees (C). Heterologous elements/differentiation may occur; examples here include (D) rhabdomyosarcomatous differentiation and (E) angio-sarcomatoid differentiation. (F) Poorly differentiated urothelial carcinoma remains in 2022 WHO classification to encompass undifferentiated carcinoma with osteoclastic giant cells and any other tumors in which a substantial component of the neoplasm does not show a definitive line of differentiation.

squamous, neuroendocrine neoplasms.[107,109] Recent genomic profiling of urachal adenocarcinomas identified frequent *TP53, KRAS,* and *SMAD4* mutations; while no mutations were detected in *TERT* promoter or chromatin-modifying genes.[26,110,111] Urachal adenocarcinomas have a 5-year survival rate ranging from 40% to 70% despite the locally advanced stage at presentation. In a nonmetastatic setting, wide/en bloc resection with negative soft tissue and bladder margins is generally curative.[26,112–116]

SUMMARY

Identifying the histologic subtypes and divergent differentiation in bladder cancer is important to establish the correct diagnosis and classification and may also be clinically relevant and dictates clinical management in certain subtypes. More work is needed to delineate the molecular biology driving these morphologic subtypes and identify predictive and prognostic biomarkers to devise novel and efficacious therapeutic approaches.

Due to the rarity of most of these subtypes, multi-institutional collaborative studies may be needed to produce adequate cohorts and generate meaningful and potentially transformative data.

REFERENCES

1. Bray F, Ferlay J, Soerjomataram I, et al. Global cancer statistics 2018: GLOBOCAN estimates of incidence and mortality worldwide for 36 cancers in 185 countries. CA Cancer J Clin 2018;68(6): 394–424.

2. Saginala K, Barsouk A, Aluru JS, et al. Epidemiology of Bladder Cancer. Med Sci (Basel) 2020;8(1).

3. Siegel RL, Miller KD, Jemal A. Cancer statistics, 2020. CA Cancer J Clin 2020;70(1):7–30.

4. Wasco MJ, Daignault S, Zhang Y, et al. Urothelial carcinoma with divergent histologic differentiation (mixed histologic features) predicts the presence of locally advanced bladder cancer when detected at transurethral resection. Urology 2007;70(1): 69–74.

5. Cai T, Tiscione D, Verze P, et al. Concordance and clinical significance of uncommon variants of bladder urothelial carcinoma in transurethral resection and radical cystectomy specimens. Urology 2014;84(5):1141–6.

6. Moch H, Humphrey PA, Ulbright TM, et al. Urinary and male genital tumours. Lyon (France): International Agency for Research on Cancer; 2016, (WHO classification of tumours series, 4th ed.; vol. 8). Available at: https://publications.iarc.fr.

7. Comperat E, Oszwald A, Wasinger G, et al. Updated pathology reporting standards for bladder cancer: biopsies, transurethral resections and radical cystectomies. World J Urol 2022;40(4): 915–27.

8. Comperat E, Amin MB, Epstein JI, et al. The Genitourinary Pathology Society Update on Classification of Variant Histologies, T1 Substaging, Molecular Taxonomy, and Immunotherapy and PD-L1 Testing Implications of Urothelial Cancers. Adv Anat Pathol 2021;28(4):196–208.

9. Board. WCoTE. Urinary and male genital tumours. Lyon (France): International Agency for Research on Cancer; 2022, (WHO classification of tumours series, 5th ed.; vol. 8). Available at: https://publications.iarc.fr.

10. Amin MB. Histological variants of urothelial carcinoma: diagnostic, therapeutic and prognostic implications. Mod Pathol 2009;22(Suppl 2):S96–118.

11. Kim SP, Frank I, Cheville JC, et al. The impact of squamous and glandular differentiation on survival after radical cystectomy for urothelial carcinoma. J Urol 2012;188(2):405–9.

12. Robertson AG, Kim J, Al-Ahmadie H, et al. Comprehensive Molecular Characterization of Muscle-Invasive Bladder Cancer. Cell 2017; 171(3):540–556 e25.

13. Warrick JI, Sjodahl G, Kaag M, et al. Intratumoral Heterogeneity of Bladder Cancer by Molecular Subtypes and Histologic Variants. Eur Urol 2019; 75(1):18–22.

14. Bontoux C, Rialland T, Cussenot O, et al. A four-antibody immunohistochemical panel can distinguish clinico-pathological clusters of urothelial carcinoma and reveals high concordance between primary tumor and lymph node metastases. Virchows Arch 2021;478(4):637–45.

15. Al-Ahmadie H, Netto GJ. Molecular Pathology of Urothelial Carcinoma. Surg Pathol Clin 2021;14(3): 403–14.

16. Ehdaie B, Maschino A, Shariat SF, et al. Comparative outcomes of pure squamous cell carcinoma and urothelial carcinoma with squamous differentiation in patients treated with radical cystectomy. J Urol 2012;187(1):74–9.

17. Xylinas E, Rink M, Robinson BD, et al. Impact of histological variants on oncological outcomes of patients with urothelial carcinoma of the bladder treated with radical cystectomy. Eur J Cancer 2013;49(8):1889–97.

18. Park S, Reuter VE, Hansel DE. Non-urothelial carcinomas of the bladder. Histopathology 2019;74(1): 97–111.

19. Blochin EB, Park KJ, Tickoo SK, et al. Urothelial carcinoma with prominent squamous differentiation in the setting of neurogenic bladder: role of human papillomavirus infection. Mod Pathol 2012;25(11): 1534–42.

20. Rogers CG, Palapattu GS, Shariat SF, et al. Clinical outcomes following radical cystectomy for primary nontransitional cell carcinoma of the bladder compared to transitional cell carcinoma of the bladder. J Urol 2006;175(6):2048–53, [discussion: 2053].

21. El-Bolkainy MN, Mokhtar NM, Ghoneim MA, et al. The impact of schistosomiasis on the pathology of bladder carcinoma. Cancer 1981;48(12):2643–8.

22. el-Sebai I, Sherif M, el-Bolkainy MN, et al. Verrucose squamous carcinoma of bladder. Urology 1974;4(4):407–10.

23. Batta AG, Engen DE, Reiman HM, et al. Intravesical condyloma acuminatum with progression to verrucous carcinoma. Urology 1990;36(5): 457–64.

24. Walther M, O'Brien DP 3rd, Birch HW. Condylomata acuminata and verrucous carcinoma of the bladder: case report and literature review. J Urol 1986;135(2):362–5.

25. Vail E, Zheng X, Zhou M, et al. Telomerase reverse transcriptase promoter mutations in glandular lesions of the urinary bladder. Ann Diagn Pathol 2015;19(5):301–5.

26. Almassi N, Whiting K, Toubaji A, et al. Clinical and genomic characterization of bladder carcinomas with glandular phenotype. JCO Precis Oncol 2022;6:e2100392.

27. Wang HL, Lu DW, Yerian LM, et al. Immunohistochemical distinction between primary adenocarcinoma of the bladder and secondary colorectal adenocarcinoma. Am J Surg Pathol 2001;25(11):1380–7.

28. Raspollini MR, Nesi G, Baroni G, et al. Immunohistochemistry in the differential diagnosis between primary and secondary intestinal adenocarcinoma of the urinary bladder. Appl Immunohistochem Mol Morphol 2005;13(4):358–62.

29. Roy S, Pradhan D, Ernst WL, et al. Next-generation sequencing-based molecular characterization of primary urinary bladder adenocarcinoma. Mod Pathol 2017;30(8):1133–43.

30. Lughezzani G, Sun M, Jeldres C, et al. Adenocarcinoma versus urothelial carcinoma of the urinary bladder: comparison between pathologic stage at radical cystectomy and cancer-specific mortality. Urology 2010;75(2):376–81.

31. Oliva E, Amin MB, Jimenez R, et al. Clear cell carcinoma of the urinary bladder: a report and comparison of four tumors of mullerian origin and nine of probable urothelial origin with discussion of histogenesis and diagnostic problems. Am J Surg Pathol 2002;26(2):190–7.

32. Sung MT, Zhang S, MacLennan GT, et al. Histogenesis of clear cell adenocarcinoma in the urinary tract: evidence of urothelial origin. Clin Cancer Res 2008;14(7):1947–55.

33. Kosem M, Sengul E. Clear cell adenocarcinoma of the urinary bladder. Scand J Urol Nephrol 2005;39(1):89–92.

34. Ortiz-Bruchle N, Wucherpfennig S, Rose M, et al. Molecular Characterization of Muellerian Tumors of the Urinary Tract. Genes (Basel). 2021;12(6):880.

35. Chan EO, Chan VW, Poon JY, et al. Clear cell carcinoma of the urinary bladder: a systematic review. Int Urol Nephrol 2021;53(5):815–24.

36. Taylor AS, Mehra R, Udager AM. Glandular Tumors of the Urachus and Urinary Bladder: A Practical Overview of a Broad Differential Diagnosis. Arch Pathol Lab Med 2018;142(10):1164–76.

37. Balbas-Martinez C, Rodriguez-Pinilla M, Casanova A, et al. ARID1A alterations are associated with FGFR3-wild type, poor-prognosis, urothelial bladder tumors. PLoS One 2013;8(5):e62483.

38. Lin CY, Saleem A, Stehr H, et al. Molecular profiling of clear cell adenocarcinoma of the urinary tract. Virchows Arch 2019;475(6):727–34.

39. Rammal R, Toubaji A, Sarungbam J, et al. Molecular Profiling of Clear Cell Adenocarcinoma of the Urinary Tract. Abstracts from USCAP 2021: Genitourinary Pathology (Including Renal Tumors) (422-531). Mod Pathol 2021;34:647–766.

40. Chang MT, Penson A, Desai NB, et al. Small-Cell Carcinomas of the Bladder and Lung Are Characterized by a Convergent but Distinct Pathogenesis. Clin Cancer Res 2018;24(8):1965–73.

41. Veskimae E, Espinos EL, Bruins HM, et al. What Is the Prognostic and Clinical Importance of Urothelial and Nonurothelial Histological Variants of Bladder Cancer in Predicting Oncological Outcomes in Patients with Muscle-invasive and Metastatic Bladder Cancer? A European Association of Urology Muscle Invasive and Metastatic Bladder Cancer Guidelines Panel Systematic Review. Eur Urol Oncol 2019;2(6):625–42.

42. Chen JF, Yang C, Sun Y, et al. Expression of novel neuroendocrine marker insulinoma-associated protein 1 (INSM1) in genitourinary high-grade neuroendocrine carcinomas: An immunohistochemical study with specificity analysis and comparison to chromogranin, synaptophysin, and CD56. Pathol Res Pract 2020;216(6):152993.

43. Kim IE Jr, Amin A, Wang LJ, et al. Insulinoma-associated Protein 1 (INSM1) Expression in Small Cell Neuroendocrine Carcinoma of the Urinary Tract. Appl Immunohistochem Mol Morphol 2020;28(9):687–93.

44. Baine MK, Hsieh MS, Lai WV, et al. SCLC Subtypes Defined by ASCL1, NEUROD1, POU2F3, and YAP1: A Comprehensive Immunohistochemical and Histopathologic Characterization. J Thorac Oncol 2020;15(12):1823–35.

45. Akbulut D, Jia L, Ozcan GG, et al. Comprehensive Profiling of Neuroendocrine Carcinomas of the Bladder with Expanded Neuroendocrine Markers ASCL1, NEUROD1, POU2F3, YAP1 and DLL3. US-CAP 2022 Abstracts: Genitourinary Pathology (including renal tumors) (522-659). Mod Pathol 2022;35:657–806.

46. Yang G, Bondaruk J, Cogdell D, et al. Urothelial-to-Neural Plasticity Drives Progression to Small Cell Bladder Cancer. iScience 2020;23(6):101201.

47. Hoffman-Censits J, Choi W, Pal S, et al. Urothelial Cancers with Small Cell Variant Histology Have Confirmed High Tumor Mutational Burden, Frequent TP53 and RB Mutations, and a Unique Gene Expression Profile. Eur Urol Oncol 2021;4(2):297–300.

48. Zheng X, Zhuge J, Bezerra SM, et al. High frequency of TERT promoter mutation in small cell carcinoma of bladder, but not in small cell carcinoma of other origins. J Hematol Oncol 2014;7:47.

49. Lynch SP, Shen Y, Kamat A, et al. Neoadjuvant chemotherapy in small cell urothelial cancer improves pathologic downstaging and long-term outcomes: results from a retrospective study at the MD Anderson Cancer Center. Eur Urol 2013;64(2):307–13.

50. Guercio BJ, Gandhi J, Teo MY, et al. Large cell neuroendocrine carcinoma of the urothelial tract (LNEC): The MSKCC experience. J Clin Oncol 2021;39(15_suppl):4526.

51. Cheng HL, Chou LP, Tsai HW, et al. Urothelial carcinoma with trophoblastic differentiation: Reappraisal of the clinical implication and immunohistochemically features. Urol Oncol 2021;39(10):732.e17-23.

52. Przybycin CG, McKenney JK, Nguyen JK, et al. Urothelial Carcinomas With Trophoblastic Differentiation, Including Choriocarcinoma: Clinicopathologic Series of 16 Cases. Am J Surg Pathol 2020; 44(10):1322–30.

53. Martin JE, Jenkins BJ, Zuk RJ, et al. Human chorionic gonadotrophin expression and histological findings as predictors of response to radiotherapy in carcinoma of the bladder. Virchows Arch A Pathol Anat Histopathol 1989;414(3):273–7.

54. Sangoi AR, Beck AH, Amin MB, et al. Interobserver reproducibility in the diagnosis of invasive micropapillary carcinoma of the urinary tract among urologic pathologists. Am J Surg Pathol 2010;34(9): 1367–76.

55. Sangoi AR, Cox RM, Higgins JP, et al. Non-invasive papillary urothelial carcinoma with 'micropapillary' architecture: clinicopathological study of 18 patients emphasising clinical outcomes. Histopathology 2020;77(5):728–33.

56. Guo CC, Dadhania V, Zhang L, et al. Gene Expression Profile of the Clinically Aggressive Micropapillary Variant of Bladder Cancer. Eur Urol 2016;70(4): 611–20.

57. Isharwal S, Huang H, Nanjangud G, et al. Intratumoral heterogeneity of ERBB2 amplification and HER2 expression in micropapillary urothelial carcinoma. Hum Pathol 2018;77:63–9.

58. Kamoun A, de Reynies A, Allory Y, et al. A Consensus Molecular Classification of Muscle-invasive Bladder Cancer. Eur Urol 2020;77(4): 420–33.

59. Ross JS, Wang K, Gay LM, et al. A high frequency of activating extracellular domain ERBB2 (HER2) mutation in micropapillary urothelial carcinoma. Clin Cancer Res 2014;20(1):68–75.

60. Tschui J, Vassella E, Bandi N, et al. Morphological and molecular characteristics of HER2 amplified urothelial bladder cancer. Virchows Arch 2015; 466(6):703–10.

61. Fairey AS, Daneshmand S, Wang L, et al. Impact of micropapillary urothelial carcinoma variant histology on survival after radical cystectomy. Urol Oncol 2014;32(2):110–6.

62. Mitra AP, Fairey AS, Skinner EC, et al. Implications of micropapillary urothelial carcinoma variant on prognosis following radical cystectomy: A multi-institutional investigation. Urol Oncol 2019;37(1): 48–56.

63. Wang JK, Boorjian SA, Cheville JC, et al. Outcomes following radical cystectomy for micropapillary bladder cancer versus pure urothelial carcinoma: a matched cohort analysis. World J Urol 2012; 30(6):801–6.

64. Nigwekar P, Tamboli P, Amin MB, et al. Plasmacytoid urothelial carcinoma: detailed analysis of morphology with clinicopathologic correlation in 17 cases. Am J Surg Pathol 2009;33(3):417–24.

65. Teo MY, Al-Ahmadie H, Seier K, et al. Natural history, response to systemic therapy, and genomic landscape of plasmacytoid urothelial carcinoma. Br J Cancer 2021;124(7):1214–21.

66. Keck B, Wach S, Stoehr R, et al. Plasmacytoid variant of bladder cancer defines patients with poor prognosis if treated with cystectomy and adjuvant cisplatin-based chemotherapy. BMC Cancer 2013;13:71.

67. Al-Ahmadie HA, Iyer G, Lee BH, et al. Frequent somatic CDH1 loss-of-function mutations in plasmacytoid variant bladder cancer. Nat Genet 2016; 48(4):356–8.

68. Sangoi AR, Chan E, Stohr BA, et al. Invasive plasmacytoid urothelial carcinoma: A comparative study of E-cadherin and P120 catenin. Hum Pathol 2020;102:54–9.

69. Penson A, Camacho N, Zheng Y, et al. Development of Genome-Derived Tumor Type Prediction to Inform Clinical Cancer Care. JAMA Oncol 2020;6(1):84–91.

70. Drew PA, Furman J, Civantos F, et al. The nested variant of transitional cell carcinoma: an aggressive neoplasm with innocuous histology. Mod Pathol 1996;9(10):989–94.

71. Comperat E, McKenney JK, Hartmann A, et al. Large nested variant of urothelial carcinoma: a clinicopathological study of 36 cases. Histopathology 2017;71(5):703–10.

72. Cox R, Epstein JI. Large nested variant of urothelial carcinoma: 23 cases mimicking von Brunn nests and inverted growth pattern of noninvasive papillary urothelial carcinoma. Am J Surg Pathol 2011; 35(9):1337–42.

73. Wasco MJ, Daignault S, Bradley D, et al. Nested variant of urothelial carcinoma: a clinicopathologic and immunohistochemical study of 30 pure and mixed cases. Hum Pathol 2010;41(2):163–71.

74. Dhall D, Al-Ahmadie H, Olgac S. Nested variant of urothelial carcinoma. Arch Pathol Lab Med 2007; 131(11):1725–7.

75. Volmar KE, Chan TY, De Marzo AM, et al. Florid von Brunn nests mimicking urothelial carcinoma: a morphologic and immunohistochemical comparison to the nested variant of urothelial carcinoma. Am J Surg Pathol 2003;27(9):1243–52.

76. Weyerer V, Weisser R, Moskalev EA, et al. Distinct genetic alterations and luminal molecular subtype

in nested variant of urothelial carcinoma. Histopathology 2019;75(6):865–75.

77. Weyerer V, Eckstein M, Comperat E, et al. Pure Large Nested Variant of Urothelial Carcinoma (LNUC) Is the Prototype of an FGFR3 Mutated Aggressive Urothelial Carcinoma with Luminal-Papillary Phenotype. Cancers (Basel) 2020;12(3).

78. Johnson SM, Khararjian A, Legesse TB, et al. Nested Variant of Urothelial Carcinoma Is a Luminal Bladder Tumor With Distinct Coexpression of the Basal Marker Cytokeratin 5/6. Am J Clin Pathol 2021;155(4):588–96.

79. Taylor AS, McKenney JK, Osunkoya AO, et al. PAX8 expression and TERT promoter mutations in the nested variant of urothelial carcinoma: a clinicopathologic study with immunohistochemical and molecular correlates. Mod Pathol 2020;33(6):1165–71.

80. Legesse T, Matoso A, Epstein JI. PAX8 positivity in nested variant of urothelial carcinoma: a potential diagnostic pitfall. Hum Pathol 2019;94:11–5.

81. Zhong M, Tian W, Zhuge J, et al. Distinguishing nested variants of urothelial carcinoma from benign mimickers by TERT promoter mutation. Am J Surg Pathol 2015;39(1):127–31.

82. Young RH, Zukerberg LR. Microcystic transitional cell carcinomas of the urinary bladder. A report of four cases. Am J Clin Pathol 1991;96(5):635–9.

83. Lopez-Beltran A, Henriques V, Montironi R, et al. Variants and new entities of bladder cancer. Histopathology 2019;74(1):77–96.

84. Zukerberg LR, Harris NL, Young RH. Carcinomas of the urinary bladder simulating malignant lymphoma. A report of five cases. Am J Surg Pathol 1991;15(6):569–76.

85. Manocha U, Kardos J, Selitsky S, et al. RNA Expression Profiling of Lymphoepithelioma-Like Carcinoma of the Bladder Reveals a Basal-Like Molecular Subtype. Am J Pathol 2020;190(1):134–44.

86. Amin MB, Ro JY, Lee KM, et al. Lymphoepithelioma-like carcinoma of the urinary bladder. Am J Surg Pathol 1994;18(5):466–73.

87. Williamson SR, Zhang S, Lopez-Beltran A, et al. Lymphoepithelioma-like carcinoma of the urinary bladder: clinicopathologic, immunohistochemical, and molecular features. Am J Surg Pathol 2011;35(4):474–83.

88. Leroy X, Gonzalez S, Zini L, et al. Lipoid-cell variant of urothelial carcinoma: a clinicopathologic and immunohistochemical study of five cases. Am J Surg Pathol 2007;31(5):770–3.

89. Lopez-Beltran A, Amin MB, Oliveira PS, et al. Urothelial carcinoma of the bladder, lipid cell variant: clinicopathologic findings and LOH analysis. Am J Surg Pathol 2010;34(3):371–6.

90. Borzacchiello G, Ambrosio V, Leonardi L, et al. Rare tumours in domestic animals: a lipid cell variant of urothelial carcinoma of the urinary bladder in a cow and a case of vesical carcinosarcoma in a dog. Vet Res Commun 2004;28(Suppl 1):273–4.

91. Mai KT, Bateman J, Djordjevic B, et al. Clear Cell Urothelial Carcinoma. Int J Surg Pathol 2017;25(1):18–25.

92. Lopez-Beltran A, Blanca A, Montironi R, et al. Pleomorphic giant cell carcinoma of the urinary bladder. Hum Pathol 2009;40(10):1461–6.

93. Wijesinghe HD, Malalasekera A. Giant Cell Urothelial Carcinoma of Bladder. Case Rep Urol 2021;2021:8021947.

94. Samaratunga H, Delahunt B, Egevad L, et al. Pleomorphic giant cell carcinoma of the urinary bladder: an extreme form of tumour de-differentiation. Histopathology 2016;68(4):533–40.

95. Samaratunga H, Delahunt B. Recently described and unusual variants of urothelial carcinoma of the urinary bladder. Pathology 2012;44(5):407–18.

96. Sanfrancesco J, McKenney JK, Leivo MZ, et al. Sarcomatoid Urothelial Carcinoma of the Bladder: Analysis of 28 Cases With Emphasis on Clinicopathologic Features and Markers of Epithelial-to-Mesenchymal Transition. Arch Pathol Lab Med 2016;140(6):543–51.

97. Lopez-Beltran A, Pacelli A, Rothenberg HJ, et al. Carcinosarcoma and sarcomatoid carcinoma of the bladder: clinicopathological study of 41 cases. J Urol 1998;159(5):1497–503.

98. Cheng L, Zhang S, Alexander R, et al. Sarcomatoid carcinoma of the urinary bladder: the final common pathway of urothelial carcinoma dedifferentiation. Am J Surg Pathol 2011;35(5):e34–46.

99. Mori K, Abufaraj M, Mostafaei H, et al. A Systematic Review and Meta-Analysis of Variant Histology in Urothelial Carcinoma of the Bladder Treated with Radical Cystectomy. J Urol 2020;204(6):1129–40.

100. Genitsch V, Kollar A, Vandekerkhove G, et al. Morphologic and genomic characterization of urothelial to sarcomatoid transition in muscle-invasive bladder cancer. Urol Oncol 2019;37(11):826–36.

101. Guo CC, Majewski T, Zhang L, et al. Dysregulation of EMT Drives the Progression to Clinically Aggressive Sarcomatoid Bladder Cancer. Cell Rep 2019;27(6):1781–1793 e4.

102. Almassi N, Vertosick EA, Sjoberg DD, et al. Pathological and oncological outcomes in patients with sarcomatoid differentiation undergoing cystectomy. BJU Int 2022;129(4):463–9.

103. Baydar D, Amin MB, Epstein JI. Osteoclast-rich undifferentiated carcinomas of the urinary tract. Mod Pathol 2006;19(2):161–71.

104. Bruins HM, Visser O, Ploeg M, et al. The clinical epidemiology of urachal carcinoma: results of a large, population based study. J Urol 2012;188(4):1102–7.

105. Molina JR, Quevedo JF, Furth AF, et al. Predictors of survival from urachal cancer: a Mayo Clinic study of 49 cases. Cancer 2007;110(11):2434–40.

106. Pinthus JH, Haddad R, Trachtenberg J, et al. Population based survival data on urachal tumors. J Urol 2006;175(6):2042–7, [discussion: 2047].

107. Gopalan A, Sharp DS, Fine SW, et al. Urachal carcinoma: a clinicopathologic analysis of 24 cases with outcome correlation. Am J Surg Pathol 2009; 33(5):659–68.

108. Amin MB, Smith SC, Eble JN, et al. Glandular neoplasms of the urachus: a report of 55 cases emphasizing mucinous cystic tumors with proposed classification. Am J Surg Pathol 2014;38(8):1033–45.

109. Paner GP, Lopez-Beltran A, Sirohi D, et al. Updates in the Pathologic Diagnosis and Classification of Epithelial Neoplasms of Urachal Origin. Adv Anat Pathol 2016;23(2):71–83.

110. Reis H, van der Vos KE, Niedworok C, et al. Pathogenic and targetable genetic alterations in 70 urachal adenocarcinomas. Int J Cancer 2018;143(7):1764–73.

111. Collazo-Lorduy A, Castillo-Martin M, Wang L, et al. Urachal Carcinoma Shares Genomic Alterations with Colorectal Carcinoma and May Respond to Epidermal Growth Factor Inhibition. Eur Urol 2016;70(5):771–5.

112. Henly DR, Farrow GM, Zincke H. Urachal cancer: role of conservative surgery. Urology 1993;42(6): 635–9.

113. Herr HW, Bochner BH, Sharp D, et al. Urachal carcinoma: contemporary surgical outcomes. J Urol 2007;178(1):74–8, [discussion: 78].

114. Sheldon CA, Clayman RV, Gonzalez R, et al. Malignant urachal lesions. J Urol 1984;131(1):1–8.

115. Siefker-Radtke AO, Gee J, Shen Y, et al. Multimodality management of urachal carcinoma: the M. D. Anderson Cancer Center experience. J Urol 2003;169(4):1295–8.

116. Wright JL, Porter MP, Li CI, et al. Differences in survival among patients with urachal and nonurachal adenocarcinomas of the bladder. Cancer 2006; 107(4):721–8.

Urothelial Carcinoma
Update on Staging and Reporting, and Pathologic Changes Following Neoadjuvant Chemotherapies

Manju Aron, MD[a,b,*], Ming Zhou, MD, PhD[c]

KEYWORDS

• Urinary tract • Bladder • Urothelial carcinoma • AJCC staging • Pathologic staging • Grading
• Reporting • Neoadjuvant chemotherapy

Key points

- pT1 substaging has prognostic implications and is recommended in transurethral resections. However, the optimal method for substaging has yet to be agreed upon.
- Further refinements in the pT4 staging of bladder cancer, pT3 renal pelvic tumors, and revising staging criteria of urethral tumors in females are likely to improve the current staging schemata.
- The recognition of potential pitfalls in the accurate diagnosis of urothelial carcinomas especially its subtypes are important to avoid clinically significant mishaps.
- Pathologic response in radical cystectomies following neoadjuvant chemotherapy has important prognostic values for patients with muscle-invasive bladder cancer.
- Tumor regression score is a simple, reproducible histopathologic measurement of response to neoadjuvant chemotherapy in muscle-invasive bladder cancer.

ABSTRACT

Staging and reporting of cancers of the urinary tract have undergone major changes in the past decade to meet the needs for improved patient management. Substantial progress has been made. There, however, remain issues that require further clarity, including the substaging of pT1 tumors, grading and reporting of tumors with grade heterogeneity, and following NAC. Multi-institutional collaborative studies with prospective data will further inform the accurate diagnosis, staging, and reporting of these tumors, and in conjunction with genomic data will ultimately contribute to precision and personalized patient management.

OVERVIEW

Pathologic stage is one of the most important prognostic and predictive factors in carcinomas of the urinary tract. These tumors are currently staged according to the 2018 (8th edition) American Joint Committee on Cancer (AJCC) tumor-node-metastasis (TNM) staging system,[1] and the major changes in bladder cancer staging are highlighted in Table 1. As in most organs, the pathologic tumor stage (pT) in the urinary tract is determined by the extent of cancer invasion into the wall of the involved viscera and the adjacent organs and is one of the most important data elements incorporated in pathology reports. Despite standardized staging and reporting guidelines,

[a] Department of Pathology, Keck School of Medicine, University of Southern California; [b] Department of Urology, Keck School of Medicine, University of Southern California; [c] Department of Anatomic and Clinical Pathology, Tufts University School of Medicine and Tufts Medical Center, 800 Washington St., Box 802, Boston, MA 02111
* Corresponding author. 1500 San Pablo Street, HC4, Room 2409, Los Angeles, CA 90033-5313.
E-mail address: manjuaro@med.usc.edu

Surgical Pathology 15 (2022) 661–679
https://doi.org/10.1016/j.path.2022.08.003
1875-9181/22/© 2022 Elsevier Inc. All rights reserved.

Table 1
Updates in the 8th edition of the American Joint Committee on Cancer Staging of bladder cancer

Stage Category	Description
T1	Attempt of substaging recommended
T2	Diverticular cancers have no T2
T4	Transmural prostatic involvement; subepithelial prostatic stromal invasion to be staged as urethral pT2
N1	Perivesical lymph node added into the category of regional lymph node
M1	Divided into nonregional lymph nodes (M1a) and nonlymph nodal distant metastasis (M1b)

challenges remain due to unresolved staging issues and pathologic pitfalls, secondary to both preanalytical (for example tissuefragmentation, crush/cautery artifacts, fibrosis, and lack of standardized specimen processing protocols) and analytical (failure to identify benign mimics, differentiate between muscularis mucosae and muscularis propria, and so forth) factors.[2] This review highlights the current updates and issues in the staging of urothelial carcinomas, recommendations in their reporting and pathologic changes secondary to neoadjuvant chemotherapies.

STAGING OF BLADDER CANCER

The changes in the 8th edition of the AJCC staging system (8e AJCC) of bladder cancer pertain only to the N and M categories and corresponding stage groups. Perivesical lymph nodes constitute the primary lymphatic drainage of the bladder and are identified in 16% to 47% of cystectomies.[3] Despite this, they were not included in the category of regional lymph nodes (pN) in the 7th edition of the AJCC. These lymph nodes may be positive in up to 7% to 10% of cases and have been shown to be an independent predictor of survival,[4] similar in significance to other nonperivesical regional lymph nodes.[5] As a result of these findings, perivesical lymph nodes were included in the pN of the 8e AJCC.

Visceral metastasis in bladder cancer is an independent predictor of poor prognosis even in patients treated with systemic chemotherapy.[6–8] In patients with locally advanced or metastatic bladder cancer treated with chemotherapy, the reported 5-year survival rates for patients with and without visceral metastasis (bone, lung, liver) are 20.9% and 6.8%, respectively.[6] Patients with metastasis limited to nonregional lymph nodes, however, fare significantly better than those with visceral and bone metastasis, with some patients even experiencing complete radiologic response after systemic chemotherapy.[8] In view of these findings, lymph node metastasis beyond the regional lymph nodes (common iliac) is classified as M1a and visceral metastasis as M1b.

There have been no changes in the pathologic staging of bladder cancer (pT) in the 8e AJCC.,However, summarized below are some of the updates, and persistent areas of ambiguity that need further clarification.

Substaging of pT1 Tumors

The 8e AJCC and other authorities including the College of American Pathologists (CAP) recommend substaging of T1 tumors on biopsy and transurethral resection (TUR) specimens. T1 tumors are a heterogeneous group of tumors with variable risk for tumor recurrence and progression.[9,10] Substaging of these tumors on the basis of the extent of invasion can provide prognostic information similar to other known risk factors including tumor size, carcinoma in situ (CIS), multifocality, and lymphovascular invasion.[3] A recent meta-analysis on substaging has shown a strong association with both disease recurrence and disease progression after adjusting for the effects of established confounding factors (eg, tumor grade, CIS and multifocality) in pT1 tumors.[11]

The pathologic approaches to T1 substaging include either using histoanatomic landmarks in the bladder wall or quantitative methods including micrometric measurements for the depth of invasion, extent of invasion (focal vs nonfocal) (Fig. 1A, B), and estimations of volume, and so forth.[2,11] The histoanatomical landmarks that have been traditionally used for substaging include the muscularis mucosae (MM) and/or vascular plexus (VP).[12–17] MM/VP substratification has been performed using either a two-tier system (above and below MM) or a three-tier system (above, into, and beyond MM).[14,18–22] The problem with this method is that MM/VP may be an inconsistent finding in TURBT specimens, since it is appreciable as a continuous layer in only ~40% of cystectomy specimens.[23] MM also shows anatomic variations within different regions of the bladder wall, being more appreciable in the

Fig. 1. High-grade urothelial carcinoma with focal (*A*) and extensive lamina propria invasion (*B*) on transurethral resection specimens. Tumor invading papillary stalk

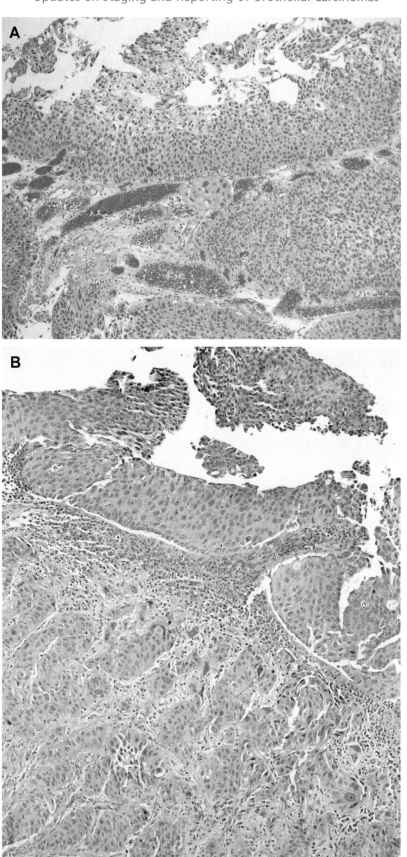

C

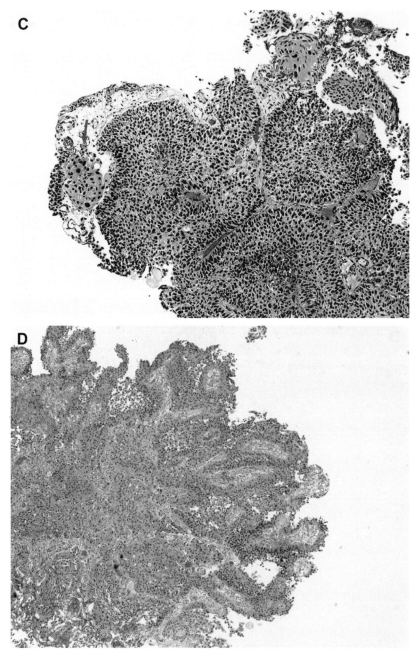

D

Fig. 1. (continued). (*C, red arrow indicating invasive nest*) and base (*D*).

dome than in the trigone (70% vs 10%). Although VP is often used as a surrogate landmark for MM, its location can also vary with respect to the level of MM and therefore cannot be reliably used for the purposes of substaging. This assessment can be further impeded in cases of repeat resections, which may lead to scarring or hyperplasia of the MM. Histoanatomic substaging has limited utility in these situations and is therefore not recommended.[18,21,24–26] In view of these

pitfalls, this method of T1 substaging has not garnered much favor among pathologists.

Quantitative approaches include measuring the extent of lamina propria (LP) invasion using either an ocular micrometer or microscopic field.[16–18,21,27–29] Using these methods, various cutoffs like 0.5 mm, 1 mm, ≥ 1.5 mm have been proposed to distinguish microinvasive and extensive disease with prognostic significance.[16,21,27,30–33] Other approaches include

Fig. 2. Urothelial carcinoma of the bladder invades the prostate either by transmucosal spread (A), which is staged as a separate pT2 urethral carcinoma or by transmural spread (B), which is staged as pT4a.

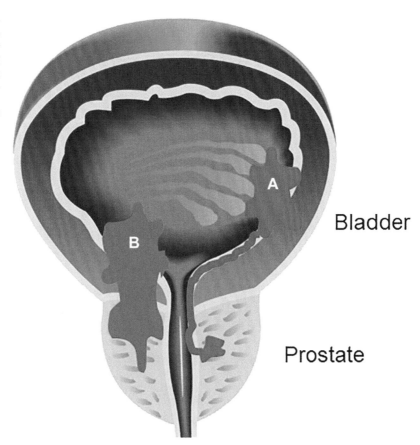

Bladder

Prostate

using the aggregate linear length of invasive carcinoma (ALLICA), with Lievo and colleagues recommending a cutoff of ≥ 2.3 mm as the best predictor of progression.[15] A recent study recommended largest contiguous focus of invasive carcinoma of 3.6 mm or greater and >3 foci of invasive carcinoma as statistically significant and a relatively simpler method of predicting progression.[34] Attempts have also been made to substratify lamina propria invasion in papillary tumors. Lawless and colleagues showed a significant association with lower progression-free survival in patients with base-extensive lamina propria invasion compared to those with stalk-only and base-focal lamina propria invasion[35] (**Fig. 1C, D**).

The quantitative methods appear to be more applicable and reproducible[18,30] and in some studies with head-to-head comparison with histoanatomic substaging techniques, the quantitative methods were more predictive of outcome (83% vs 50%), remaining predictive in multivariate analysis in 50%.[14,16,17,21,27,31] However, in the absence of well-designed prospective studies comparing the various methods of pT1 substaging (micrometric and histoanatomic) there is no consensus at present regarding the optimal method for substaging T1 tumors. AJCC and World Health Organization (WHO) both recommend T1 substaging using consistent methods within a practice.

Prostatic Involvement by Bladder Cancer

The prostate can be involved by urothelial carcinoma of the bladder either by transmucosal spread (extension from the bladder to prostate along the urothelium), or by transmural spread (bladder neck involvement or extravesical invasion) (**Fig. 2**)[36–38]; transmural spread is associated with significantly worse outcome.[37,39–43] Although the 7th edition of the AJCC had excluded transmucosal spread to the prostate from being staged as pT4a bladder carcinoma, the 8e AJCC has further clarified such involvement of the prostatic stroma to be staged as a separate pT2 urethral carcinoma.

Seminal Vesicle Invasion in Bladder Cancer

Seminal vesicle invasion by urinary bladder cancer is staged by the 8e AJCC as pT4 without further

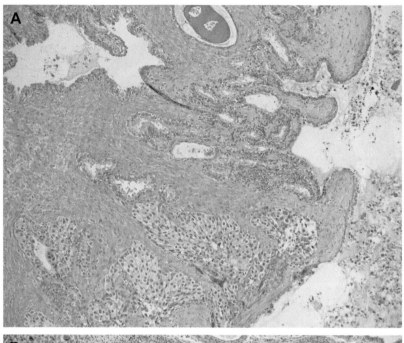

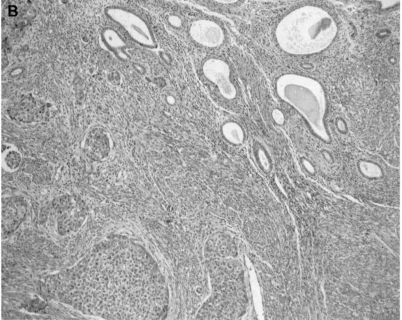

Fig. 3. High-grade urothelial carcinoma of the bladder involving seminal vesicle (*A*) and uterus (*B*).

subclassification into either pT4a or pT4b categories (**Fig. 3**A). There is some evidence in the literature that seminal vesicle invasion has worse prognosis than transmural prostatic stromal invasion (pT4a).[44–47] In a study of 1682 patients, the 5-year survival for patients with seminal vesicle invasion was similar to patients with pT4b (10% vs 7%) tumors and significantly worse than those with prostatic stromal invasion (pT4a - 38%).[44] These studies indicate that seminal vesicle

invasion portends a poor prognosis and perhaps should be subclassified as pT4b.

Invasion of the Female Genital Tract

Direct invasion of the female genital tract by bladder cancer is uncommon and is documented in 3% to 6% of radical cystectomies.[48–52] The commonly involved organs in this situation are the uterus (**Fig. 3**B) and the vagina.[53] Invasion of the female genital tract is staged pT4a, analogous to prostatic stromal invasion. However, studies have shown that the recurrence-free survival and cancer-specific survival for pT4a tumors following radical cystectomy in females is worse, compared to males.[54–56] In addition to direct invasion of the vagina, pagetoid involvement of the vaginal mucosa can also occur and the staging of tumors in these rare instances still requires clarification.

Urothelial Carcinoma in Bladder Diverticula

Bladder diverticula are mostly acquired and usually do not contain muscularis propria.[57] The 8e AJCC clarifies the exclusion of a T2 category in tumors arising in the bladder diverticulum. Studies on the staging of bladder diverticular tumors are limited, but the existing data suggest comparable outcomes to corresponding bladder tumor staging categories.[58–61]

Pathologic Pitfalls in Staging Bladder Cancers

The optimal staging of bladder cancers in pathologic specimens is fraught with pitfalls due to issues inherent to the limitations of the submitted sample, ambiguity in diagnostic criteria, and inter-observer variability. Lamina propria invasion in biopsy and TUR specimens maybe difficult to diagnose due to surgical procedural artifacts (crush/cautery), tissue processing artifacts (tangential sectioning/poor orientation), and stromal changes like inflammation at the tumor interface.[56,62] Even among genitourinary pathologists the interobserver variability may be high, with one study on pT1 tumors showing agreement in only 47% of the cases.[63] Some invasive urothelial carcinoma variants with bland morphology maybe difficult to distinguish from benign proliferative entities like florid von Brunn nests.[64–66] Distinguishing muscularis mucosa from splayed muscularis propria in biopsy/TUR specimens can be challenging making the distinction between pT1 and pT2 tumors difficult.[2] The distinction of pT2 tumors from pT3 tumors may also be problematic in cystectomy specimens because of the poor demarcation between the outer layer of the muscularis propria and perivesical fat. Interobserver variability has been documented even among experts.[2,67] Distinction of macroscopic extravesical mass (pT3b) in cystectomy specimens from desmoplastic reaction due to a microscopic focus of invasion can also be challenging and requires accurate gross assessment and extensive sampling.[1,68] Staging of tumors beyond pT2 is not recommended on biopsy/TUR specimens because of the presence of microscopic fat throughout the thickness of the bladder wall.

UROTHELIAL CARCINOMA OF THE URETHRA

The current 8e AJCC staging system, unlike the 7th edition does not separate carcinoma in situ involving the prostatic urethra according to its location in either the urethral mucosa (previous Tis pu), ducts (previous Tis pd), or prostatic acini. It also clarifies pT1 to involve tumor invasion into the connective tissue underlying the urothelium. Tumors involving prostatic stroma around ducts and acini are categorized as pT2 tumors and tumors invading the bladder wall are considered pT4. However, the current staging of urethral carcinoma in females is grouped with the staging of non-prostatic male urethra and does not take into account the histologic landmarks that are unique to the female urethra. Some of the limitations of the current staging system includes the lack of inclusion of staging of anterior urethral tumors beyond pT2 and the inclusion of anterior vaginal wall involvement as pT3 disease instead of considering the vagina as a separate organ (and hence pT4). A recent study has tried to address this issue by proposing a new staging system for female urethral cancers based on the histoanatomy of the female urethra that provided outcome-related information.[69] Larger multi-institutional prospective studies are required to further validate the findings of this study.

STAGING OF UROTHELIAL CARCINOMA OF THE UPPER URINARY TRACT

Staging of urothelial carcinomas of the renal pelvis and ureter, in large part, parallels that of bladder cancer. Accurate grading and staging are important in identifying patients for neoadjuvant chemotherapy (NAC) and definitive surgical therapy. Information regarding staging on ureteroscopic biopsies can be challenging because of technical difficulties in obtaining an adequate deep biopsy;[70] therefore, a multidisciplinary approach relying on imaging, biopsy, and urine cytology is often used in the risk stratification of these patients. The visual appearance of the tumor taken into account with the histologic grade has been found to correlate with stage 70% of the time.[71] A simplified model for risk stratification using tumor grade and imaging stage has been reported to better identify patients with localized tumors.[72]

The pathologic staging of urothelial carcinomas of the upper urinary tract has not undergone many updates. pT3 tumors of the renal pelvis encompass tumors involving the peripelvic fat, renal parenchyma, or both. However, there is evidence to suggest that renal pelvic pT3 tumors are a clinically heterogeneous group, with variable survival of patients within this category.[73–75] Studies have documented that tumors with peripelvic fat invasion have worse disease-specific survival than those without peripelvic fat invasion,[76–78] with some studies showing better overall survival, similar to pT2 tumors in cases with renal parenchymal invasion.[76,79] These studies suggest the potential utility of further stratifying the pT3 category in renal pelvic tumors, and possibly incorporating renal parenchymal invasion into pT2 disease. Studies of larger multi-institutional cohorts may further validate these findings.

The other change in the 8e AJCC relates to the nodal staging of upper tract urothelial carcinomas. Since there is no relevant data to substantiate the existence of the three N categories of the 7th AJCC edition, the category of N3(metastasis in a lymph node greater than 5 cm) is now included as N2.

REPORTING OF UROTHELIAL CARCINOMA

The standards for reporting urothelial carcinoma in the bladder and other portions of the urinary tract are continually reviewed and revised by pathology organizations like CAP and the International Collaboration on Cancer Reporting (ICCR).[80–82] These reporting standards are integrated into guidelines, which aid in the optimal management of patients. Despite the presence of these standards, challenges remain in their uniform application and adoption due to various factors including lack of adequate clinical information, guidelines for grossing certain specimens (large TURBT, lymphadenectomy specimens, and so forth), and pathologic pitfalls, especially in biopsy specimens.

The required and recommended features to report in bladder specimens, according to the current ICCR dataset is enumerated in **Table 2**. Similar datasets are also available for specimens of the upper urinary tract and the urethra and incorporate similar recommendations.

Clinical History

Clinical history and the location of the lesion are critical in the optimal evaluation of specimens. Information regarding the history of chemotherapy and radiation is extremely useful to prevent potential misdiagnosis of malignancy.[83,84] Nephrogenic adenoma arising in the setting of previous resections can also mimic carcinoma.[85,86] Pertinent history of carcinoma elsewhere in the body such as prostatic adenocarcinoma, colorectal carcinoma and squamous cell carcinoma of the cervix, especially in biopsy/TUR specimens can prevent diagnostic misadventures that can potentially be catastrophic. Cystoscopic findings can further inform the pathologist to evaluate additional levels of the tissue sections, if for instance a papillary lesion seen on cystoscopy is not identified on

Table 2
The International Collaboration on Cancer Reporting dataset for bladder cancer (www.ICCR-cancer.org), required and recommended features

Required	Recommended
Specimen Site	Clinical information including the history of previous therapy
Operative procedure	Block identification key
Histologic tumor type; subtype and divergent differentiation	Tumor focality[a]
Histologic grade	Substaging T1(TURBT)
Lymphovascular invasion	Associated epithelial lesions
Presence of invasive cancer, extent of invasion	Coexistent pathology
Macroscopic and microscopic extent of invasion for pT3 disease[a]	Ancillary studies
Noninvasive carcinoma (coexistent CIS)	Tumor location[a]
Margin status[a]	Response to neoadjuvant chemotherapy[a]
Lymph node status with histologically confirmed metastasis[a]	
Pathologic stage[a]	
Status of muscularis propria (TURBT)	

[a] For cystectomy and cystoprostatectomy specimens; TURBT: transurethral resection of bladder tumor.

initial pathologic evaluation. The location of the lesion can also be important for the pathologist to not only entertain the appropriate differential diagnosis but also for staging purposes.

Updated Terminologies, Urothelial Subtypes, and Divergent Differentiation

In addition to the updated staging systems, the pathology reports should include standardized terminology for both flat and papillary lesions and invasive urothelial carcinomas as included in the recent WHO 2022 classification systems.[87] Some of the changes include the exclusion of the category of the urothelial proliferation of undetermined malignant potential (UPUMP), which is now believed to represent early low-grade noninvasive papillary carcinoma or a lateral extension of such tumors.

In the invasive urothelial carcinoma category, the updates pertain predominantly to the substitution of the term "variants" with "subtypes" to distinguish the association of the term "variant" with genomic alterations. Invasive urothelial carcinoma is characterized by its propensity to show variable morphologic features due to divergent differentiation and histologic subtypes. The presence of any urothelial component including urothelial carcinoma in situ within a malignant lesion qualifies the tumor to be classified as urothelial carcinoma.[80,81,87] An exception to this rule is for cases with any amount of neuroendocrine component (small cell neuroendocrine carcinoma or large cell neuroendocrine carcinoma), which qualifies it to be classified as a neuroendocrine carcinoma and treated accordingly. The presence of subtypes and/or divergent differentiation is important as the percentage of a subtype in a sample may inform clinicians to tailor treatment protocols based on the prognostic and/or therapeutic implications associated with that specific subtype. Clinical trials may exclude urothelial carcinomas with a significant subtype component. Although the documentation of the percentage of each subtype within a specimen is recommended, the significance of the exact percentage of a particular subtype/divergent differentiation is as yet unclear.[87,88] Also, as previously mentioned from the pathologist's perspective some subtypes mimicking benign proliferations (nested variant) and/or resembling metastasis from other sites can potentially cause clinically significant diagnostic mishaps.[89]

Squamous differentiation is the most common histologic differentiation seen in urothelial carcinomas of the bladder and is reported in up to 40% of the tumors.[90] Urothelial carcinoma with extensive squamous differentiation on biopsy and TUR specimens may be difficult to differentiate from pure squamous cell carcinoma in the absence of an unidentifiable/unsampled urothelial carcinoma component. Tumors in the basal-squamous molecular subtype tend to display squamous morphology.[91]

Glandular differentiation is seen in up to 18% of urothelial carcinomas[90] and is the second most common type of divergent differentiation. The morphology of the glandular differentiation most commonly is the intestinal type and may be indistinguishable from colorectal adenocarcinoma. Both squamous and glandular differentiation are often associated with higher stage at presentation; however, their presence does not influence prognosis once the stage is accounted for.[90,92]

Micropapillary subtype of urothelial carcinoma is characterized by multiple small clusters of tumor cells within a lacunar space. These tumors usually show lymphovascular invasion and have aggressive behavior. Radical cystectomy is a consideration in patients with nonmuscle-invasive disease if they have a significant component of this subtype.[93,94] However, evidence regarding the oncologic outcome of micropapillary urothelial carcinoma and benefit from neoadjuvant chemotherapy (NAC) in this subtype is unclear.[95,96] On transcriptomic analysis most of these tumors showed a luminal subtype.[97]

Plasmacytoid urothelial carcinoma is an aggressive subtype with a propensity to spread extensively along tissue planes and peritoneal surfaces.[98,99] There is very little data regarding the treatment of this tumor subtype, and the benefits of newer adjuvant chemotherapy in plasmacytoid urothelial carcinoma is unclear.

The new WHO classification separates nested and the large nested variant of urothelial carcinoma into two different subgroups. They are distinguished from each other by the size of the infiltrating tumor nests. Both of these tumor subtypes are characterized by bland cytologic features and are often diagnosed at a higher stage. 70% of patients with large nested subtype present with pT2 tumors and 58% have extravesical disease (>pT3 and or lymph node metastasis), with almost a quarter dying of the disease in one published study.[64,100–103] Pure large nested variant of urothelial carcinoma has been shown to be associated with FGFR3 mutations and a luminal-papillary phenotype.[103]

Grading of Urothelial Carcinomas

The tumor grade of the tumor is a required parameter in the reporting of urothelial tumors and the current practice is to use a two-tier system (high and low). There is controversy regarding the reporting of rare cases of low-grade urothelial carcinoma that invade the lamina propria, with many pathologists reporting these tumors as high-grade based on their presumed clinical behavior.[104] The Genitourinary Pathology society (GUPS) recommends adding a note in such cases to highlight the similar prognosis based on stage for these cases compared with tumors having a high-grade morphology, and to clarify that there is insufficient data to suggest any difference in therapy based on the grade of the invasive component.[105] Grade heterogeneity within noninvasive papillary urothelial carcinoma is seen in up to a third of the tumors.[106] Tumors with ≥ 5% high-grade morphology were classified as high-grade tumors in the WHO 2016 classification, and this remains the recommendation in the 2022 WHO classification. However, there are studies to suggest that tumors with less than 10% high-grade morphology show significantly better 5-year progression-free and disease-specific survival than high-grade carcinomas.[107] GUPS recommends that mixed tumors with less than 10% high-grade component be diagnosed as noninvasive low-grade papillary carcinoma. Larger prospective studies are required to determine the optimal cut-off to distinguish low-grade carcinomas in cases with grade heterogeneity. Although not routinely used immunohistochemical markers and/or molecular biomarkers may find more widespread application as surrogate markers or complementary tests for optimal grading of urothelial carcinomas.[108,109] In the future, the use of deep learning and artificial intelligence may become mainstream in the fully automated detection and grading of urothelial carcinomas. Tumor regression grade following neoadjuvant chemotherapy characterized by stromal and epithelial changes is discussed in the section on pathologic changes following neoadjuvant chemotherapy.

Lymphovascular Invasion

Lymphovascular invasion (LVI) in urothelial carcinomas on radical cystectomies and resection specimens of the upper urinary tract is a highly significant predictor of outcome.[110–113] In contrast, there is less data regarding the clinical significance of LVI in bladder biopsy or TUR specimens and even less so in biopsies of the upper urinary tract and urethra. LVI identified in biopsy and TUR specimens has been correlated with upstaging in radical cystectomy in some studies. Based on the convincing evidence on resection specimens of the bladder and upper tract, the reporting of LVI is a required element in urothelial carcinomas of all sites in the urinary tract. Despite this requirement, the identification and reporting of LVI in bladder biopsies and TUR specimens can vary

anywhere from <10% to as high as 67%. Although IHC may help, it is not recommended as a routine practice in the detection of LVI.[114]

Lymph Nodes

The updates regarding lymph node staging for bladder cancer is mentioned in the section on staging. However, there remains considerable debate regarding the ideal extent of lymph node dissection and the minimal number of lymph nodes to be submitted for pathologic evaluation for urothelial cancer of the bladder and the upper urinary tract.[115–117] The pathologic assessment of lymph nodes is also fraught with issues regarding smallest lymphoid structure eligible for counting, separation of spatially related structures and the differences between counts on gross and microscopic assessment.[118] This was highlighted by a survey of pathologists from 23 countries, which showed considerable variation in the reporting of lymph node dissection specimens.[119] Therefore, there still remains significant challenges in the handling and reporting of lymph nodes that need to be resolved. Although serial sectioning and IHC may increase the chance of detection of lymph node metastasis, this is not currently recommended for routine reporting.

Urothelial Carcinoma In Situ

Urothelial carcinoma in situ (CIS) often coexists with high-grade papillary urothelial carcinoma and is seen in up to 65% of invasive urothelial carcinomas.[81] Concomitant CIS is associated with ureteral involvement, but not with significant differences in mortality or recurrence-free survival. However, in organ-confined bladder cancer, CIS is associated with worse recurrence-free survival and greater cancer-specific mortality.[120] The recognition and reporting of concomitant CIS in TUR specimens is easy if CIS is present on a separate fragment; however, if a severely atypical flat intraurothelial lesion is seen in the same fragment as a high-grade papillary tumor then it may be difficult to distinguish CIS from a "shoulder lesion" of the papillary tumor. There are no accepted criteria for making this clinically significant distinction, but generally speaking, if there is normal urothelium between the papillary lesion and the atypical flat lesion, most genitourinary pathologists would report it as CIS.

Surgical Margins

Surgical margin evaluation in radical cystectomy includes the evaluation of the ureteral, urethral, and soft tissue margins, with the first two specimens often submitted as frozen sections, although the American Urology Association (AUA) and European

Association of Urology (EAU) guidelines do not recommend the routine use of frozen sections for evaluating ureteral margins. A recent meta-analysis of 14 studies with 8208 patients showed a pooled sensitivity and specificity of frozen section analysis (FSA) for urethral margins on radical cystectomy to be 0.83 (95% CI of 0.38–0.97) and 0.95 (95% CI 0.91–0.97), respectively. The FSA for ureteral margins on radical cystectomy showed a pooled sensitivity and specificity of 0.77 (95% CI 0.67–0.84) and 0.97 (95% CI 0.95–0.98), respectively. This analysis highlights the role of FSA during radical cystectomies and raises the need perhaps for its continual use until quality-of-life-based cost-effectiveness studies identify patients who are unlikely to benefit from it.[121]

EVALUATION AND REPORTING OF RADICAL CYSTECTOMIES AFTER NEOADJUVANT CHEMOTHERAPY

Pathologic Response in Bladder Cancer Following Neoadjuvant Chemotherapy

The standard management of muscle-invasive bladder cancers (MIBC) is cisplatin-based neoadjuvant chemotherapy (NAC) followed by radical cystectomy and bilateral lymph node dissection, which has been shown to provide overall survival benefits compared with radical cystectomy (RC) alone[122] in eligible patients. However, approximately 40% of patients develop disease recurrence after RC despite NAC.[123,124] For chemo-resistant tumors, NAC not only exposes patients to possible toxic effects associated with chemotherapy but also increases the risk of cancer progression before surgery. Many clinical, imaging, and pathologic factors have been investigated for their predictive values of NAC response. Patient and imaging characteristics have minimal utility to predict NAC response.[125] Molecular biomarkers associated with tumor aggressiveness determined in urine, blood, and tumor tissues are promising in predicting treatment response and survival.[125] Pathologic features of the bladder cancer and response following NAC may also have prognostic values and are the focus of this portion of the review. Two important issues will be discussed, including whether pathologic features of bladder cancer in transurethral resection specimens (TUR) predict response to NAC and postcystectomy survival, and whether pathologic response and lymph node status at RC following NAC provide prognostic value.

The pathologic features in TUR that may significantly impact the pathologic response to NAC are not well understood. High mitotic rate (median: 4/ high-power field) was found to correlate with complete pathologic response.[126] A recent study found artificial intelligence models were able to integrate histologic features and clinical factors to predict responders to NAC, suggesting that computational approaches applied to routine TUR specimens of MIBC may distinguish between responders and nonresponders to NAC.[127]

The impact of the histologic subtypes and divergent differentiation on the pathologic response and survival after NAC is not entirely clear and data in the literature are conflicting. An early study found pure urothelial carcinoma is associated with greater rates of pT0 at RC than those with mixed histologic subtypes including squamous, glandular differentiation, small cell, micropapillary, sarcomatoid, nested component, lymphoepithelioma-like, and plasmacytoid variants.[128] More studies, however, reached opposite conclusions, that is, subtypes and divergent differentiation diagnosed in TUR had survival benefits that were greater than pure UC[129] or were associated with pathologic downstaging with NAC.[130,131] In micropapillary bladder cancers, NAC resulted in pathologic downstaging in a significant number of patients, with complete pathologic response (ypT0) ranged from 11% to 55%, although no survival improvement was reported.[132] However, another study found no significant difference in pathologic response to NAC between micropapillary and conventional urothelial carcinoma.[133] Plasmacytoid urothelial carcinoma is an aggressive subtype with overall poor outcomes. Pathologic downstaging after NAC has been reported in a small number of patients. However, there were no survival benefits between patients treated with NAC or initial surgery.[99] Another study, however, found plasmacytoid urothelial carcinoma had a poor pathologic response to NAC when compared with conventional urothelial carcinomas.[134] In small cell carcinoma of the bladder, NAC is associated with a high rate of pathologic downstaging with long-term survival benefits compared with historical expectations.[135] Nonmetastatic small cell carcinoma of the bladder is chemo-sensitive and patients have excellent long-term survival if responsive to NAC. However, patients with metastatic disease have poor survival despite systemic therapy.[136] Further studies are needed to better understand the role of NAC in bladder cancer histologic subtypes and divergent differentiation.

Evaluation of Pathologic Response in Bladder Cancer in Radical Cystectomies Following Neoadjuvant Chemotherapy

Pathologic response and lymph node status in RC following NAC have been shown to be significant prognosticators of disease course.[122] When the treatment is effective, the tumor regresses and leaves behind "zone of regression," which is indicated by dense fibrosis or myofibroblastic responses (Fig. 4A–C). Mixed inflammatory infiltrates, including macrophages, lymphocytes, and rarely eosinophils and neutrophils, are often seen. Zones of tissue necrosis are sometimes seen. Although TUR procedures may cause similar pathologic findings as NAC, such as fibroblastic reaction and necrosis, hyalinization is specific for NAC,[137] and the regressive changes associated with TUR would be limited to the bladder wall and would not involve the perivesical fat. Histopathologic tumor regression grade (TRG) was proposed by Fleischmann and colleagues to evaluate the pathologic response of MIBC following NAC.[126] It is based on the microscopic estimation of % of viable tumor cells in relation to the macroscopically identifiable tumor bed. At gross examination, the tumor bed should be adequately sampled, especially when a tumor is grossly not evident. TRG has 3 grades, TRG 1 to 3. TRG1 is defined as a complete absence of viable tumor cells, TRG2 as residual tumor cells occupying <50% of the tumor bed, and TRG3 as no regressive changes or residual tumor cells outgrowing the tumor bed ($\geq$50%) (see Fig. 4C).[126] Noninvasive papillary tumors or carcinomas in situ present in the specimens are not considered for the purpose of tumor regression evaluation. Lymph node dissection specimens without metastasis or with fibrotic zones indicative of completely regressed metastasis are assigned TRG1. The TRG grades for primary tumor and lymph nodes may be different. The higher TRG of primary tumor and lymph nodes is reported for the entire case. TRG is an excellent prognostic factor and better predictor of survivals than ypT stage. Multivariate analysis that included TRG, ypN-stage ypT-stage, and diameter of residual tumor showed the dominant TRG was the only independent risk factor for overall survival. This grading method was validated by 2 additional studies to be a simple, reproducible histopathologic measurement of response to NAC in MIBC,[138,139] including a study of 389 patients who underwent cisplatin-based chemotherapy before radical cystectomy in 8 centers.[139] ypTNM and TRG were combined to formulate final response categories: major response ($\leq$ypT1 and pN0), partial response

($\geq$ypT2 or pN+ and TRG2) and no response ($\geq$ypT2 or pN+ and TRG3). This combined ypTNM and TRG grade could discriminate the overall survival and was superior to ypTNM staging alone. However, the conclusions in the aforementioned studies were different from several other studies[137,140] which identified TRGs as a prognostic parameter in univariable analyses, but not in multivariable analysis, although other traditional parameters, including T stage, N stage, lymphovascular invasion, and margin status, correlated with the cancer-related death. The differences in the study design between these studies included smaller sample size and inclusion of histologic subtypes in the latter studies. The value of TRG needs to be validated and the grading method is standardized in further studies. We hold the opinion that information to determine TRG can be obtained during routine pathologic examination of the cystectomy specimen and can be useful, especially when combined with ypTNM, in assessing the response to NAC and providing guidance for additional therapy in the adjuvant setting.

Evaluation of Radical Cystectomy Specimens Following Neoadjuvant Chemotherapy

Protocols for gross examination, dissection, sampling and reporting of radical cystectomies have been published[141,142] and revised periodically (chrome-extension://efaidnbmnnnibpcajpcglclefindmkaj/https://documents.cap.org/protocols/Bladder_4.1.0.0.REL_CAPCP.pdf). Special attention should be paid for RC specimens in the post-NAC setting. The specimen should be immediately evaluated when possible. In some cases, it may be preferable to evaluate the fresh specimen before fixation. If no lesions are identified on initial evaluation, it may help to gently palpate the bladder wall to identify areas of induration or nodularity. A detailed section/block key should be provided to include reference to the originating anatomic location, disease state (tumor, scar, suspicious lesion, normal appearing, and so forth), and contents of each submitted tissue cassette.

If any lesions (tumor, scar, or ulcer) are grossly identified, each separate lesion should be amply sampled and submitted. The entire area (including adjacent induration) should be submitted with at least 1 cm margins around the periphery of the lesion. If no lesions are identified after a thorough examination of the bladder, a minimum of 15 sections of representative bladder should be submitted, including, but not limited to, anterior wall, posterior wall, trigone, dome, left lateral wall, right lateral wall, longitudinal section of each ureteral orifice, and urethral margin.

Fig. 4. A cystectomy specimen shows complete tumor regression following neoadjuvant chemotherapy with no residual tumor and dense fibrosis (*A*) and scattered mixed inflammation (*B*) involving the perivesical fat. Another cystectomy shows urothelial carcinoma invading muscularis propria without significant regressive changes following chemotherapy (*C*).

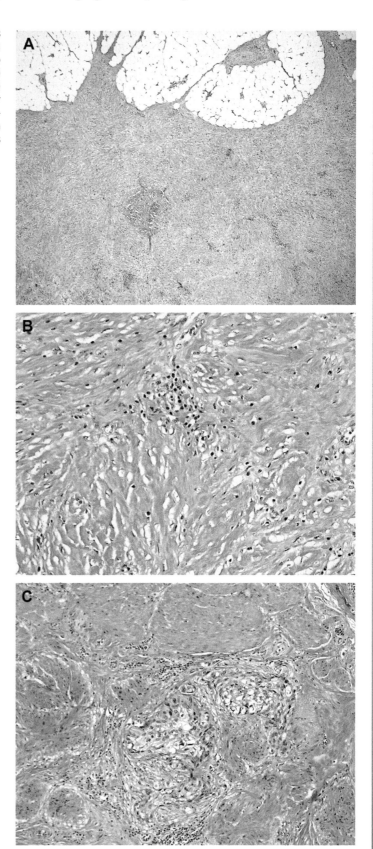

Identification of lymph nodes in the posttherapy setting may be challenging. Furthermore, there may be variability in the extent of lymph node dissection performed and in the subsequent recovery of lymph nodes from the specimen. Lymph node packets should be carefully examined and searched. If upon microscopic evaluation fewer than 3 lymph nodes are identified, an attempt should be made to go back to the specimen and submit the entirely remaining fibroadipose tissue in each packet.

SUMMARY

The staging and reporting of urothelial carcinoma of the urinary tract have undergone major changes in the past decade due to the collaboration between pathologists, urologists, and oncologists. There, however, remain issues that require further clarity, including the substaging of pT1 tumors, grading and reporting of tumors with grade heterogeneity and following NAC, and the role of molecular classification of urothelial carcinoma, to name just a few. Despite these lacunae, substantial progress has been made that has greatly helped in the accurate diagnosis and management of patients with urothelial carcinoma. Multi-institutional collaborative studies with prospective data will further inform the accurate diagnosis, staging, and reporting of these tumors.

DISCLOSURE

Authors have no conflicts of interest to declare that are relevant to the content of this article.

REFERENCES

1. Amin MB, Edge SB, Greene FL, et al. AJCC cancer staging manual. New York, NY: Springer; 2017.
2. Paner GP, Montironi R, Amin MB. Challenges in pathologic staging of bladder cancer: proposals for fresh approaches of assessing pathologic stage in light of recent studies and observations pertaining to bladder histoanatomic variances. Adv Anat Pathol 2017;24:113–27.
3. Paner GP, Stadler WM, Hansel DE, et al. Updates in the 8th edition of the tumor-node-metastasis staging classification for urologic cancers. Eur Urol 2018;73:560–9.
4. Bella AJ, Stitt LW, Chin JL, et al. The prognostic significance of metastatic perivesical lymph nodes identified in radical cystectomy specimens for transitional cell carcinoma off the bladder. J Urol 2003;170: 2253–7.
5. Hu B, Satkunasivam R, Schuckman A, et al. Significance of perivesical lymph node in radical cystectomy for bladder cancer. Urol Oncol 2014;32: 1158–65.
6. von der Maase H, Sengelov L, Robert JT, et al. Long term survival results of a randomized trial comparing gemcitabine plus cisplatin, with methotrexate, vinblastine, doxorubicin, plus cisplatin in patients with bladder cancer. J Clin Oncol 2005;23:4602–8.
7. Apolo AB, Ostrovnaya I, Halabi S, et al. Prognostic model for predicting survival of patients with metastatic urothelial cancer treated with cisplatin-based chemotherapy. J Natl Cancer Inst 2013;105:499–503.
8. Galsky MD, Moshier E, Krege S, et al. Nomogram for predicting survival in patients with unresectable and/or metastatic urothelial cancer who are treated with cisplatin- based chemotherapy. Cancer 2013; 119:3012–9.
9. Babjuk M, Burger M, Comperat EM, et al. European Association of Urology guidelines on nonmuscle invasive bladder cancer (Ta/T1 and carcinoma in situ)- 2019 update. Eur Urol 2019;76:639–57.
10. Klassen Z, Kamat AM, Kassouf W, et al. Treatment strategy for newly diagnosed T1 high grade bladder urothelial carcinoma: new insights and updated recommendations. Eur Urol 2018;74:597–608.
11. Parizi M, Enikeev D, Glybochko PV, et al. Prognostic value of T1 substaging on oncological outcomes in patients with non-muscle-invasive bladder urothelial carcinoma: a systematic literature review and meta-analysis. World J Urol 2020; 38:1437–49.
12. Younes M, Sussman J, True LD. The usefulness of the level of the muscularis mucosae in the staging of invasive transitional cell carcinoma off the urinary bladder. Cancer 1990;66:543–8.
13. Rouperet M, Seisen T, Comperat E, et al. Prognostic interest in discriminating muscularis mucosa invasion (T1a vs T1b) in nonmuscle invasive bladder carcinoma: French national multicenter study with central pathology review. J Urol 2013; 189:2069–76.
14. Fransen van de Putte EE, Behrendt MA, Pigot GLS, et al. Prognostic significance of substage and WHO classification systems in T1 urothelial carcinoma of the bladder. Curr Opin Urol 2015;25:427–35.
15. Leivo MZ, Sahoo D, Hamilton Z, et al. Analysis of T1 bladder cancer on biopsy and transurethral resection specimens: comparison and ranking of T1 quantification approaches to predict progression to muscularis propria invasion. Am J Surg Pathol 2018;42:e1–10.
16. DE Marco V, Cerruto MA, D'Elia C, et al. Prognostic role of sub staging in T1 G 3 transitional cell carcinoma of the urinary bladder. Mol Clin Oncol 2014;2: 575–80.
17. Brimo F, Wu C, Zeizafoun N, et al. Prognostic factors in D1 bladder urothelial carcinoma: the value of recording millimetric depth of invasion, diameter

of invasive carcinoma, and muscularis mucosae invasion. Hum Pathol 2013;44:95–102.

18. Colombo R, Hurle E, Moschini M, et al. Feasibility and clinical roles of different sub staging systems at 1st and 2nd transurethral resection in patients with T1 high-grade bladder cancer. Eur Urol Focus 2018;4(1):87–93.

19. Lee JY, Joo HJ, Cho DS, et al. Prognostic significance of sub staging according to the depth of lamina propria invasion in primary T1 transitional cell carcinoma of the bladder. Korean J Urol 2012;53:317–23.

20. Olsson H, Hultman P, Rosell J, et al. Population based study on prognostic factors for recurrence and progression in primary stage T1 bladder tumors. Scand J Urol 2013;47(3):188–95.

21. Patriarca C, Hurle R, Moschini M, et al. Usefulness of PT1 sub staging in papillary urothelial bladder carcinoma. Diagn Pathol 2016;11:6.

22. Patschan O, Sjodahl G, Chebil G, et al. A molecular pathologic framework for risk stratification of stage T1 urothelial carcinoma. Eur Urol 2015;68(5): 824–32.

23. Paner GP, Ro JY, Wojcik EM, et al. Further characterization of the muscle layers and laminar propria of the urinary bladder by systematic histologic mapping: implications for pathologic staging of invasive urothelial carcinoma. Am J Surg Pathol 2007;31:1420–9.

24. Angulo JZ, Lopez JI, Grignon DJ, et al. Muscularis mucosa differentiates two populations with different prognosis stage T1 bladder cancer. Urology 1995; 45:47–53.

25. Sozen S, Akbal C, Sokmensuer C, et al. Microstaging of pT1 transition cell carcinoma of the bladder. Does it really differentiate two populations with different prognosis? (pT1 subcategory). Urol Int 2002;69:200–6.

26. Cheng L, Jones TD, McCarthy RP, et al. Molecular genetic evidence for a common clonal origin of urinary bladder small cell carcinoma and coexisting urothelial carcinoma. Am J Pathol 2005;166: 1533–9.

27. van Rhijn BWG, van der Kwast TH, Alkhateeb SS, et al. A new and highly prognostic system to discern T1 bladder cancer substage. Eur Urol 2012;61:378–84.

28. Hu Z, Mudaliar K, Quek ML, et al. Measuring the dimension of invasive component in pT1 urothelial carcinoma in transurethral resection specimens can predict time to recurrence. Ann Diagn Pathol 2014;18:49–52.

29. Otto W, van Rhijn BW, Breyer J, et al. Infiltrative lamina propria invasion pattern as an independent predictor for cancer- specific and overall survival of instillation treatment-naive stage T1 high-grade urothelial bladder cancer. Int J Urol 2018;25:442–9.

30. van der Aa MN, van Leenders GJ, Steyerberg EW, et al. A new system for substaging PT1 papillary bladder cancer: prognostic evaluation. Hum Pathol 2005;36:981–6.

31. Bertz S, Denzinger S, Otto W, et al. Substaging by estimating the size of invasive tumor can improve risk stratification in pT1 urothelial bladder cancer evaluation of a large hospital- based single- center series. Histopathology 2011;59:722–32.

32. Chang WC, Chang YH, Pan CC. Prognostic significance in substaging of T1 urinary bladder urothelial carcinoma on transurethral resection. Am J Surg Pathol 2012;36:454–61.

33. Nishiyama N, Kitamura H, Maeda T, et al. Clinical pathological analysis of patients with non- muscle-invasive bladder cancer: prognostic value and clinical reliability of the 2004 WHO classification system. Jpn J Clin Oncol 2013;43:1124–31.

34. Budina A, Farahani SJ, Lal P, et al. Subcategorization of T1 bladder cancer on biopsy and transurethral specimens for predicting progression. Arch Pathol Lab Med 2021. https://doi.org/10.5858/ arpa.2021-0175-OA. Online ahead of print.

35. Lawless M, Gulati R, Tretiakova M. Stalk versus base invasion in pT1 papillary cancers of the bladder: improved substaging system predicting the risk of progression. Histopathology 2017;71: 406–14.

36. Donat SM, Genega EM, Herr HW, et al. Mechanisms of prostatic stromal invasion in patients with bladder cancer: clinical significance. J Urol 2001; 165:1117–20.

37. Esrig D, Freeman JA, Elmajian DA, et al. Transitional cell carcinoma involving the prostate with the proposed staging classification for stromal invasion. J Urol 1996;15:1071–6.

38. Montironi R, Cheng L, Mazzucchelli R, et al. Critical evaluation of the prostate from cystoprostatectomy for bladder cancer: insights from a complete sampling with the whole mount technique. Eur Urol 2009;55:1305–9.

39. Knoedler JJ, Boorjian SA, Tollefson K, et al. Urothelial carcinoma involving the prostate: association of revised tumor stage and coexistent bladder cancer with survival after radical cystectomy. BJU Int 2014; 1114:832–6.

40. Njinou Ngninkeu B, Lorge F, Moulin P, et al. Transitional cell carcinoma involving the prostate: a clinicopathological retrospective study of 76 cases. J Urol 2003;169:149–52.

41. Ayyathurai R, Gomez P, Luongo T, et al. Prostatic involvement by urothelial carcinoma bladder: clinicopathological features and outcome after radical cystectomy. BJU Int 2007;100:1021–5.

42. Vallo S, Gilfrich C, Burger M, et al. Comparative analysis of the effect of prostatic invasion patterns on cancer- specific mortality after radical

cystectomy in pT4 a urothelial carcinoma of the bladder. Urol Oncol 2016;34:432.e1–8.

43. Patel AR, Cohn JA, Abd El Latif A, et al. Validation of new AJCC exclusion criteria for subepithelial prostatic stromal invasion from pT4a bladder urothelial carcinoma. J Urol 2013;189:53–8.

44. Daneshmand S, Stein JP, Lesser T, et al. Prognosis of seminal vesicle involvement by transitional cell carcinoma of the bladder. J Urol 2004;172(1):81–4.

45. Volkmer BG, Kufer R, Maier S, et al. Outcome in patients with seminal vesicle invasion after radical cystectomy. J Urol 2003;169:1299–302.

46. May M, Brookman-May S, Burger M, et al. Concomitant seminal vesicle invasion in pT4a urothelial carcinoma of the bladder with contiguous prostatic infiltration is an adverse prognosticator for cancer-specific survival after radical cystectomy. Ann Surg Oncol 2014;21:4034–40.

47. You D, Kim SC, Jeong IG, et al. Urothelial carcinoma of the bladder with seminal vesicle invasion: prognostic significance. BJU Int 2010;106:1657–61.

48. Chen ME, Pisters LL, Malpica A, et al. Risk of urethral, vaginal and cervical involvement in patients undergoing radical cystectomy for bladder cancer: results of a contemporary cystectomy series from MD Anderson Cancer Center. J Urol 1997;157:2120–3.

49. Salem H, El-Mazny A. Clinicopathologic study of gynecologic organ involvement at radical cystectomy for bladder cancer. Int J Gynecol Obstet 2011;115:188–90.

50. Varkaris IM, Pinggera G, Antoniou N, et al. Pathological review of internal genitalia after anterior exenteration for bladder cancer in women. Evaluating risk factors for female organ involvement. Int Urol Nephrol 2007;39:1015–21.

51. Ali-El-Dein B, Abdel-Latif M, Mosbah A, et al. Secondary malignant involvement of gynecological organs in radical cystectomy specimens in women: is it mandatory to remove these organs routinely? J Urol 2004;172:885–7.

52. Groutz A, Gillon G, Konichezky M, et al. involvement of internal genitalia in female patients undergoing radical cystectomy for bladder cancer: a clinico pathological study of 37 cases. Int J Gynecol Cancer 1999;9:302–6.

53. Ghoneim MA, Abdel-Latif M, el-Mekresh M, et al. Radical cystectomy for carcinoma the bladder: 2,720 consecutive cases five years later. J Urol 2008;180:121–7.

54. Tilki D, Reich O, Svatek RS, et al. Characteristics and outcomes of patients with clinical carcinoma in situ only treated with radical cystectomy: an international study of 243 patients. J Urol 2010;183:1757–63.

55. Aziz A, Shariat SF, Roghmann F, et al. Prediction of cancer- specific survival after radical cystectomy in pT4a urothelial carcinoma of the bladder: development of a tool for clinical decision-making. BJU Int 2016;117:272–9.

56. May M, Bastian PJ, Brookman-May S, et al. Gender specific differences in cancer- specific survival after radical cystectomy for patients with urothelial carcinoma of the urinary bladder in pathologic tumor stage T4a. Urol Oncol 2013;31:1141–7.

57. Magers MJ, Lopez-Beltran A, Montironi R, et al. Staging of bladder cancer. Histopathology 2019;74:112–34.

58. Hansel DE, Paner GP, Nese N, et al. Limited smoothelin expression within the muscularis mucosa: validation in bladder diverticula. Hum Pathol 2011;42:1770–6.

59. Goliajinin D, Yossepowitch O, Beck SD, et al. Carcinoma in a bladder diverticulum: presentation and treatment outcome. J Urol 2003;170:1761–4.

60. Tamas EF, Stephenson AJ, Campbell SC, et al. Histological features and clinical outcomes in 71 cases of bladder diverticula. Arch Pathol Lab Med 2009;133:791–6.

61. Hu B, Satkunasivam R, Schuckman A, et al. Urothelial carcinoma in bladder diverticula: outcomes after radical cystectomy. World J Urol 2015;33:1397–402.

62. Cheng L, Montironi R, Davidson DD, et al. Staging and reporting of urothelial cancers of the urinary bladder. Mod Pathol 2009;22(Suppl.2):70–95.

63. Comperat E, Egevad L, Lopez-Beltran A, et al. An interobserver reproducibility study on invasiveness of bladder cancer using virtual microscopy and heat maps. Histopathology 2013;63:756–66.

64. Beltran AL, Cheng L, Monitroni R, et al. Clinicopathological characteristics and outcome of nested carcinoma of the urinary bladder. Virchows Arch 2014;465:199–205.

65. Volmar KE, Chan TY, DeMarzo AM, et al. Florid von Brunn nests mimicking urothelial carcinoma: a morphologic and immunohistochemical comparison to the nested variant of urothelial carcinoma. Am J Surg Pathol 2003;27:1243–52.

66. Wasco MJ, Diagnault S, Bradley D, et al. Nested variant of urothelial carcinoma: a clinicopathologic and immunohistochemical study of 30 pure and mixed cases. Hum Pathol 2010;41:163–71.

67. Ananthanarayan V, Pan Y, Tretiakova M, et al. Influence of histologic criteria and confounding factors in staging of equivocal cases for microscopic perivesical invasion (pT3a): an interobserver study among genitourinary pathologists. Am J Surg Pathol 2014;38:167–75.

68. Tretter EM, Ebel JJ, Pohar KS, et al. Does the gross prosector impact pT3 subclassification or lymph node counts in bladder cancer? Hum Pathol 2017;61:190–8.

69. Aron M, Park S, Lowenthal BM, et al. Primary female urethral carcinoma proposed staging

modifications based on assessment of female ure-thra Histology and analysis of a large series of female urethral carcinomas. Am J Surg Pathol 2020;44:1591–2.

70. Vashistha V, Shabsigh A, Zynger DL. Utility and diagnostic accuracy of uretroscopic biopsy in upper tract urothelial carcinoma. Arch Pathol Lab Med 2013;137:400–7.

71. El-Hakim A, Weiss GH, Lee BR, et al. Correlation of ureteroscopic appearance with histologic grade of upper tract transitional cell carcinoma. Urology 2004;63:647–50.

72. Katayama S, Mori K, Schuettfort VM, et al. Accuracy and clinical utility offer tumor grade- and stage- based predictive model in localized upper tract urothelial carcinoma. Eur Urol Focus 2021; S2405-4569(21):00154–61. Online ahead of print.

73. van der Poel HG, Antonini N, van Tinteren H, et al. Upper urinary tract cancer: location is correlated with prognosis. Eur Urol 2005;48:438–44.

74. Kikuchi E, Marguilis V, Karakiewicz PI, et al. Lymphovascular invasion predicts clinical outcomes in patients with node- negative upper tract urothelial carcinoma. J Clin Oncol 2009;27:612–8.

75. Raman JD, Ng CK, Scherr DS, et al. Impact of tumor location on prognosis for patients with upper tract urothelial carcinoma managed by radical nephroureterectomy. Eur Urol 2010;57:1072–9.

76. Cho KS, Cho NH, Park SY, et al. Prognostic impact of peripelvic fat invasion in pT3 renal pelvic transitional cell carcinoma. J Korean Med Sci 2008;23:434–8.

77. Park J, Ha SH, Min GE, et al. The protective role of renal parenchyma as a barrier to local tumor spread of upper tract transitional cell carcinoma and its impact on patient survival. J Urol 2009; 182:894–9.

78. Park J, Park S, Song C, et al. Peripelvic/periureteral fat invasion is independently associated with worse prognosis in pT3 upper tract urothelial carcinoma. World J Urol 2014;32:157–63.

79. Wu D, Lee CT, Zynger DL, et al. Reclassifying pT3 renal pelvic urothelial carcinoma with renal parenchyma invasion to pT2 improves correlation with overall survival. Hum Pathol 2022;125:79–86.

80. Cancer protocol templates (Internet). College of American Pathologists. 2022. https://www.cap.org/protocols-and-guidelines/cancer-reporting- tools/cancer-protocol-templates. Accessed September 12, 2022.

81. Comperat E, Srigley JR, Brimo F, et al. Dataset for the reporting of carcinoma of the bladder- cystectomy, cystoprostatectomy and diverticulectomy specimens: recommendations from the International Collaboration on Cancer Reporting (ICCR). Virchows Arch 2020;476:521–34.

82. Varma M, Srigley JR, Brimo F, et al. Data set for the reporting of urinary tract carcinoma- biopsy and transurethral resection specimen: recommendations from the International Collaboration on Cancer Reporting (ICCR). Mod Pathol 2020;33:700–12.

83. Lopez-Beltran A, Luque RJ, Mazzucchelli R, et al. Changes produced in the urothelium by traditional and newer therapeutic procedures for bladder cancer. J Clin Pathol 2002;55:641–7.

84. Chan TY, Epstein JI. Radiation or chemotherapy cystitis with "pseudocarcinomatous" features. Am J Surg Pathol 2004;28:909–13.

85. Lopez JI, Schiavo-Lena M, Corominas-Cishek A, et al. Nephrogenic adenoma of the urinary tract: clinical, histological and immunohistochemical characteristics. Virchows Arch 2013;463:819–25.

86. Pina-Oviedo S, Shen SS, Truong LD, et al. Flat pattern of nephrogenic adenoma: previously unrecognized pattern unveiled using PAX2 and PAX 8 immunohistochemistry. Mod Pathol 2013;26:792–8.

87. Williamson SR, Al-Ahmadie HA, Cheng L, et al. Invasive urothelial carcinoma. In: WHO classification of Tumors editorial Board. Urinary and male genital tumors. 5th edition. Lyon(France): International Agency for Research on Cancer; 2022. p. 157.

88. Meeks JJ, Al-Ahmadie H, Faltas BM, et al. Genomic heterogeneity in bladder cancer: challenges and possible solutions to improve outcomes. Nat Rev Urol 2020;17:259–70.

89. Hansel DE, Amin MB, Comperat E, et al. A contemporary update on pathology standards for bladder cancer: transurethral resection and radical cystectomy specimens. Eur Urol 2013; 623:321–32.

90. Wasco MJ, Daignault S, Zhang Y, et al. Urothelial carcinoma with divergent histologic differentiation (mixed histologic features) predicts the presence of locally advanced bladder cancer when detected at transurethral resection. Urology 2007;70:69–74.

91. Kamoun A, de Reynies A, Allory Y, et al. A consensus molecular classification of muscle-invasive bladder cancer. Eur Urol 2020;77:420–33.

92. Kim SP, Frank I, Cheville JC, et al. The impact of squamous and glandular differentiation and survival after radical cystectomy for urothelial carcinoma. J Urol 2012;188:405–9.

93. Willis DL, Flaig TW, Hansel DE, et al. Micropapillary bladder cancer: current treatment patterns and review of the literature. Urol Oncol 2014;32:826–32.

94. Bertz S, Wach S, Taubert H, et al. Micropapillary morphology is an indicator of poor prognosis in patients with urothelial carcinoma treated with transurethral resection and radiochemotherapy. Virchows Arch 2016;469:339–44.

95. Meeks JJ, Taylor JM, Matsushita K, et al. Pathologic response to neoadjuvant chemotherapy for muscle- invasive micropapillary bladder cancer. BJU Int 2013;111:325–30.

96. Sui W, Matulay JT, James MB, et al. Micropapillary bladder cancer: insights from the National Cancer database. Bladder Cancer 2016;2:415–23.

97. Guo CC, Dhadhania V, Zhang I, et al. Gene expression profile of the clinically aggressive micropapillary variant of bladder cancer. Eur Urol 2016;70:611–20.

98. Kaimaklioitis HZ, Monn MF, Cheng L, et al. Plasmacytoid bladder cancer: variant histology with aggressive behavior and a new mode of invasion along fascial planes. Urology 2014;83:1112–6.

99. Dayyani F, Czerniak BA, Sircar K, et al. Plasmacytoid urothelial carcinoma, a chemosensitive cancer with poor prognosis, and peritoneal carcinomatosis. J Urol 2013;189:1656–61.

100. Comperat E, McKenney JK, Hartmann A, et al. Large nested variant of urothelial carcinoma: a clinicopathological study of 36 cases. Histopathology 2017;71:703–10.

101. Cox R, Epstein JI. Large nested variant: 23 cases mimicking von Brunn nests and inverted growth pattern of non invasive papillary urothelial carcinoma. Am J Surg Pathol 2011;35:1337–42.

102. Linder BJ, Frank I, Cheville JC, et al. Outcomes following radical cystectomy for nested variant of urothelial carcinoma: a matched cohort analysis. J Urol 2013;189:1670–5.

103. Wayerer V, Eckstein M, Comperat E, et al. The large nested variant of urothelial carcinoma (LUNC) is the prototype of an FGFR 3 mutated aggressive urothelial carcinoma with luminal-papillary phenotype. Cancers (Basel) 2020;12:763.

104. Pan CC, Chang YH, Chen KK, et al. Prognostic significance of the 2004 WHO/ISUP classification for prediction of recurrence, progression, and cancer-specific mortality of non-muscle- invasive urothelial tumors of the urinary bladder: a clinical pathologic study of 1515 cases. Am J Clin Pathol 2010;133:788–95.

105. Amin MB, Comperat E, Epstein JI, et al. The Genitourinary Pathology Society update on classification and grading of flat and papillary urothelial neoplasia with new reporting recommendations and approach to lesions with mixed and early patterns of neoplasia. Adv Anat Pathol 2021;28:179–95.

106. Cheng L, Neumann RM, Nehra A, et al. Cancer heterogeneity and its biologic implications in the grading of urothelial carcinoma. Cancer 2000;88:163–70.

107. Gofrit ON, Pizov G, Shapiro A, et al. Mixed high and low grade bladder tumors; are they clinically high or low grade? J Urol 2014;191:1693–6.

108. Comperat E, Varinot J, Moroch J, et al. A practical guide to bladder cancer pathology. Nat Rev Urol 2018;15:143–54.

109. van Rhijn BW, Musquera M, Liu L, et al. Molecular and clinical support for a four tiered grading system for bladder cancer based on the WHO1973 and 2004 classifications. Mod Pathol 2015;28:695–705.

110. Eisenberg MS, Boorjian SA, Cheville JC, et al. The SPARC score: a multifactorial outcome prediction model for patients undergoing radical cystectomy for bladder cancer. J Urol 2013;190:2005–10.

111. von Rundstedt FC, Mata DA, Groshen S, et al. Significance of lymphovascular invasion in organ-confined, node- negative urothelial cancer of the bladder: data from the prospective p53 -MVAC trial. BJU Int 2015;116:44–9.

112. Cha EK, Shariat SF, Kormaksson M, et al. Predicting clinical outcomes after radical nephroureterectomy for upper tract urothelial carcinoma. Eur Urol 2012;61:818–25.

113. Hurel S, Rouperat M, Ouzzane A, et al. Impact of lymphovascular invasion on oncological outcomes in patients with upper tract urothelial carcinoma after radical nephroureterectomy. BJU Int 2013;111:1199–207.

114. Amin MB, Trpkov K, Lopez-Beltran A, et al. Best practices recommendations in the application of immunohistochemistry in bladder lesions: report from the International Society of Urologic Pathology consensus conference. Am J Surg Pathol 2014;38:e20–34.

115. Leissner J, Hohenfaellner R, Thuroff JW, et al. Lymphadenectomy in patients with transitional cell carcinoma of the unary bladder; significance for staging and prognosis. BJU Int 2000;85:817–23.

116. Herr HW, Bochner BH, Dalbangi G, et al. Impact of the number of lymph nodes retrieved on outcome in patients with muscle invasive bladder cancer. J Urol 2002;167:1295–8.

117. Wright JL, Din DW, Porter MP. The association between extended lymphadenectomy and survival among patients with lymph node metastasis undergoing radical cystectomy. Cancer 2008;112:2401–8.

118. Parkash V, Bifulco C, Feinn R, et al. To count and how to count that is the question: interobserver and intraobserver variability among pathologists in lymph node counting. Am J Clin Pathol 2010;134:42–9.

119. Prendeville S, Berney DM, Bubendorf L, et al. Handling and reporting of pelvic lymphadenectomy specimens in prostate and bladder cancer: a web- based survey by the European network of Europe pathology. Histopathology 2019;74:844–52.

120. Kimura S, Mari A, Foerster B, et al. Prognostic value of concomitant carcinoma in situ in the radical cystectomy specimen: systematic review and meta-analysis. J Urol 2019;201:46–53.

121. Laukhtina E, Rajwa P, Mori K, et al. Accuracy of frozen section analysis of urethral and ureteral margins during radical cystectomy for bladder

cancer: a systematic review and diagnostic meta analysis. Eur Urol Focus 2021;S2405-4569(21): 00162-70. https://doi.org/10.1016/j.euf.2021.05. 010.

122. Grossman HB, Natale RB, Tangen CM, et al. Neo-djuvant chemotherapy plus cystectomy compared with cystectomy alone for locally advanced bladder cancer. N Engl J Med 2003;349:859–66.

123. Shariat SF, Krakiewicz PI, Palapattu GS, et al. Out-comes of radical cystectomy for transitional cell carcinoma of the bladder: a contemporary series from the Bladder Cancer Research Consortium. J Urol 2006;176:2414–22.

124. Stein JP, Lieskovsky G, Cote R, et al. Radical cys-tectomy in the treatment of invasive bladder can-cer: long- term results in 1,054 patients. J Clin Oncol 2001;19:666–75.

125. Motterle G, Andrews JR, Morlacco A, et al. Predict-ing response to neoadjuvant chemotherapy in bladder cancer. Eur Urol Focus 2020;6:642–9.

126. Fleischmann A, Thalmann GN, Perren A, et al. Tu-mor regression grade of urothelial bladder cancer after neoadjuvant chemotherapy: a novel and suc-cessful strategy to predict survival. Am J Surg Pathol 2014;38:325–32.

127. Mi H, Bivalacqua TJ, Kates M, et al. Predictive models of response to neoadjuvant chemotherapy in muscle- invasive bladder cancer using nuclear morphology and tissue architecture. Cell Rep Med 2021;2:100382.

128. Pokuri VK, Syed JR, Yang Z, et al. Predictors of complete pathologic response (pT0) to neoadju-vant chemotherapy in muscle- invasive bladder carcinoma. Clin Genitourin Cancer 2016;14: e59–65.

129. Scosyrev E, Ely BW, Messing EM, et al. Do mixed histological features affect survival benefit from neo-adjuvant platinum- based combination chemo-therapy in patients with locally advanced bladder cancer? Secondary analysis of Southwest Oncology Group- Directed Intergroup Study (S8710). BJU Int 2011;108:693–9.

130. Zargar-Shoshtari K, Sverrisson EF, Sharma P, et al. Clinical outcomes after neoadjuvant chemotherapy and radical cystectomy in the presence of urothe-lial cancer of the bladder with squamous or glan-dular differentiation. Clin Genitourin Cancer 2016; 14:82–8.

131. Vetterlein MW, Wankowicz SAM, Seisen T, et al. Neoadjuvant chemotherapy prior to radical cystec-tomy for muscle- invasive bladder cancer with variant histology. Cancer 2017;123:4346–55.

132. Abufaraj M, Foerster B, Schernhammer E, et al. Mi-cropapillary urothelial cancer of the bladder: a sys-tematic review and meta- analysis of disease

characteristics and treatment outcomes. Eur Urol 2019;75:649–58.

133. Diamantopoulos LN, Holt SK, Khaki AR, et al. Response to neoadjuvant chemotherapy and sur-vival in micropapillary urothelial carcinoma: data from tertiary referral center and the surveillance, epidemiology, and end results (SEER) program. Clin Genitourin Cancer 2021;19:144–54.

134. Diamantopoulos LN, Khaki AR, Grivas P, et al. Plas-macytoid urothelial carcinoma: response to chemo-therapy and oncologic outcomes. Bladder Cancer 2020;6:71–81.

135. Lynch SP, Shen Y, Kamat A, et al. Neoadjuvant chemotherapy in small cell urothelial cancer im-proves pathologic downstaging and long- term outcomes: results from a retrospective study at the MD Anderson Cancer Center. Eur Urol 2013; 64:307–13.

136. Teo MY, Guercio BJ, Arora A, et al. Long term out-comes of local and metastatic small cell carcinoma of the urinary bladder and genomic analysis of pa-tients treated with neoadjuvant chemotherapy. Clin Genitourin Cancer 2022;S1558-7673(22):00110-20. https://doi.org/10.1016/j.clgc.2022.05.005. Online ahead of print.

137. Wang HJ, Solanki S, Traboulsi S, et al. Neoadjuvant chemotherapy- related histologic changes in radical cystectomy: assessment accuracy and pre-diction of response. Hum Pathol 2016;53:35–40.

138. Gronostaj K, Czech AK, Fronczek J, et al. The prognostic value of tumor regression grades com-bined with TNM classification in patients with mus-cle- invasive bladder cancer who underwent neoadjuvant chemotherapy followed by radical cystectomy. Clin Genitourin Cancer 2019;17: e1203–11.

139. Voskuilen CS, Oo HZ, Genitsch V, et al. Multicenter validation of histopathologic tumor regression grade after neoadjuvant chemotherapy in muscle-invasive bladder carcinoma. Am J Surg Pathol 2019;43:1600–10.

140. Brant A, Kates M, Chappidi MR, et al. Pathologic response in patients receiving neoadjuvant chemo-therapy for muscle- invasive bladder cancer: Is therapeutic effect owing to chemotherapy or TURBT? Urol Oncol 2017;35:34.e17–25.

141. Hansel DE, Amin MB, Comperat E, et al. Contem-porary update on pathology standards for bladder cancer: transurethral resection and radical cystec-tomy specimens. Eur Urol 2013;63:321–32.

142. Comperat E, Oszwald A, Wasinger G, et al. Up-dated pathology reporting standards for bladder cancer: biopsies, transurethral resection and radical cystectomies. World J Urol 2022;40: 915–27.

Molecular Taxonomy and Immune Checkpoint Therapy in Bladder Cancer

Charles C. Guo, MD*, Bogdan Czerniak, MD, PhD

KEYWORDS

- Bladder cancer • Molecular classification • Luminal subtype • Basal subtype
- Immune checkpoint therapy • Histologic variant

Key points

- Bladder cancers develop through two different oncogenic pathways—papillary/luminal and nonpapillary/basal.
- Bladder cancers are divided into different molecular subtypes based on distinct genomic expression signatures.
- Intrinsic molecular subtypes show different clinicopathologic features and therapeutic responses.
- Genomic alterations underlie the development of bladder cancer histologic subtypes.
- Biomarkers are useful in immune checkpoint therapy for bladder cancer.

ABSTRACT

Bladder cancer is a heterogeneous disease, which exhibits a wide spectrum of clinical and pathologic features. Recent genomic studies have revealed that distinct molecular alterations may underlie the diverse clinical behaviors of bladder cancer, leading to a novel molecular classification. The intrinsic molecular subtypes exhibit distinct gene expression signatures and different clinicopathologic features. Genomic alterations also underlie the development of bladder cancer histologic subtypes. Genomic characterization provides new insights to understanding the biology of bladder cancer and improves the diagnosis and treatment of this complex disease. Biomarkers can aid the selection of patients for immune checkpoint therapy.

OVERVIEW

Bladder cancer is a heterogenous disease, which shows a wide spectrum of pathologic and clinical attributes.[1,2] Approximately 90% of bladder cancers are urothelial carcinoma (UC), which is believed to develop in the urothelium along dual-track oncogenic pathways referred to as papillary and nonpapillary, leading to different but somewhat overlapping subsets of diseases with distinct pathologic manifestations and challenges for clinical management.[2–4] Most of bladder cancers are papillary UC, which is characterized by exophytic growth on the mucosal surface. Papillary UC usually does not invade the bladder wall, but it has a high tendency for recurrence after local treatment, which necessitates lifetime surveillance that is both intrusive and costly to the patient. The remaining bladder cancers are nonpapillary UC which includes invasive UC and UC in situ (UCIS). Nonpapillary UC invades the bladder wall and progresses rapidly, and a large proportion of them are lethal. For clinical management, bladder cancers are also divided into non-muscle invasive and muscle-invasive diseases. Non-muscle invasive bladder cancers (NMIBCs) are treated conservatively with a combination of transurethral resection, intravesical bacillus Calmette–Guérin

Department of Pathology, The University of Texas MD Anderson Cancer Center, 1515 Holcombe Boulevard, Unit 0085, Houston, TX 77030, USA

* Corresponding author.

E-mail address: ccguo@mdanderson.org

Surgical Pathology 15 (2022) 681–694
https://doi.org/10.1016/j.path.2022.07.004
1875-9181/22/© 2022 Elsevier Inc. All rights reserved.

(BCG), and intravesical chemotherapy. Muscle-invasive bladder cancers (MIBCs) are usually treated aggressively with radical cystectomy and/or adjuvant chemotherapy and radiation treatment. Recently immune checkpoint therapy has shown promising therapeutic potential for refractory and metastatic bladder cancers.[5,6]

The pathologic classification of bladder cancer has been traditionally based on morphologic assessment with the aid of immunohistochemistry.[2] Over the last decade, several research groups have performed comprehensive genomic analysis of bladder cancer using a multi-platform approach, which provided a detailed characterization of genetic and epigenetic alterations in this heterogenous disease.[7–10] These breakthroughs have transformed our view of bladder cancer biology, generated new hypotheses for oncogenesis and chemoresistance, and identified new potential therapeutic targets. The identification of intrinsic molecular subtypes in bladder cancers has led to improved accuracy in forecasting the clinical outcome and predicting the patient's response to therapy.[7–10] Although a comprehensive review of all the molecular alternations in bladder cancer is beyond the scope of this review, we focus on the molecular classification of bladder cancers based on the genomic mRNA expressions and its potential impacts on diagnosis, prognosis, and treatment.

DUAL-TRACK CARCINOGENIC PATHWAYS

It is currently believed that bladder cancer arises from successive genomic alterations in a specific cell clone in the urothelium, enabling its eventual escape from the regulatory mechanism for cell division and genomic integrity.[3,4,11,12] The bladder urothelium is composed of three different cell types based on their level of differentiation. The basal cells adjacent to the basement membrane are the least differentiated and express the basal keratins CK5/6 and CK14 but not CK18 and CK20, which are characteristic of more differentiated intermediate cells.[13] The basal cells also express the surface anchoring molecules, such laminin receptor, β4-integrins, and CD44.[13–15] Stem cells or uroprogenitor cells with self-renewal capacity likely reside in the basal layer.[15,16] The intermediate cells between the basal and luminal layers show moderate differentiation and express CK18, CD44, and CK5/6 at reduced levels.[16] The proliferating potential of intermediate cells is limited and similar to the so-called partially committed cells described in other tissues.[17,18] The surface or luminal cells are terminally differentiated umbrella cells that express uroplakins and CK20.[17]

The whole-organ pathologic analyses of cystectomy specimens have provided strong evidences that bladder cancers are likely to develop via two distinct but somewhat overlapping pathways, papillary and nonpapillary (**Fig. 1**).[19] Most bladder cancers are noninvasive papillary UC, which arises from a premalignant lesion, referred to as low-grade intraurothelial neoplasia or urothelial dysplasia.[1,3,4,20] The remaining bladder cancers are invasive UC, which is believed to develop from a flat precursor lesion, referred to as high-grade intraurothelial neoplasia or UCIS. Furthermore, 10% to 15% of noninvasive papillary UC may eventually progress to invasive UC, which is preceded by the development of UCIS in the adjacent urothelial mucosa. The dual-track pathogenetic concept of bladder cancer is supported by molecular studies and animal models.[21–24] Recent genomic analyses have shown that the two tracks start *de novo* from the mucosal field effects, which harbor several thousand gene mutations and alternations in several signal pathways involving immunity, differentiation, and transformation.[11,25] The bladder carcinogenesis spans 10 to 15 years and can be divided into dormant and progressive phases, which are driven by a unique set of gene mutations. The widespread genomic alterations are also present in the otherwise microscopically normal urothelium, suggesting they may present as the initiators of bladder carcinogenesis.[11,25]

MOLECULAR CLASSIFICATION OF NON-MUSCLE INVASIVE BLADDER CANCER

Most of the bladder cancers are NMIBC, which include low- and high-grade noninvasive papillary UC, as well as superficially invasive (pT1) tumors. There have been limited studies on the molecular profile of NMIBCs. Lindgren *and colleagues* proposed the first classification of NIMBC based on the genome-wide gene expression, which showed two distinct molecular subtypes named MS1 and MS2.[26] The MS1 and MS2 subtypes differed significantly in terms of genomic alterations, *FGFR3* and *TP53* mutations. Furthermore, the MS1 subtype was more common in low grade and noninvasive tumors, whereas the MS2 subtypes were associated with high grade and invasive tumors. Subsequently, Sjödahl *and colleagues* proposed that NMIBCs could be divided into four distinct molecular subtypes based on the gene expression signature, including urobasal A (UroA), urobasal B (UroB), genomically unstable (GU), and squamous cell carcinoma-like (SCCL).[27] These intrinsic molecular subtypes

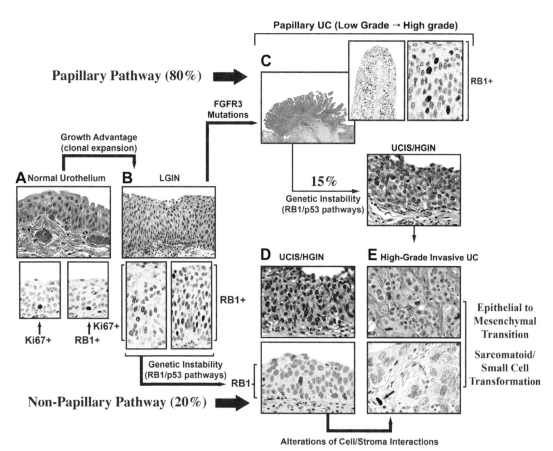

Fig. 1. Dual-track pathways in bladder carcinogenesis. The expansion of a preneoplastic clone, low-grade intra-urothelial neoplasia (LGIN), is the incipient event in bladder carcinogenesis. In the papillary pathway, LGIN progresses to low-grade papillary urothelial carcinoma (LGPUC) with FGFR3 mutations and subsequently to high-grade papillary UC. Approximately 15% of papillary UC may develop invasive UC with mutations in RB1 and p53. In the nonpapillary pathway, LGIN progresses to high-grade intraurothelial neoplasia (HGIN) or urothelial carcinoma in situ (UCIS) with mutations in p53 and RB1, which subsequently develops invasive UC with alterations of cancer cell/stromal interaction. Epithelial to mesenchymal transition may be involved in the development of UC histologic variants, such as sarcomatoid and small cell carcinoma variants. (*Adapted from* Majewski T, et. al. Understanding the development of human bladder cancer by using a whole-organ genomic mapping strategy. Lab Invest. 2008 Jul;88(7):694-721. https://doi.org/10.1038/labinvest.2008.27. Epub 2008 May 5. PMID: 18458673; PMCID: PMC2849658.)

showed distinct molecular signatures as well as significant prognostic differences (**Table 1**). Hedegaard J *et al* also performed a comprehensive transcriptional analysis of 460 NMIBCs, which revealed three distinct molecular classes with basal- and luminal-like characteristics (**Fig. 2**).[28] The three molecular classes demonstrated different clinicopathologic features and showed a close association with the other molecular classifications.[27]

Immunohistochemical (IHC) study of NMIBC has provided strong evidence to support the distinct gene expression patterns in the molecular subtypes.[29] The UroA subtype shows similar features to the normal urothelium, with the expression of KRT5, P-cadherin (P-Cad), and epidermal growth factor receptor (EGFR) confined to the basal cells. In contrast, the SCCL subtype expresses KRT5, P-Cad, EGFR, and CK14 uniformly throughout all the tumor cells (TCs). The GU subtype shows high levels of ERBB2 and E-Cad expression but absence of KRT5, P-Cad, and EGFR expression. UroB tumors show features shared by both UroA and SCCL subtypes. Recently, a three-antibody (GATA3, KRT5, and p16) IHC panel was proposed for the molecular classification of NMIBC.[30] NMIBCs were divided into basal (GATA3-/KRT5+) and luminal (GATA3+/KRT5 variable). The luminal subtype was further divided into urothelial-like (p16 low), URO-KRT5+, and GU (p16 high) subtypes. Although uncommon in NMIBCs, the basal subtype (3%) showed higher cancer

Table 1
Molecular classification of non-muscle invasive bladder cancer by the Lund group

Subtype	Urothelial-like (UroA and UroB)[a]	Genomically Unstable	Basal/Squamous-Like
Marker gene expression	Express FGFR3, CCND1 and cell adhesion proteins	Express FOXM1 and ERBB2, but not KRT5 and cell adhesion proteins	Express KRT5, KRT14, and cell adhesion genes, but not FOXA1 and GATA3
Genetic/genomic alteration	Frequent loss of 9p21 (CDKN2A)	Frequent mutations in *TP53* and *RB1*. Show an increased activity of late G1 phase.	Frequent mutations in *CCNB1*, *Ki-67*, and *EGFR* genes. Show an increased cell proliferation.
Morphology	Low-grade papillary UC	High-grade papillary UC and UCIS	High-grade papillary UC, UCIS, and squamous differentiation
Clinical features	Indolent tumor	Associated with cancer recurrence, progression, and positive cytology	More common in women
Prognosis	Good	Intermediate	Worst

[a] UroB expresses higher level of KRT14, CCNB1, and MKI67 and lower level of CDKN2A than UroA. KRT5-expressing cells are not restricted to the basal and suprabasal cell layers in Uro B.

grade and stage and rapid progression to muscle invasion. URO, the most common subtype (46%), showed rapid recurrence compared with its GU counterpart (29%). URO-KRT5+ tumors (22%) were typically low grade and recurred slowly. Therefore, this three-antibody panel can identify clinically relevant molecular subtypes in NMIBCs and may be useful in optimizing surveillance and treatment strategy.[30]

MOLECULAR CLASSIFICATION OF MUSCLE INVASIVE BLADDER CANCER

A small subset of bladder cancers are MIBC, which invades the muscularis propria or beyond (pT2-pT4). Several research groups have used different strategies to subclassify MIBC into different molecular subtypes based on the genomic analyses of DNA, RNA, and protein. By performing a whole-genome mRNA expression profiling, we found that MIBC could be divided into two distinct intrinsic molecular subtypes: basal and luminal (**Fig. 3**).[8] The molecular markers used in our profiling analysis generally reflected the gene expression signatures of normal basal (such as CK5/6, CK14, and p63) and luminal (such as uroplakins, CK18, CK20, and GATA3) layers. In addition to the distinct signatures of gene expressions, the molecular subtypes also showed different clinicopathologic features. The basal subtype was typically enriched with squamous and sarcomatoid features, and patients

often presented with advanced or metastatic diseases. Although it was intrinsically aggressive, basal UC was highly sensitive to cisplatin-based chemotherapy. Luminal UC was enriched with papillary morphology, *FGFR3* mutations and *ERBB2* amplifications, and their gene expression profiles were controlled by peroxisome proliferator activator receptor γ (PPARγ) pathway. To assess the use of IHC in the molecular classification of MIBC, we evaluated a panel of antibodies based on the genomic expression profiles.[31] Parallel analyses of genomic expression profiles and IHC expression patterns found that a small set of IHC biomarkers, including CK5/6, CK14, CK20, GATA-3, and uroplakin II, could be used to classify bladder cancer into different molecular subtypes. Furthermore, we found that the IHC expression levels of just two signature markers, GATA3 and CK5/6, were sufficient to classify bladder cancers into luminal and basal categories with more than 80% accuracy.[32] Reciprocal positivity and negativity for GATA3 and CK5/6 was a strong discriminatory feature for luminal and basal subtypes. However, luminal tumors might occasionally show a few scattered positive KRT5/6 cells or a linear layer of KRT5/6-positive cells outlining the tumor nests (see **Fig. 3**).

The most comprehensive molecular characterization of MIBCs was conducted under the auspices of The Cancer Genome Atlas (TCGA) and the International Cancer Genome Consortium (ICGC).[9] The analyses included somatic

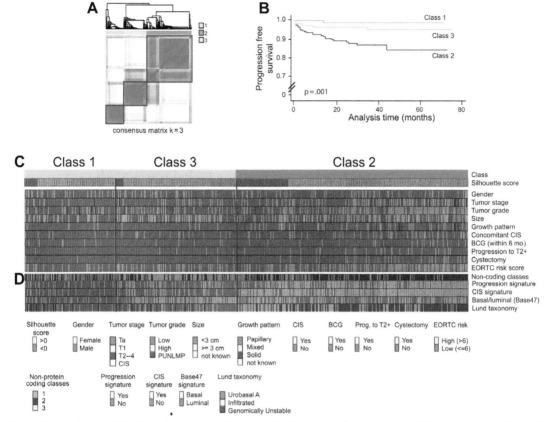

Fig. 2. Molecular classification of non-muscle invasive bladder cancer by genomic mRNA expression analysis. (*A*) Unsupervised consensus clustering matrix heatmap of gene expressions in the three distinct molecular classes. Values range from 0 (no correlation, white) to 1 (perfect correlation, dark blue). (*B*) Kaplan–Meier plot of progression-free survival as a function of the molecular class. (*C*) Different clinicopathologic features in the molecular classes. (*D*) Classification of the tumor samples using other algorithms. (*From* Hedegaard J,et al,. Comprehensive Transcriptional Analysis of Early-Stage Urothelial Carcinoma. Cancer Cell. 2016 Jul 11;30(1):27-42. https://doi.org/10.1016/j.ccell.2016.05.004. Epub 2016 Jun 16. PMID: 27321955.)

mutations, DNA copy number variation, mRNA and microRNA expression, protein and phosphoproteins, and DNA methylation analyses. MIBC showed one of the highest somatic mutation rates in all human cancers, only after lung cancer and melanoma.[9,10] Based on the genomic analysis, the TCGA group divided MIBCs into five distinct molecular subtypes, including luminal-papillary, luminal-infiltrated, luminal, basal-squamous, and neuronal (Table 2).[9] These molecular subtypes showed not only distinct signatures of mRNA expressions but also different clinicopathologic features, which may lead to a novel therapeutic approach to this complex disease.

Several other research groups, including those at the Lund University, University of North Carolina, Baylor College of Medicine, and CIT Consortium, also proposed different molecular classification systems of MIBC.[7–10,33–35] It is evident from these studies that bladder cancer is

a molecularly heterogeneous disease. Although the names and numbers of subtypes are somewhat different in these classification systems, they show striking similarities to the intrinsic basal and luminal subtypes identified in human breast cancers. An international meta-analysis of 1750 MIBC transcriptomic profiles from 18 published datasets proposed a consensus classification with six distinct molecular subtypes: luminal papillary (24%), luminal nonspecified (8%), luminal unstable (15%), stroma-rich (15%), basal/squamous (35%), and neuroendocrine-like (3%) (Fig. 4).[36] There is a general consensus that the top-level separation occurs at the basal and luminal differentiation checkpoint.[36] The luminal UC appears to evolve through the papillary track, whereas the basal UC develops via the nonpapillary track (see Fig 1).[3,4,12] The superficial papillary tumors are almost exclusively luminal, whereas the invasive bladder cancers are equally divided into

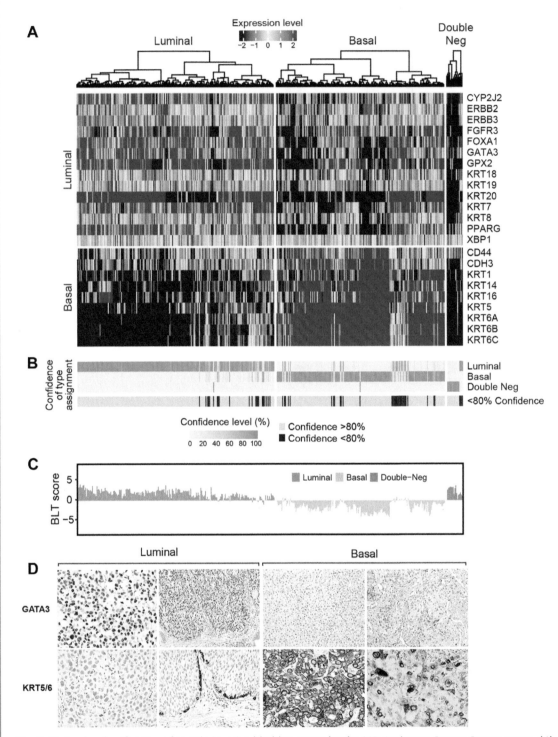

Fig. 3. Molecular classification of muscle-invasive bladder cancer by the MD Anderson Cancer Center group. (*A*) Hierarchical clustering with luminal and basal markers. (*B*) Prediction strengths of molecular subtypes. (*C*) Basal to luminal transition (BLT) scores in molecular subtypes of bladder cancer. (*D*) Examples of immunohistochemical expression patterns of signature luminal (GATA3) and basal (KRT5/6) markers. (*From* Guo, C.C., Bondaruk, J., Yao, H. et al. Assessment of Luminal and Basal Phenotypes in Bladder Cancer. Sci Rep 10, 9743 (2020). https://doi.org/10.1038/s41598-020-66747-7, http://creativecommons.org/licenses/by/4.0/.)

Table 2
The molecular classification of MIBC by the TCGA group

Subtype	Luminal Papillary	Luminal Non-specified	Luminal Infiltrated	Basal/Squamous	Neuroendocrine-Like
Frequency	35%	6%	19%	35%	5%
Clinical features	Present at lower stage and affects younger patients (<60 y)	Affects older patients (>80 y)	Present at lower stage	Present at higher stage. More common in women	Present at higher stage. Most aggressive
Therapy	Respond poorly to cisplatin-based chemotherapy. May be sensitive to FGFR3 inhibitors	Respond poorly to cisplatin-based chemotherapy	Respond poorly to cisplatin-based chemotherapy, but may be sensitive to immune checkpoint therapy and radiation therapy	Respond well to cisplatin-based chemotherapy. May be sensitive to immune checkpoint therapy and EGFR-targeted therapy	Respond well to etoposide/cisplatin-based chemotherapy like lung small cell carcinoma. May respond to radiation therapy
Medium Survival	4 y	1.8 y	2.9 y	1.2 y	1 y
Histology	Papillary	May be associated with micropapillary variant	Strong stromal reaction with a proliferation of lymphocytes, smooth muscle and myofibroblasts	Associated with squamous differentiation. Enriched with CD8 T cells and NK cells.	May show small cell carcinoma or high-grade neuroendocrine carcinoma features, but not always present. Numerous mitoses
Marker gene expression	Express high levels of luminal markers (GATA3, FOXA1, and PPARG)	Express high levels of luminal markers	Express high levels of luminal markers, immune checkpoint markers (PD-L1, PD-1, and CTLA-4)	Express high levels of basal markers (CD44, KRT5, KRT6, KRT14), immune checkpoint markers, squamous differentiation markers (TGM1, DSC3, PI3), and EGFR	Express high levels of both neuroendocrine and neuronal genes by mRNA-seq or IHC
Gene mutations	Mutations in *FGFR3* and *KDM6A* genes	Mutations in *ELF3* and *PPARG*	The highest number of gene mutations	Mutations in *EGFR*	Mutations in *TP53* and *RB1*

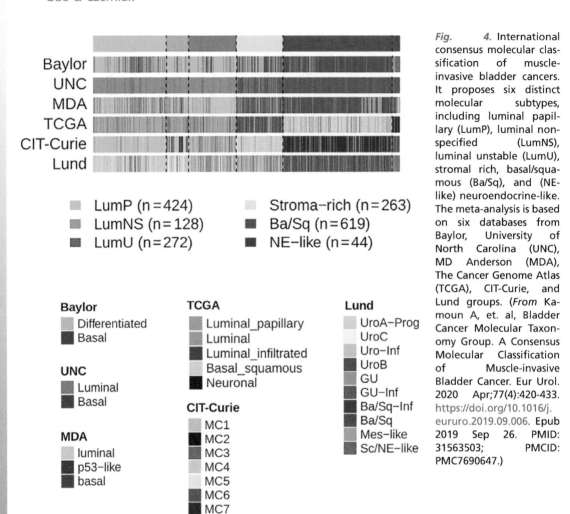

Baylor
- Differentiated
- Basal

UNC
- Luminal
- Basal

MDA
- luminal
- p53–like
- basal

TCGA
- Luminal_papillary
- Luminal
- Luminal_infiltrated
- Basal_squamous
- Neuronal

CIT-Curie
- MC1
- MC2
- MC3
- MC4
- MC5
- MC6
- MC7

Lund
- UroA–Prog
- UroC
- Uro–Inf
- UroB
- GU
- GU–Inf
- Ba/Sq–Inf
- Ba/Sq
- Mes–like
- Sc/NE–like

Legend:
- LumP (n=424)
- LumNS (n=128)
- LumU (n=272)
- Stroma–rich (n=263)
- Ba/Sq (n=619)
- NE–like (n=44)

Fig. 4. International consensus molecular classification of muscle-invasive bladder cancers. It proposes six distinct molecular subtypes, including luminal papillary (LumP), luminal non-specified (LumNS), luminal unstable (LumU), stromal rich, basal/squamous (Ba/Sq), and (NE-like) neuroendocrine-like. The meta-analysis is based on six databases from Baylor, University of North Carolina (UNC), MD Anderson (MDA), The Cancer Genome Atlas (TCGA), CIT-Curie, and Lund groups. (*From* Kamoun A, et. al, Bladder Cancer Molecular Taxonomy Group. A Consensus Molecular Classification of Muscle-invasive Bladder Cancer. Eur Urol. 2020 Apr;77(4):420-433. https://doi.org/10.1016/j.eururo.2019.09.006. Epub 2019 Sep 26. PMID: 31563503; PMCID: PMC7690647.)

luminal and basal types. The invasive tumors that show luminal expression signatures likely evolve from the preexisting papillary disease and represent a progression of superficial papillary tumors (see **Fig. 1**).

MOLECULAR CLASSIFICATION OF BLADDER CANCER HISTOLOGIC SUBTYPES

Bladder UC, particularly invasive UC, shows a high tendency for divergent differentiation, leading to several distinct histologic subtypes.[2] Several histologic subtypes, such as sarcomatoid, small-cell carcinoma (SCC), micropapillary, and plasmacytoid, show highly aggressive clinical behavior that may require a different treatment strategy from that for conventional UC. It has been hypothesized that enrichment of gene mutations and activation of distinct molecular pathways may underlie the aggressive behavior of UC subtypes.[3,37–40]

Micropapillary UC is characterized by small morula-like tumor nests surrounded by empty spaces. It has a high propensity for metastasis to regional lymph nodes and distant organs. Our genomic expression analysis revealed that the micropapillary subtype showed differential expressions in a large number of genes when compared with conventional UC.[38] The expression profile was characterized by dysregulation of multiple oncogenic pathways converging on transformation, cell cycle regulation, DNA damage repair, and signal transduction. Interestingly, the micropapillary expression signature was also present in conventional UC with no apparent micropapillary features, suggesting that the micropapillary subtype arises from a unique subset of conventional UC. Micropapillary UCs were almost exclusively of luminal type. It also showed significant downregulation of miR-296 and activation of chromatin-remodeling complex RUVBL1.

Plasmacytoid subtype is characterized by discohesive malignant cells with eccentric nuclei in a loose stroma with minimal stromal reaction.

Plasmacytoid UC typically displays a diffuse growth pattern with a high tendency for peritoneal spread, leading to the positive margin at cystectomy. Recent analysis by next-generation sequencing identified the presence of *CDH1* truncating mutations, and less frequently *CDH1* promoter hypermethylation, as the defining molecular signature of the plasmacytoid subtype.[41] The *CDH1* alterations resulted in loss of E-cadherin protein expression, and negative IHC staining represented a good surrogate marker for this subtype of bladder cancer. The patterns of other altered genes were similar in the plasmacytoid subtype and co-existent conventional UC, suggesting that both histologic subtypes may evolve from a common cell of origin.[40]

SCC is a rare neuroendocrine subtype of bladder cancer, which is associated with a particularly dismal prognosis. It frequently coexists with conventional UC, suggesting a progression of the preexisting tumor to a poorly differentiated small cell malignancy.[42] Our recent comprehensive genomic analysis showed that SCC was characterized by a double-negative molecular subtype with downregulation of both luminal and basal markers.[39] SCCs displayed a lineage plasticity driven by urothelial-to-neural phenotypic switch with dysregulated epithelial-to-mesenchymal transition (EMT) network. SCCs were depleted of immune cells, and expressed high levels of the immune checkpoint receptor, adenosine receptor A2A (ADORA2A), which is a potent inhibitor of immune infiltration.

Sarcomatoid subtype displays a biphasic tumor with epithelial and mesenchymal components. It shows a high propensity for metastasis and is associated with short survival. We also analyzed the genomic expression of sarcomatoid UC and found that it was related to the basal molecular subtype (Fig. 5).[37] Sarcomatoid UC was characterized by downregulation of homotypic adherence genes and dysregulation of the EMT network. Our quantitative assessment of EMT showed that basal and double-negative SARCs had intermediate and low EMT scores, respectively, which reflected their partial and complete EMT states, and the purely mesenchymal, or double-negative, SARC was the most aggressive variant of the disease.

IMMUNE CHECKPOINT THERAPY IN BLADDER CANCER

Over the past decade, immune-checkpoint therapy has changed the therapeutic landscape of bladder cancer.[5,6,43–46] Immune checkpoint therapy induces an antitumor response by reinvigorating the function of T cells, which is regulated by a complex interplay of immune checkpoint points, such as programmed death-1 (PD-1), its ligand (PD-L1), and cytotoxic T lymphocyte-associated protein (CTLA-4) (Fig. 6). Immune checkpoint inhibitors (ICIs) block the inhibitory effect of immune checkpoints and promote the activation and proliferation of T cells, which reinforce the cytotoxic effect on cancer cells.

ICIs have achieved profound and durable responses in a subset of patients with metastatic bladder cancer as well as localized disease.[5,6,44,45,47–50] Intravesical treatment with BCG has been used in the management of NMIBC for decades. However, up to 40% of patients with NMIBC will recur after BCG immunotherapy. Recently the US Food and Drug Administration (FDA) has approved the use of pembrolizumab in patients with high-risk, BCG-unresponsive NMIBC who are ineligible for cystectomy.[5] In metastatic bladder cancer, platinum-based chemotherapy (PBC) with cisplatin is preferred as the first-line standard of treatment. In patients who are ineligible for PBC, pembrolizumab and atezolizumab have shown a promising response as the first-line treatment, which resulted in an accelerated approval by the FDA.[51,52] Although ICIs induce dramatic, sometimes durable, responses in bladder cancers, they are however not universally effective in all patients, supporting the need for predictive biomarkers.

Several biomarkers have been used to select patients for ICI treatment in bladder cancer.[44,53] PD-L1 has been the most widely used biomarker in immune checkpoint therapy. Different PD-L1 assays have been used in clinical trials, such as the 28 to 8 pharmDx (Nivolumab), the 22C3 pharmDx (Pembrolizumab), Ventana SP142 (Atezolizumab), and Ventana PD-L1 SP263 (Durvalumab), but there are questions about their interchangeability and comparability and diagnostic use.[45,53] The expression of PD-L1 expression on immune cells (IC), but not TCs, is associated with a response to anti-PD-1/L1 ICI in a subset of patients.[6] The combined positive score (CPS), defined as the percentage of TCs and infiltrating immune cells with positive PD-L1 expression over the total number of TCs, provides greater positive and negative predictive value than TC evaluation alone.[45] Currently, the first-line treatment with Atezolizumab and Pembrolizumab in platinum-ineligible patients requires IHC PD-L1 testing. In the second-line setting, all drugs are approved without PD-L1 testing.[44,45]

The molecular classification of bladder UC has recently been assessed in several trials as a

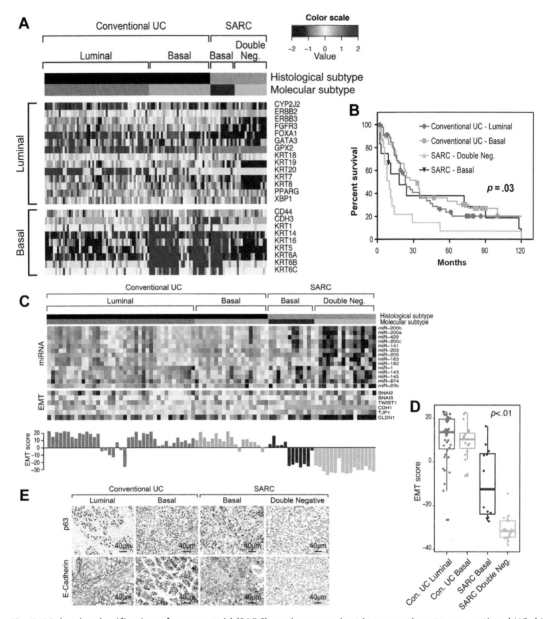

Fig. 5. Molecular classification of sarcomatoid (SARC) carcinoma variant in comparison to conventional UC. (*A*) The expression of luminal and basal markers in molecular subtypes. (*B*) Kaplan–Meier analysis of molecular subtypes and log-rank testing. (*C*) Expression patterns of epithelial-mesenchymal transition (EMT) genes with EMT scores. (*D*) Boxplot of EMT scores in different molecular subtypes. (*E*) Examples of immunohistochemical expression of E-cadherin (epithelial) and p63 (basal) in different molecular subtypes (from *CC*. (*From* Guo CC, et. al,. Dysregulation of EMT Drives the Progression to Clinically Aggressive Sarcomatoid Bladder Cancer. Cell Rep. 2019   May   7;27(6):1781-1793.e4.   https://doi.org/10.1016/j.celrep.2019.04.048.   PMID: 31067463;   PMCID: PMC6546434.)

predictor of the response to ICI therapy.[9,36] In comparison to the luminal subtype, the basal subtype showed a higher level of PD-L1 expression in TCs (39% vs 4%) as well as enrichment of PD-L1-positive immune cells (60% vs 23%), indicating a favorable response to ICI therapy.[9,10] We evaluated

the expressions of immune checkpoint genes in sarcomatoid UC in comparison to conventional UC (see **Fig. 6**).[37] Our analysis revealed that sarcomatoid UC had an infiltrated immune phenotype with upregulation of PD-L1, suggesting that immune checkpoint therapy may be an attractive therapeutic option in

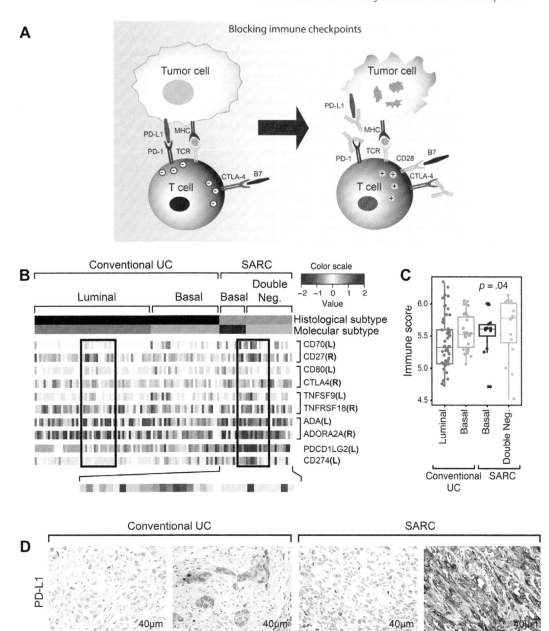

Fig. 6. Immune checkpoint therapy in bladder cancer. (*A*) CTLA4 and PD-1 bind to B7 and PD-L1, respectively, leading to the inhibition of T cells. Immune checkpoint inhibitors targeting CTLA4 (ipilimumab), PD-1 (pembrolizumab and nivolumab), or PD-L1 (atorolimumab) block the inhibitory effect and reactivate T cells. (*B*) Expression of immune checkpoint genes in conventional and sarcomatoid (SARC) urothelial carcinoma. The black boxes indicate the cases with enrichment for the immune profile. (*C*) Boxplot of immune scores calculated using the gene expression profile. (*D*) Examples of immunohistochemical expression of PD-L1. (*From* Sweis RF, Luke JJ. Mechanistic and pharmacologic insights on immune checkpoint inhibitors. Pharmacol Res. 2017 Jun;120:1-9. https://doi.org/10.1016/j.phrs.2017.03.012. Epub 2017 Mar 18. PMID: 28323141; PMCID: PMC5419683; and Guo CC, et. al,. Dysregulation of EMT Drives the Progression to Clinically Aggressive Sarcomatoid Bladder Cancer. Cell Rep. 2019 May 7;27(6):1781-1793.e4. https://doi.org/10.1016/j.celrep.2019.04.048. PMID: 31067463; PMCID: PMC6546434.)

this aggressive subtype.[37] Tumor mutation burden (TMB) may also be associated with a durable response to ICI in multiple cancer types, including bladder cancer.[52,54] Microsatellite instability (MSI) has been associated with a high sensitivity to ICI, regardless of the histologic type and organ of origin. Pembrolizumab has been approved by the FDA for the first tissue/site agnostic ICI therapy, and it may be used as the first-line treatment in cisplatin-ineligible patients.[55,56,57]

SUMMARY

Bladder cancer is a heterogenous disease that is likely to arise from the uroprogenitor cells through papillary/luminal and nonpapillary/basal tracks. Recent comprehensive genomic analyses of bladder cancers have revealed distinct molecular subtypes that recapitulate the differentiation patterns of the normal urothelium. Molecular diversity underlies a wide spectrum of clinical behaviors of bladder cancer and their different responses to conventional and targeted therapies. Bladder cancer histologic subtypes show distinct gene expression signatures, which may underlie their aggressive behaviors. Immune checkpoint therapy has become an effective treatment in a selective subset of bladder cancers, necessitating the predictive biomarker test. The new molecular paradigm of bladder cancer has improved our understanding of this heterogenous disease and expanded the diagnostic and therapeutic options.

CLINICS CARE POINTS

- Bladder cancer is a heterogenous disease with diverse clinicopathologic features.

- Distinct molecular subtypes show different clinical behaviors and differential responses to targeted therapy.

- Genomic alterations may aid the diagnosis and treatment of bladder cancer histologic subtypes.

- Biomarkers may be useful in the selection of patients for immune checkpoint therapy.

DISCLOSURE

The authors have nothing to disclose.

FUNDING STATEMENT

The study was supported in part by the NIH/NCI under award number P30 CA016672.

REFERENCES

1. Kamat AM, Hahn NM, Efstathiou JA, et al. Bladder cancer. Lancet 2016;388(10061):2796–810.
2. Grignon DJAAH, Algaba F, Amin MB, et al. Tumors of the urinary tract. 4 ed. Lyon, France: IARC Press; 2016.
3. Guo CC, Czerniak B. Bladder cancer in the genomic era. Arch Pathol Lab Med 2019;143(6):695–704.
4. Spiess PE, Czerniak B. Dual-track pathway of bladder carcinogenesis: practical implications. Arch Pathol Lab Med 2006;130(6):844–52.
5. Balar AV, Kamat AM, Kulkarni GS, et al. Pembrolizumab monotherapy for the treatment of high-risk non-muscle-invasive bladder cancer unresponsive to BCG (KEYNOTE-057): an open-label, single-arm, multicentre, phase 2 study. Lancet Oncol 2021; 22(7):919–30.
6. Sharma P, Retz M, Siefker-Radtke A, et al. Nivolumab in metastatic urothelial carcinoma after platinum therapy (CheckMate 275): a multicentre, single-arm, phase 2 trial. Lancet Oncol 2017;18(3): 312–22.
7. Damrauer JS, Hoadley KA, Chism DD, et al. Intrinsic subtypes of high-grade bladder cancer reflect the hallmarks of breast cancer biology. Proc Natl Acad Sci U S A 2014;111(8):3110–5.
8. Choi W, Porten S, Kim S, et al. Identification of distinct basal and luminal subtypes of muscle-invasive bladder cancer with different sensitivities to frontline chemotherapy. Cancer Cell 2014;25(2): 152–65.
9. Robertson AG, Kim J, Al-Ahmadie H, et al. Comprehensive molecular characterization of muscle-invasive bladder cancer. . Cell. 2017;171(3):540–556 e525.
10. Cancer Genome Atlas Research N. Comprehensive molecular characterization of urothelial bladder carcinoma. Nature 2014;507(7492): 315–22.
11. Majewski T, Yao H, Bondaruk J, et al. Whole-organ genomic characterization of mucosal field effects initiating bladder carcinogenesis. Cell reports. 2019;26(8):2241–56.e2244.
12. Czerniak B, Dinney C, McConkey D. Origins of bladder cancer. Annu Rev Pathol 2016;11:149–74.
13. Kurzrock EA, Lieu DK, Degraffenried LA, et al. Label-retaining cells of the bladder: candidate urothelial stem cells. Am J Physiol Renal Physiol 2008; 294(6):F1415–21.
14. He X, Marchionni L, Hansel DE, et al. Differentiation of a highly tumorigenic basal cell compartment in urothelial carcinoma. Stem Cells (Dayton, Ohio) 2009; 27(7):1487–95.
15. Chan KS, Espinosa I, Chao M, et al. Identification, molecular characterization, clinical prognosis, and therapeutic targeting of human bladder tumor-initiating cells. Proc Natl Acad Sci U S A 2009; 106(33):14016–21.
16. Brandt WD, Matsui W, Rosenberg JE, et al. Urothelial carcinoma: stem cells on the edge. Cancer Metastasis Rev 2009;28(3-4):291–304.
17. Farsund T. Cell kinetics of mouse urinary bladder epithelium. II. Changes in proliferation and nuclear DNA content during necrosis regeneration, and hyperplasia caused by a single dose of

cyclophosphamide. Virchows Arch B Cell Pathol 1976;21(4):279–98.

18. Reya T, Morrison SJ, Clarke MF, et al. Stem cells, cancer, and cancer stem cells. Nature 2001; 414(6859):105–11.

19. Koss LG, Tiamson EM, Robbins MA. Mapping cancerous and precancerous bladder changes. A study of the urothelium in ten surgically removed bladders. JAMA 1974;227(3):281–6.

20. Czerniak BHF. Molecular biology of common genito-urinary tumors. In: LG K, editor. Diagnostic cytology of the urinary tract with histopathologic and clinical correlation. Philadelphia, PA: Lippincott-Raven; 1995. p. 345–64.

21. Zhang ZT, Pak J, Huang HY, et al. Role of Ha-ras activation in superficial papillary pathway of urothelial tumor formation. Oncogene 2001;20(16): 1973–80.

22. Mo L, Zheng X, Huang HY, et al. Hyperactivation of Ha-ras oncogene, but not Ink4a/Arf deficiency, triggers bladder tumorigenesis. J Clin Invest 2007; 117(2):314–25.

23. Zhang ZT, Pak J, Shapiro E, et al. Urothelium-specific expression of an oncogene in transgenic mice induced the formation of carcinoma in situ and invasive transitional cell carcinoma. Cancer Res 1999; 59(14):3512–7.

24. Cheng J, Huang H, Pak J, et al. Allelic loss of p53 gene is associated with genesis and maintenance, but not invasion, of mouse carcinoma in situ of the bladder. Cancer Res 2003;63(1):179–85.

25. Bondaruk J, Jaksik R, Wang Z, et al. The Origin of Bladder Cancer from Mucosal Field Effects. bioRxiv 2021, 2021.2005.2012.443785.

26. Lindgren D, Frigyesi A, Gudjonsson S, et al. Combined gene expression and genomic profiling define two intrinsic molecular subtypes of urothelial carcinoma and gene signatures for molecular grading and outcome. Cancer research 2010;70(9):3463–72.

27. Sjodahl G, Lauss M, Lovgren K, et al. A molecular taxonomy for urothelial carcinoma. Clin Cancer Res 2012;18(12):3377–86.

28. Hedegaard J, Lamy P, Nordentoft I, et al. Comprehensive transcriptional analysis of early-stage urothelial carcinoma. Cancer Cell 2016;30(1):27–42.

29. Sjodahl G, Lovgren K, Lauss M, et al. Toward a molecular pathologic classification of urothelial carcinoma. Am J Pathol 2013;183(3):681–91.

30. Jackson CL, Chen L, Hardy CS, et al. Diagnostic and prognostic implications of a three-antibody molecular subtyping algorithm for non-muscle invasive bladder cancer. J Pathol Clin Res 2021.

31. Dadhania V, Zhang M, Zhang L, et al. Meta-analysis of the luminal and basal subtypes of bladder cancer and the identification of signature immunohistochemical markers for clinical use. EBioMedicine 2016;12:105–17.

32. Guo CC, Bondaruk J, Yao H, et al. Assessment of luminal and basal phenotypes in bladder cancer. Sci Rep 2020;10(1):9743.

33. Rebouissou S, Bernard-Pierrot I, de Reyniès A, et al. EGFR as a potential therapeutic target for a subset of muscle-invasive bladder cancers presenting a basal-like phenotype. Sci Transl Med 2014;6(244): 244ra291.

34. Eriksson P, Rovira C, Liedberg F, et al. A validation and extended description of the Lund taxonomy for urothelial carcinoma using the TCGA cohort. Scientific Reports 2018;8(1):1–12.

35. Mo Q, Nikolos F, Chen F, et al. Prognostic power of a tumor differentiation gene signature for bladder urothelial carcinomas. J Natl Cancer Inst 2018;110(5): 448–59.

36. Kamoun A, de Reyniès A, Allory Y, et al. A consensus molecular classification of muscle-invasive bladder cancer. Eur Urol 2020;77(4):420–33.

37. Guo CC, Majewski T, Zhang L, et al. Dysregulation of EMT drives the progression to clinically aggressive sarcomatoid bladder cancer. Cell reports 2019; 27(6):1781–93.e1784.

38. Guo CC, Dadhania V, Zhang L, et al. Gene expression profile of the clinically aggressive micropapillary variant of bladder cancer. Eur Urol 2016;70(4): 611–20.

39. Yang G, Bondaruk J, Cogdell D, et al. Urothelial-to-neural plasticity drives progression to small cell bladder cancer. iScience 2020;23(6):101201.

40. Al-Ahmadie HA, Iyer G, Lee BH, et al. Frequent somatic CDH1 loss-of-function mutations in plasmacytoid variant bladder cancer. Nat Genet 2016;48(4): 356–8.

41. Fox MD, Xiao L, Zhang M, et al. Plasmacytoid urothelial carcinoma of the urinary bladder: a clinicopathologic and immunohistochemical analysis of 49 cases. Am J Clin Pathol 2017;147(5): 500–6.

42. Chang MT, Penson A, Desai NB, et al. Small-cell carcinomas of the bladder and lung are characterized by a convergent but distinct pathogenesis. Clin Cancer Res 2018;24(8):1965–73.

43. Ribas A, Wolchok JD. Cancer immunotherapy using checkpoint blockade. Science 2018;359(6382): 1350–5.

44. Lopez-Beltran A, Cimadamore A, Blanca A, et al. Immune checkpoint inhibitors for the treatment of bladder cancer. Cancers (Basel) 2021;13(1).

45. Schulz GB, Todorova R, Braunschweig T, et al. PD-L1 expression in bladder cancer: which scoring algorithm in what tissue? Urologic oncology 2021; 39(10), 734.e731-734.e710.

46. Sharma P, Allison JP. Immune checkpoint targeting in cancer therapy: toward combination strategies with curative potential. Cell 2015;161(2): 205–14.

47. Rijnders M, de Wit R, Boormans JL, et al. Systematic review of immune checkpoint inhibition in urological cancers. Eur Urol 2017;72(3):411–23.

48. Tang C, Ma J, Liu X, Liu Z. Identification of four immune subtypes in bladder cancer based on immune gene sets. Front Oncol 2020;10:544610.

49. Seiler R, Gibb EA, Wang NQ, et al. Divergent biological response to neoadjuvant chemotherapy in muscle-invasive bladder cancer. Clin Cancer Res 2018.

50. De Simone M, Arrigoni A, Rossetti G, et al. Transcriptional landscape of human tissue lymphocytes unveils uniqueness of tumor-infiltrating T regulatory cells. Immunity 2016;45(5):1135–47.

51. Balar AV, Castellano D, O'Donnell PH, et al. First-line pembrolizumab in cisplatin-ineligible patients with locally advanced and unresectable or metastatic urothelial cancer (KEYNOTE-052): a multicentre, single-arm, phase 2 study. Lancet Oncol 2017;18(11):1483–92.

52. Balar AV, Galsky MD, Rosenberg JE, et al. Atezolizumab as first-line treatment in cisplatin-ineligible patients with locally advanced and metastatic urothelial carcinoma: a single-arm, multicentre, phase 2 trial. Lancet 2017;389(10064):67–76.

53. Eckstein M, Cimadamore A, Hartmann A, et al. PD-L1 assessment in urothelial carcinoma: a practical approach. Ann Transl Med 2019;7(22):690.

54. Samstein RM, Lee CH, Shoushtari AN, et al. Tumor mutational load predicts survival after immunotherapy across multiple cancer types. Nat Genet 2019;51(2):202–6.

55. Lemery S, Keegan P, Pazdur R. First FDA approval agnostic of cancer site - when a biomarker defines the indication. N Engl J Med 2017;377(15):1409–12.

56. Majewski T, Lee S, Jeong J, et al. Understanding the development of human bladder cancer by using a whole-organ genomic mapping strategy. Lab Invest 2008;88(7):694–721.

57. Sweis RF, Luke JJ. Mechanistic and pharmacologic insights on immune checkpoint inhibitors. Pharmacol Res 2017;120:1–9.

FURTHER READINGS

Robertson A G, et al. Comprehensive Molecular Characterization of Muscle-Invasive Bladder Cancer. Cell 2017;171(3):540–56.

Eckstein M, et al. Hartmann A, et al. PD-L1 assessment in urothelial carcinoma: a practical approach. Ann Transl Med. 2019;7(22):690. 2019;7(22):690. https://doi.org/10.21037/atm.2019.10.24.

Kamoun A, et al. A Consensus Molecular Classification of Muscle-invasive Bladder Cancer 2020;77(4):420-433. Eur Urol 2020;77(4):420–33.

Bondaruk J, et al. The origin of bladder cancer from mucosal field effects. iSceince 2022;25(7):104551. https://doi.org/10.1016/j.isci.2022.104551.

Lindskrog SV, et al. An integrated multi-omics analysis identifies prognostic molecular subtypes of non-muscle-invasive bladder cancer. Nat Commun. 2021;12(1):2301. https://doi.org/10.1038/s41467-021-22465-w.

How New Developments Impact Diagnosis in Existing Renal Neoplasms

Mahmut Akgul, MD[a], Sean R. Williamson, MD[b],*

KEYWORDS

- Renal cell carcinoma • Clear cell renal cell carcinoma • Chromophobe renal cell carcinoma
- Oncocytoma • Papillary renal cell carcinoma

Key points

- Clear cell RCC is known for alterations of *VHL* and chromosome 3p25 loss; however, *BAP1*, *PBRM1*, and *SETD2* are genes more recently recognized as having key roles in this tumor type.

- Oncocytic renal neoplasm of low malignant potential, not further classified, has been proposed as a category for tumors in the gray zone borderline between oncocytoma and chromophobe RCC.

- The release of the 2022 World Health Organization classification of urologic relabels clear cell papillary RCC as clear cell papillary renal cell tumor, considering its highly favorable behavior.

- Papillary RCC type 1 seems to be a very consistent distinct entity; however, distinguishing type 1 versus 2 tumors is no longer favored because type 2 is now thought to contain a mixture of several diagnostic entities.

- Infiltrative high-grade renal tumors include urothelial carcinoma, SMARCB1-deficient medullary carcinoma, fumarate hydratase-deficient carcinoma, and metastases from other cancers. Collecting duct carcinoma is a diagnosis of exclusion for primary renal cell carcinoma, after which these have been excluded.

ABSTRACT

In recent years, several emerging diagnostic entities have been described in renal cell carcinoma (RCC). However, our understanding of well-known and established entities has also grown. Clear cell papillary RCC is now relabeled as a tumor rather than carcinoma in view of its nonaggressive behavior. Renal tumors with a predominantly infiltrative pattern are very important for recognition, as most of these have aggressive behavior, including fumarate hydratase-deficient RCC, SMARCB1-deficient medullary carcinoma, collecting duct carcinoma, urothelial carcinoma, and metastases from other cancers.

OVERVIEW

In a recent review on the developments of the renal neoplasia in the last half century; MacLennan and Cheng rightfully liken the changes on this topic to the acceleratingly enlarging universe.[1] The number of recognized kidney epithelial tumors by the World Health Organization (WHO) has increased from 3 to 14 between 1973 and 2004 to 19 in 2016, and several more entities are introduced in the fifth edition (Fig. 1). Fueled by the recognition of distinct immunohistochemical (IHC) profiles and genomic signatures, this rapid change does

[a] Department of Pathology and Laboratory Medicine, Albany Medical Center, 47 New Scotland Ave, Room F110S, MC81 Albany, NY 12208, USA; [b] Department of Pathology, Robert J. Tomsich Pathology and Laboratory Medicine Institute, Cleveland Clinic Foundation, 9500 Euclid Avenue, Mail Code L25 Cleveland, OH 44195, USA
* Corresponding author. 9500 Euclid Avenue, Mail Code L25, Cleveland, OH 44195, USA
E-mail address: williamson.sean@outlook.com

Surgical Pathology 15 (2022) 695–711
https://doi.org/10.1016/j.path.2022.07.005
1875-9181/22/© 2022 Elsevier Inc. All rights reserved.

not only provide introduction of new entities but also better understanding of the currently available subtypes. This review intends to serve as a practical and concise overview of the existing renal tumors.

RENAL TUMORS WITH CLEAR CELL CYTOLOGY

Clear Cell Renal Cell Carcinoma: Refining the Morphologic and Molecular Spectrum

Clear cell renal cell carcinoma (CCRCC) is the most common malignant tumor of the adult kidney, accounting for more than 60% of renal cell carcinoma (RCC),[2] and implicates a higher risk of adverse outcomes just by the histologic subtype.[3] Approximately 30% of RCC has regional lymph node spread or distant metastasis, most of them being CCRCC.[2,4] In most cases, characteristic histologic features including clusters and acini of tumor cells with clear cytoplasm wrapped by delicate vascular network—"sinusoidal pattern"—coupled with a limited IHC panel (diffuse, strong, and membranous carbonic anhydrase 9 [CA9] expression, negative or focal keratin 7 [KRT7] expression),[5] are sufficient for the diagnosis. However, CCRCC have a range of heterogeneous morphology including eosinophilic cytology (Fig. 2A),[5] syncytial type giant cells or low-grade multinucleation (Fig. 2B, C),[6] hemangioma-like vascular proliferation,[7] clear cell papillary carcinoma (tumor)-like or TFE3 RCC-like features (Fig. 2D),[8] tumor cells with hyaline globules,[9] or stromal fibrosis resembling

RCC with fibromyomatous stroma.[10–12] These features frequently overlap with existing and emerging renal tumors including melanocyte inducing transcription factor family gene rearrangement-associated RCC, clear cell papillary tumor, RCC with fibromyomatous stroma, and ELOC1-mutated RCC. Generous sampling of the tumor is often required to find representative sections depicting classic CCRCC features. For instance, definitive subtype of an RCC with fibromatous stroma may only be determined by the documentation of an entity-defining mutation.[11–14] It is unclear whether these aberrant histologic subtypes affect outcome, although at least some of them, for instance CCRCC with syncytial type giant tumor cells, may provide prediction about the behavior of the cancer. Several other histologic features including higher International Society of Urologic Pathology (ISUP)/WHO nuclear grade, coagulative necrosis, and the presence of rhabdoid and sarcomatoid differentiation are validated in CCRCC to suggest aggressive disease. Sarcomatoid differentiation in CCRCC may also be associated with susceptibility to immunotherapy.

The arm level loss of chromosome 3p is found more than 90% of CCRCC,[15] and this locus includes tumor suppressor gene VHL. Its mutation is a canonical and early event in CCRCC oncogenesis, both in hereditary and sporadic settings.[14,16–18] The VHL protein functions as part of the E3 ligase complex, which is ubiquitinating certain proteins.[18,19] This complex manages the adaptation of the oxidative stress by degrading

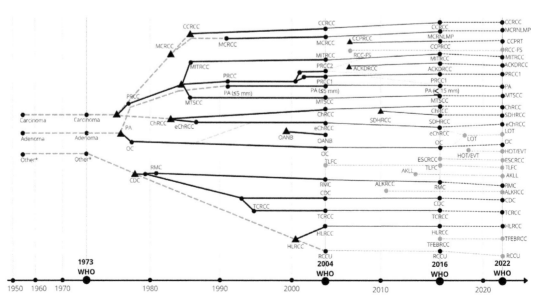

Fig. 1. Timeline of the evolution of renal neoplasm classification. *Other classification included renal cell carcinoma with high-grade features (e.g. renal medullary carcinoma, collecting duct carcinoma) and/or mesenchymal neoplasms of the kidney.

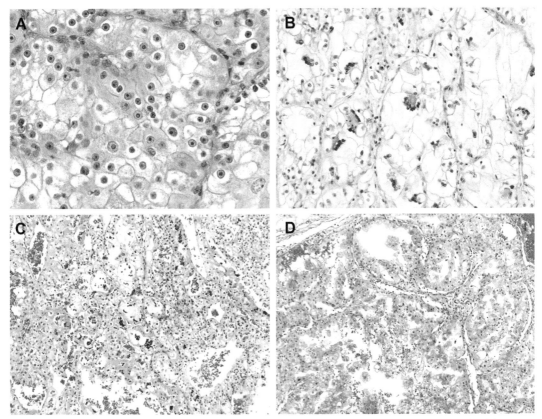

Fig. 2. CCRCC may present with predominantly eosinophilic features (*A*). Rarely, syncytial giant cells (*B*) or multi-nucleated cells (*C*) are present. These atypical morphological features may resemble other RCC variants such as TFE3 RCC (*D*). All photomicrographs are taken with 200× magnification.

HIF1a and HIF1b proteins, inhibiting their stimulation of multiple pathways in response to hypoxia including glycolytic energy production and angiogenesis.[20,21] *VHL* gene mutation disrupts this inhibition.[20,21] *VHL* mutations' oncogenic effects also result from non-HIF interactions including (but not limited to) microtubule stability and mitotic spindle functions, and PI3K signaling.[14]

Recent comprehensive genomic interrogations of RCC[13,17,22] have identified frequent gene mutations whose products are mainly responsible for histone remodeling including *PBRM1*, *SETD2*, and *BAP1*, and these seem to involve in the evolution and the subclonality and potentially treatment response of the CCRCC.[14,23] *PBRM1* gene mutations, seen in up to 40% of CCRCC, are usually absent in sarcomatoid CCRCC, and also associated with less T-cell infiltration and increased angiogenesis. Furthermore, *PBRM1*-mutated CCRCCs seem to have increased response to sunitinib with diminished response to atezolizumab (monotherapy or in combination). *BAP1* gene mutations (10%–20% of RCC) are associated with the poor outcomes, regardless of the stage. *BAP1* mutations are found to have distinct morphologic features, strikingly resembling MITF family rearrangement RCC, including large tumor cells with abundant cytoplasm and papillary architecture.[24] They also exhibit racemase and KRT7 positivity, which is uncommon in otherwise normal CCRCC.[24] *SETD2* mutations may contribute to the disruption of homologous recombination repair process of the double-stranded DNA.[19] Several other chromosome-level events, such as losses of 9p or 14q, are associated with metastatic disease.[19] The genomic profile of CCRCC, although not currently widely used in diagnostic practice, may increasingly affect the daily practice of pathologists, and may change diagnostic algorithms by introducing mutational landscape-driven prognostic and predictive markers.

Key Features–Clear Cell Renal Cell Carcinoma

- Clear cytoplasm is prototypical but eosinophilic cells are not unusual with higher grade
- CA9 typically shows diffuse membranous staining but may be decreased with higher grade
- KRT7 is usually minimal or negative
- Molecular features include *VHL* gene alterations, chromosome 3p25 loss, and alterations of *BAP1, SETD2, PBRM1*, and others

Chromophobe Renal Cell Carcinoma: How to Detect the Rare Aggressive Behavior

Chromophobe RCC (ChRCC) is the second most common renal tumor with clear cell cytology, accounting for roughly 5% of RCC. The variable proportions of 2 cell types; "classical" type with abundant clear cytoplasm with "cell wall-like" prominent membranes and nuclear membrane irregularity, and smaller eosinophilic cells with perinuclear halos are diagnostic in most cases (**Fig. 3**A). ChRCC does not usually share the wide morphologic range of CCRCC, although unusual presentations of ChRCC including eosinophilic (**Fig. 3**B)[25] or pigmented microcystic variants[26] may be seen. Papillary architecture in chromophobe RCC was also recently reported.[27] Sarcomatoid and/or rhabdoid differentiation rate is similar to that of CCRCC. About 95% of ChRCC are indolent, although cases with local and distant metastases do occur (**Fig. 3**C). Conventional ISUP/WHO nuclear grading scheme is not validated in ChRCC[28] and is considered inappropriate for ChRCC[29,30]; therefore, attempts to correlate histologic features and the outcome have been made.[31–33] Nuclear crowding, anaplasia, coagulative tumor necrosis, and sarcomatoid differentiation are consistently associated with adverse disease[31,32]; however, the utility of these parameters are still debated.[34,35] IHC typically shows positivity for KIT, negative vimentin, negative/minimal CA9, and often substantial membranous KRT7 (however, we have encountered classic ChRCC that is entirely negative).[36]

Key Features–Chromophobe Renal Cell Carcinoma

- Cells with clear to eosinophilic cytoplasm, often prominent cell borders resembling plant cells
- Immunohistochemistry positive for KIT, often KRT7 (but not always), and negative for vimentin
- Behavior is typically favorable but aggressive tumors may contain vascular invasion, necrosis, or sarcomatoid change

It is surprising that a tumor, with characteristic (and often diagnostic) multiple somatic chromosomal losses (particularly chromosomes 1, 2, 6, 10, 13, 17, and 21), shows metastatic potential, let alone cell viability. In a landmark study, Casuscelli and colleagues[37] showed that primary tumors of the metastatic chromophobe RCC had "imbalanced chromosome duplication (ICD)," that is, additional chromosome copies in 3 or more somatic chromosomes. The presence of ICD in primary ChRCC increased the likelihood of metastasis by 2.6 to 5.3 times when compared with ChRCC with primary tumors not demonstrating ICD. *PTEN* and *TP53* gene mutations were more common in ChRCC with metastasis and were unsurprisingly associated with poor survival.

Clear Cell Papillary Renal Cell Tumor (Carcinoma): No Recurrence, No Metastasis, No Carcinoma

Clear cell papillary renal cell tumor (carcinoma) entered into the official WHO tumor classification in 2016,[38] a decade after its first identification in patients with end-stage renal disease.[39] Characteristic morphologic features include well-circumscribed and often encapsulated tumor with cells with clear cytoplasm and low-grade nuclei predominantly forming tubules and papilla, and suprabasal positioning of the nuclei (**Fig. 3**D).[39–41] Diffuse CA9 expression with less prominence on the luminal caps (**Fig. 3**E), diffuse KRT7 expression (**Fig. 3**F), negative immunoreactivity with proximal tubule markers such as racemase and CD10, with frequent expression of markers related to distal tubules including GATA3 or high molecular weight cytokeratin are very specific for these tumors.[40] It may have striking morphologic resemblance to RCC with fibromatous stroma,[11] and other differential diagnoses include clear cell RCC and papillary RCC with clear cell features.[40,42] Clear cell papillary renal cell tumor (carcinoma) has distinct mutational profile including lack of *VHL* mutations in the vast majority of tumors and lack of chromosome 7 and 17 gains[43] with mutations in *MET, PTEN, ERBB4*, and *STK11* genes.[44–46]

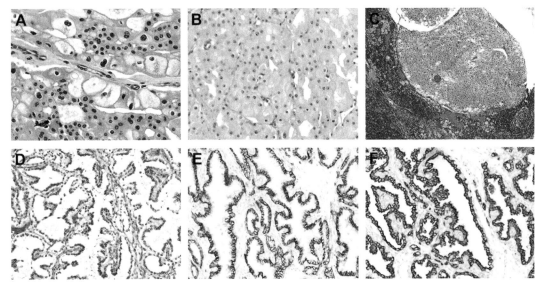

Fig. 3. Classic ChRCC shows 2 distinct cell populations and innate nuclear atypia (*A*; 200×), whereas eosinophilic variant may not have the cells with clear cytoplasm and "vegetable-like" cytology (*B*; 100×). About 5% of chromophobe RCC shows aggressive disease such as lymph node metastasis (*C*, 40×). Clear cell papillary tumor (*D*; 100×) characteristically exhibits diffuse CA9 expression with luminal clearing (*E*; 100×) and KRT7 expression (*F*; 100×).

Data from single institutions[47] as well as meta-analysis[45] indicate that this tumor does not exhibit recurrence or metastatic potential, therefore, it likely warrants reclassification as a benign or low malignant potential tumor. Clear cell papillary cystadenoma,[40] clear cell papillary adenomatoid tumor,[45] and clear cell papillary renal tumor are among the proposed terminologies. The fifth edition of WHO classification renames it as clear cell papillary renal tumor.[48]

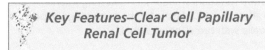

> **Key Features–Clear Cell Papillary Renal Cell Tumor**
>
> - Branching glands lined by cells with clear cytoplasm, variable papillae
> - Often prominent nuclear alignment
> - Consistent diffuse KRT7 and CA9 (sometimes lacking the apical membrane)
> - Often positive GATA3 and high molecular weight keratin
> - Negative/minimal CD10/AMACR

MIT Family Translocation-Associated Renal Cell Carcinoma: Expanding Spectrum of Morphology, Immunoprofile, and Genetics

Although grouped under one subtype "MIT family translocation renal cell carcinoma," these cancers are probably different entities with distinct outcome implications. The *TFE3* gene is the most commonly rearranged in this group,[49] and *TFE3* gene rearrangement was the first identified translocation event in RCC.[50] Other genes with documented gene rearrangements include *TFEB*[51] and rarely *MITF* itself.[52,53] *TFE3* gene rearranged RCC (TFE3 RCC) accounts for approximately 90% of all MIT family translocation-associated RCC,[54] and it is the most common RCC in pediatric patients, responsible for 40% of RCC in this age group.[49] Several single-institutional and multi-institutional studies[55–60] clearly demonstrate that it can be seen in any age, including adults, and may make up as much as 4% of adult RCC.[61] TFE3 RCC is morphologically heterogeneous, including classical morphology of tumor cells with abundant clear or eosinophilic cytoplasm and papillary formation (**Fig. 4**A), as well as eosinophilic tumors with low-grade nuclei (**Fig. 4**B), clear or chromophobe RCC-like (**Fig. 4**C), clear cell papillary renal cell tumor-like (**Fig. 4**D), or high-grade infiltrative features.[55]

Some of the translocation partners of *TFE3* include *PRCC* (common),[62] *ASPSCR1* (common),[63] *SFPQ*,[64] *NONO*,[64] *RBM10*,[65] *ARID1B*,[66] *EWSR1*,[67] *NEAT1*,[68] *KAT6A*,[68] and *MED15*,[69] and these gene partners have important implications in many aspects. *ASPSCR1::TFE3* translocation is associated with the classical TFE3 RCC morphology.[59] *NONO::TFE3* and *SFPQ::TFE3* gene rearranged RCC are associated with tumor cells with subnuclear

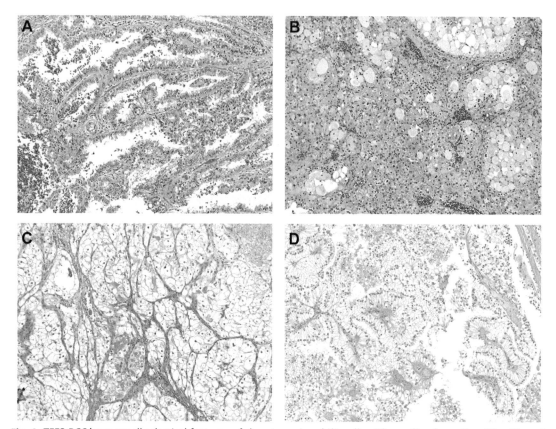

Fig. 4. TFE3 RCC have usually classical features of clear to eosinophilic cells with papillae formation (*A*); although low-grade eosinophilic (*B*), CCRCC (*C*), or clear cell papillary RCC/tumor-like (*D*) morphology (All photomicrographs are 100×).

vacuolization,[59] whereas *PRCC::TFE3* is associated with CCRCC-like morphology and consistent positive cathepsin K, contrasting to tumors with other fusion partners, which are not always positive for this marker.[59] *RBM10*, *RBMX*, *GRIPAP1*, and *NONO* are cryptic intrachromosomal translocations. These may cause a false-negative result in fluorescence in situ hybridization (FISH) assays.[59,60,65] IHC features are variable. The classic thinking is that keratins and vimentin are usually negative, including pankeratin and KRT7, although this is not absolute and positivity should not be considered to exclude the diagnosis. Occasional positivity for melanocytic markers (eg, HMB45, Melan A) or frequent positive cathepsin K (depending on fusion partner) may help support the diagnosis.[55] The most consistently immunoreactive biomarker is TFE3 protein,[55,70] although TFE3 IHC may be subject to inconsistent performance due to technical difficulties.[71] A recent multinational survey on expert urologic pathologists documented the distrust on TFE3 IHC in the diagnosis of TFE3 RCC.[70] Main concerns of the TFE3 IHC were low specificity (16/42) and unreliable performance (15/42). About half of the (23/48) respondents preferred

TFE3 FISH for the diagnosis, regardless of the IHC profile. However, the *TFE3* FISH assay is also imperfect, due to subtle or false-negative results with intrachromosomal rearrangements, and different cut-off levels for the percentage of positive cells with break-apart signal.[70]

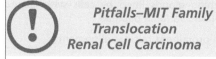

Pitfalls–MIT Family Translocation Renal Cell Carcinoma

! Morphology can overlap with other tumors, including oncocytic tumors, clear cell RCC, and clear cell papillary renal cell tumor (nuclear alignment)

! Although FISH is a useful tool, false-negative results may occur with intrachromosomal inversion, such as with partners *RBM10*, *RBMX*, *GRIPAP1*, and *NONO*

! Although RCC in young patients/children is suspicious for MIT translocation carcinoma, there are likely more tumors in older adults, due to the rarity of RCC at young age

In a recent landmark study, Bakouny and colleagues[54] reported the most comprehensive genomic interrogation on MIT family RCCs. This report showed worse outcomes in patients with MIT family RCC than clear cell RCC, and few additional somatic mutations, most notably 9p21.3 deletions and activated NRF2 pathway. Immunotherapies also seemed to be better than vascular endothelial growth factor inhibitors.[54]

TUMORS WITH EOSINOPHILIC CELLS

This section serves as a quick review on the low-grade eosinophilic renal neoplasms, which has seen one of the most dynamic changes with multiple emerging entities in recent years, including low-grade oncocytic tumor (LOT),[72–79] eosinophilic vacuolated tumor (EVT),[76,80–82] and eosinophilic solid and cystic RCC.[83–89] For more detailed discussion of the newly identified entities, the reader is directed to another article in this issue; however, these entities have profoundly affected the traditional diagnostic workup on eosinophilic renal tumors, particularly diagnosis of oncocytoma as the most common tumor in this category.

Oncocytoma: Stricter Diagnostic Criteria Amid Expanded Differential Diagnosis

Oncocytoma is the archetype of the low-grade eosinophilic renal tumors and accounts for approximately 5% of renal neoplasms in adults. Oncocytoma is a benign tumor with characteristic features of variably sized clusters and nests of tumor cells in the background of loose edematous stroma.[5,90] Tumor cells are often uniform with regular nuclear membranes and homogenous eosinophilic cytoplasm. Degenerative atypia can be seen, and sampling from the central scar may produce morphologic variation (**Fig. 5**A–C).[90–92] Oncocytoma with small cells, scant cytoplasm, and rosette formation, so-called small cell variant are rarely seen.[93–96] Typical immunohistochemistry is diffuse KIT positivity (sometimes weak, requiring high magnification) with KRT7 immunoreactivity in scattered tumor cells; diffuse KRT7 expression or no expression argue against oncocytoma.[5,92] Vimentin is typically negative, although both KRT7 and vimentin may be positive in the central scar areas for unknown reasons. "Adverse" features including vascular or perinephric/renal sinus adipose tissue extension[90–92,97,98] are well documented and do not seem to alter the benign behavior of oncocytoma. Variations in diagnostic approaches exist, although the presence of mitotic figures, frequent nuclear membrane irregularity or perinuclear halo, coagulative necrosis, and

unequivocal papilla formation are considered to most strongly argue against diagnosis of oncocytoma.[92] Morphologic and IHC nuances have become more critical with the emerging entities. Briefly, oncocytoma-like tumor cells with diffuse growth pattern and diffuse KRT7 expression with negative KIT immunoreactivity support LOT(5). Irregular nuclear membranes, perinuclear halos, and diffuse dual KRT7/KIT immunoreactivity is consistent with chromophobe RCC.[5] Intracytoplasmic vacuoles with lack of KRT7 expression should prompt the investigation of succinate dehydrogenase-deficient RCC (SDH RCC).[38]

Key Features–Oncocytoma

- Nests of eosinophilic cells with round nuclei
- KRT7 labels rare cells
- Vimentin negative
- KIT positive
- Mitotic activity should be absent

Pitfalls–Oncocytoma

! Involvement of fat or blood vessels does not indicate adverse behavior

! KRT7 and vimentin IHC may be increased in the central scar areas

! Degenerative atypia can be present and does not affect behavior

Oncocytomas often lack significant copy number alterations, although loss of chromosome 1 overlaps with ChRCC, and up to one-third are associated with *CCND1* gene rearrangements,[99] which might be helpful to distinguish it from other low-grade eosinophilic renal neoplasms. Interestingly, newly identified eosinophilic renal neoplasms, namely LOT (**Fig. 5**D), EVT, and eosinophilic solid and cystic RCC (**Fig. 5**E), have common mutations in genes in the mechanistic target of rapamycin kinase pathway.[75,76,78–80,82,85]

Hybrid Oncocytic Chromophobe Tumor: A Term to Be Used Only for the Hereditary Setting and Oncocytic Renal Neoplasm of Low Malignant Potential: A Term for Borderline Tumors

It is not unusual to encounter low-grade eosinophilic renal tumors that do not fit perfectly into

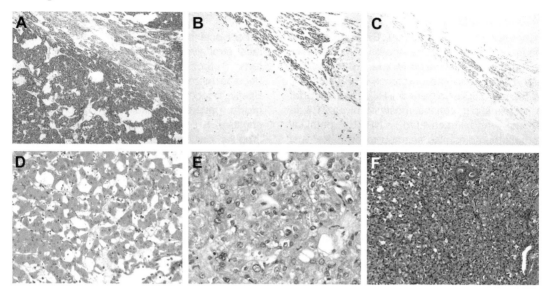

Fig. 5. Central scar in oncocytoma may not only have disrupted morphology (*A*; 40×) but also altered biomarker expression such as diffuse KRT7 (*B*, 40×) and CA9 (*C*, 40×), which may cause significant misdiagnosis in renal biopsy. LOT has similar cytology with oncocytoma (*D*, 100×) with lace-like stroma. Eosinophilic solid and cystic RCC have abundant eosinophilic cytoplasm and intracytoplasmic basophilic stippling (*E*, 200×). SDH RCC has low-grade nuclei with characteristic intracytoplasmic vacuoles (*F*, 100×).

the category of one of these established or emerging entities.[100] Particularly problematic is the gray zone between oncocytoma and chromophobe RCC.[100] Because aggressive behavior is rare even in eosinophilic ChRCC, it is hard to know exactly where the cutoff should be drawn between these 2 entities. If the other classifiable tumors are excluded (especially SDH RCC), these tumors can be labeled as "oncocytic renal neoplasm of low malignant potential, not further classified," per the latest Genitourinary Pathology Society recommendations.[100] Despite the fact that hybrid oncocytic/chromophobe tumors (HOCT) can be seen in sporadic setting,[101] the term "HOCT" is suggested to be reserved for a very distinct hereditary disorder that is almost exclusively seen in patients with germline mutations in *FLCN* gene, known as Birt-Hogg-Dube (BHD) syndrome,[102,103] or in the setting of renal oncocytosis without BHD syndrome. Patients with BHD present with skin fibrofolliculomas, pulmonary cysts and frequent pneumothorax, and kidney neoplasms, predominantly HOCT.[102,104,105] Clear cell RCC and potentially other RCC subtypes can also be seen.[105] Perhaps, not surprisingly, mutations in HOCT in patients with BHD are also linked to the MTOR pathway.[103,106]

Succinate Dehydrogenase–Deficient Renal Cell Carcinoma

SDH RCC is typically associated with a germline mutation, and it exhibits dangerously low-grade

eosinophilic features. In one study, 3 of 273 tumors (1.1%) that were previously diagnosed as oncocytoma exhibited lack of SDHB immunoreactivity, demonstrating the risk of potentially catastrophic misdiagnosis.[107] Mean age for SDH RCC is about 40 years, and although it is mostly nonaggressive, metastases have been reported.[108] Although most show characteristic morphologic features (**Fig. 5**F), up to one-fifth of them may have high-grade morphologic features and unusual papillary or other deceptive features.[109] Loss of function in the SDH enzyme complex can be demonstrated by the negative SDHB IHC. However, weak staining may be found in other tumors, such as those with clear cytoplasm, due to sparse mitochondria rather than true abnormality of the protein.[110,111]

RENAL TUMORS WITH PAPILLA FORMATION

"Type 2 Papillary Renal Cell Carcinoma": Not a Single Entity

Papillary RCC is the second most common RCC in adults, accounting for approximately 15% of all RCC.[38] Historically, it is the first subtype that was histologically separated from the rest of "renal adenocarcinoma."[112] This report identified 34 of 224 renal tumors that were predominantly well-circumscribed, extensively necrotic, and infiltrated with macrophages.[112] Detailed histologic observations revealed potentially 2 different morphologic patterns: tumors with papillary or tubular morphology, lined by a single layer of tumor cells, and a second group with pseudostratification.

Uncommonly, tumors with high-grade nuclear atypia were seen.[112]

This first definition founded the distinction of type 1 and type 2 papillary RCC, with type 2 PRCC having more adverse outcomes when compared with type 1 papillary RCC. This dichotomy was supported by numerous clinical, imaging, and morphologic studies.[113–120] Type 1 papillary RCC represents a single entity with characteristic morphologic features (**Fig. 6**A) and distinct molecular features, including recurrent chromosomal gains, in particular 7 and 17.[100,121] It is associated with *MET* gene alterations,[122] in the hereditary papillary RCC syndrome,[38] and also sporadically. However, growing evidence demonstrates the heterogeneity of so called "type 2 papillary RCC," showing a varied molecular landscape (eg, *CDKN2A* silencing, *SETD2* mutations, NRF2 antioxidant response element activity).[122] It is now recognized that the former type 2 category also contains multiple other recognizable subtypes including TFE3 RCC (**Fig. 6**B), fumarate hydratase–deficient RCC (FH RCC), *ALK* rearrangement RCC, and any other renal tumors with possible papillary growth patterns.[100,121] The fifth edition of WHO classification no longer recommends type 1 and type 2 subtyping, and type 2 papillary RCC is not considered as a distinct histologic subtype.

The issue of papillary RCC with both type 1 and type 2 histologic patterns was potentially addressed by a recent study on single-institutional cohort of 199 papillary RCC with at least focal type 1 papillary RCC features.[116] This study showed that both morphologic areas exhibited similar somatic mutations in 78% of the cases, including chromosomal gains of 7 and 17 by copy number variation analysis. Moreover, the presence of minor type 2 morphology, that is, high nucleolar grade, was not associated with significant survival difference.[116] This study suggests that papillary tumors with at least focal type 1 papillary RCC features can be designated as such.

Oncocytic Papillary Renal Cell Carcinoma: Making a Comeback

Recognizing oncocytic variant of papillary RCC as a distinct entity was discouraged at the 2013 ISUP consensus meeting,[123] because various preceding studies used different criteria for diagnosis, and it was not clear that a uniform entity existed at that time. However, in current practice, this entity seems to be a making a comeback, following refinement of the diagnostic criteria. In 2019, Al-Obaidy and colleagues[124] identified 18 renal neoplasms with branching papillae and predominantly eosinophilic cells with regular but strikingly apically located nuclei (**Fig. 6**C), which they termed papillary renal neoplasm with reverse polarity (PRNRP). This corresponds to what Saleeb and colleagues[125] described as "type 4/oncocytic low-grade" papillary RCC in another study. These tumors typically show diffuse KRT7 (**Fig. 6**D) with variable alpha-methylacyl-CoA racemase (AMACR) immunoreactivity (often more limited than typical papillary RCC). Interestingly, they are

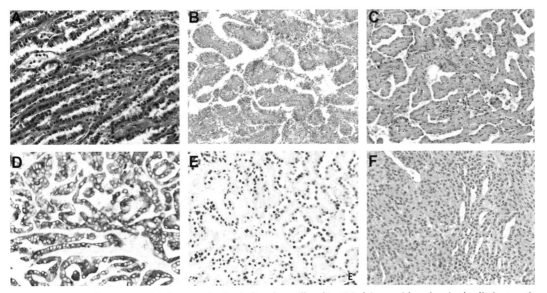

Fig. 6. Type 1 papillary RCC, with low-grade single lined papillae (*A*; 100×) is considered a single distinct entity, whereas type 2 papillary RCC is more of a histologic description that can encompass several diagnostic entities, such as TFE3 RCC (*B*; 40×). PRNRP was previously considered as a variant of papillary RCC (*C*; 100×). Interestingly, PRNRP shows diffuse KRT7 expression (*D*, 100×) and GATA3 (*E*, 100×). MTSCC (*F*; 100×) can resemble type 1 papillary RCC but often shows intercellular mucin and low-grade spindle cell proliferation.

usually negative for vimentin (resembling oncocytoma and ChRCC) but consistently positive for GATA3 (Fig. 6E).[124] This entity likely also corresponds to what was described in an earlier study as "papillary RCC with oncocytic cells and nonoverlapping low grade nuclei," although it did not gain traction in practice until recently.[126] It is now known these tumors consistently harbor *KRAS* mutations, in contrast to other existing renal neoplasms in multiple independent studies.[124,127–129] None of the PRNRP documented in the literature thus far has shown recurrence or metastasis.[128]

Key Features–Papillary Renal Neoplasm with Reverse Polarity

- Papillary structures lined by cells with eosinophilic cytoplasm and apically aligned nuclei

- Vimentin negative, similar to oncocytoma/chromophobe RCC

- AMACR variable, often less than papillary RCC

- KRT7 often diffuse, unlike other eosinophilic tumors

- GATA3 consistently positive

- *KRAS* mutations consistently present

Mucinous Tubular and Spindle Cell Carcinoma: New Genomic Insights

Mucinous tubular and spindle cell carcinoma (MTSCC) is a rare entity showing classic morphologic features including predominantly low-grade tumor cells arranged in packed papillary structures and tubules in the background of focally mucinous stroma (Fig. 6F).[130,131] Low-grade spindle cell proliferation can be present.[132,133] Although predominantly indolent tumors, they can occasionally show aggressive behavior,[133] and solid/nested growth, irregular trabeculae/single cell infiltration, tumor necrosis, increased mitotic activity, and lymphovascular invasion are associated with worse clinical outcomes.[133] Morphology is usually sufficient for this diagnosis, although some are almost indistinguishable from type 1 papillary RCC, even with IHC.[5] In the last 5 years, several genomic interrogation studies[133,134] have pointed out distinct genetic alterations including multiple chromosomal losses in chromosomes 1, 4, 6, 8, 9, 13, 14, 15, and 22 and lack chromosome 7 and 17 gains, a practical difference in challenging cases. Homozygous loss of *CDKN2A/B* was associated with locally advanced, metastatic

disease.[133] In difficult cases, overexpression of VSTM2A by in situ hybridization test can be used, because this marker is very specific for the diagnosis of MTSCC.[135]

HIGH-GRADE INFILTRATIVE TUMORS

High-grade infiltrative tumors of the kidney include a wide range of entities, spanning from primary neoplasms to high-grade urothelial carcinoma and metastatic tumors (Fig. 7A, B).[5] Complete clinical history (evidence of prior malignancy or hemoglobinopathies), extensive sampling of the tissue, and morphology-based comprehensive IHC and FISH panels are often required to resolve this differential diagnosis. Practically any recognized RCC may present with high-grade infiltrative features such as CCRCC (Fig. 7C), ChRCC, or TFE3 RCC.[5] However, several entities that are inherently infiltrative are discussed here.

FH RCC was first identified as a hereditary condition where patients develop dermal and uterine leiomyomatosis and very aggressive form of RCC (hereditary leiomyomatosis and RCC syndrome). However, it seems that FH RCC can also occur in the sporadic setting.[38] Unlike other hereditary kidney cancers, FH RCC tends to occur as solitary mass, many times presenting as advanced or metastatic disease.[38] Large tumor cells with eosinophilic or amphophilic cytoplasm with characteristic large "viral inclusion-like" nuclei (Fig. 7D) are seen at least focally. These cells usually form papillary architecture, although solid, cribriform pattern, and even with low-grade nuclei are identified.[136] Lack of KRT7 and FH IHC expression with increased labeling for 2-succino-cysteine are helpful ancillary assays.[137] Germline status should usually be tested in these patients because the majority likely occurs with a hereditary basis.[121]

SMARCB1-deficient renal medullary carcinoma (RMC) is perhaps the most devastating outcome of patients with hemoglobinopathy, most commonly patients with sickle cell trait. Due to the increased prevalence of this hemoglobinopathy, young male African Americans are disproportionately affected.[138] The outcome is dismal, 71% of patients have metastatic disease at the time of diagnosis.[138] This tumor extensively infiltrates kidney parenchyma, where tubular and cribriform pattern tumor cells and the elements of benign kidney parenchyma are often intermixed (Fig. 7E).[139] Tumor cells have abundant purplish cytoplasm and high-grade nuclei. An acute inflammatory infiltrate is often also present.[139] Characteristic negative/lost SMARCB1 (INI1) expression and OCT4 positivity aid in recognition.[5] Molecular studies identified that the most recurrent genetic alteration

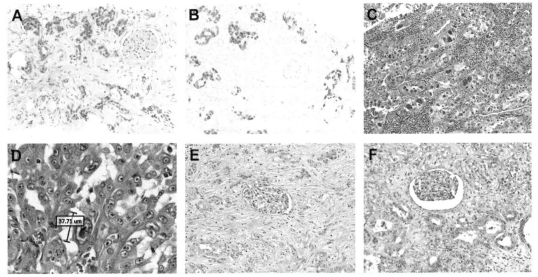

Fig. 7. Metastatic tumors, such as lung adenocarcinoma involving the kidney (*A*, 100×; *B*, TTF1, 100×), show an infiltrative pattern, overlapping with entities such as CDC. Common kidney tumors with high-grade features, such as CCRCC (*C*, 100×), can also mimic this pattern. FH RCC has characteristic large "viral inclusion like" nucleoli (*D*, 100×). RMC (*E*, 100×) and CDC (*F*, 100×) are primary renal tumors with highly infiltrative pattern, although both are rare, and the latter is a diagnosis of exclusion.

in RMC is silencing of the *SMARCB1* gene,[140] most commonly due to translocations.[141] RCC with the loss of *SMARCB1* but without known hemoglobinopathy has been reported, and terminology of RCC unclassified with medullary phenotype has been proposed in this scenario.[100] With somewhat similar morphology and the same catastrophic outcome, collecting duct carcinoma (CDC) is a diagnosis of exclusion.[38] In molecular studies, a subset of tumors have been also found to have *SMARCB1* genomic alterations,[142] suggesting that these likely in truth represent RMC or RCC unclassified with medullary phenotype. Predominantly infiltrative tubular formation by high-grade tumor cells and desmoplasia are somewhat nonspecific definitions for CDC (**Fig.** 7F), and FH RCC, RMC, *ALK* gene-rearranged RCC, *TFEB*-amplified RCC, high-grade urothelial carcinoma, and metastatic tumors should be excluded.[38]

Pitfalls–Infiltrative Renal Tumors

! Metastases to the kidney may occur many years after primary diagnosis and mimic a primary tumor (solitary, sometimes extension into the renal pelvis).

! Urothelial carcinoma may mimic infiltrative RCC–PAX8 may be positive in both RCC and urothelial carcinoma; therefore, urothelial markers such as GATA3 or p63 are helpful.

! Rare carcinomas with a SMARCB1-deficient phenotype, can occur in patients without sickle trait/hemoglobinopathy, termed RCC unclassified with medullary phenotype.

! Fumarate hydratase-deficient RCC can have multiple patterns, resembling papillary, tubulocystic, and infiltrative RCC.

! CDC is a diagnosis of exclusion, once these considerations are argued against.

SUMMARY

The number of recognized subtypes of renal neoplasms has grown dramatically over recent years. This includes a variety of potentially emerging diagnostic entities; however, we have also improved our understanding of existing entities. In addition to *VHL,* several other key genes are now known to have important roles in CCRCC. Distinguishing oncocytoma from ChRCC remains a challenge; however, refined diagnostic terminology, such as oncocytic renal neoplasm of low malignant potential, is now available for recognition of borderline tumors. Distinguishing type 1 and type 2 papillary RCC is now thought to be less critical because the former type 2 category likely included a mixture of entities that are now recognized as distinct, such as MIT family translocation RCC, FH RCC, and others. PRNRP seems to be perched for recognition as a distinct tumor type in the near future, differing from papillary RCC in several ways, such as less intense labeling for AMACR, consistent positive GATA3, and consistent *KRAS* gene mutations. Renal tumors with a predominantly infiltrative pattern are very important for recognition because most of these have aggressive behavior, including FH RCC, RMC, CDC, urothelial carcinoma, and metastases from other cancers.

CLINICS CARE POINTS

- When clear cell RCC shows unusual morphology, often with higher grade, diffuse CA9 staining or molecular testing (VHL mutation or 3p loss) can be used to support the diagnosis.

- Oncocytoma should exhibit only scattered cells positive for keratin 7, negative vimentin, and positive KIT; however, "oncocytic renal neoplasm of low malignant potential" can be used as a diagnostic term for tumors with borderline features.

- For infiltrative renal tumors, differential diagnoses to evaluate may include metastatic carcinoma to the kidney (with organ-specific markers, such as TTF1), urothelial carcinoma (with markers such as p63, or GATA3), medullary carcinoma (with SMARCB1), and fumarate hydratase-deficient RCC (with FH and 2SC IHC).

REFERENCES

1. MacLennan GT, Cheng L. Five decades of urologic pathology: the accelerating expansion of knowledge in renal cell neoplasia. Hum Pathol 2020;95: 24–45.
2. Siegel RL, Miller KD, Fuchs HE, et al. Cancer statistics, 2021. CA Cancer J Clin 2021;71:7–33.
3. Leibovich BC, Lohse CM, Crispen PL, et al. Histological subtype is an independent predictor of outcome for patients with renal cell carcinoma. J Urol 2010;183:1309–15.
4. Kluger N, Giraud S, Coupier I, et al. Birt-Hogg-Dube syndrome: clinical and genetic studies of 10 French families. Br J Dermatol 2010;162: 527–37.
5. Akgul M, Williamson SR. Immunohistochemistry for the diagnosis of renal epithelial neoplasms. Semin Diagn Pathol 2022;39:1–16.
6. Williamson SR, Kum JB, Goheen MP, et al. Clear cell renal cell carcinoma with a syncytial-type multi-nucleated giant tumor cell component: implications for differential diagnosis. Hum Pathol 2014;45: 735–44.
7. Alaghehbandan R, Limani R, Ali L, et al. Clear cell renal cell carcinoma with prominent microvascular hyperplasia: Morphologic, immunohistochemical and molecular-genetic analysis of 7 sporadic cases. Ann Diagn Pathol 2022;56:151871.
8. Ross H, Martignoni G, Argani P. Renal cell carcinoma with clear cell and papillary features. Arch Pathol Lab Med 2012;136:391–9.
9. Hes O, Benakova K, Vanecek T, et al. Clear cell type of renal cell carcinoma with numerous hyaline globules: a diagnostic pitfall. Pathol Int 2005;55: 150–4.
10. Gournay M, Dugay F, Belaud-Rotureau MA, et al. Renal cell carcinoma with leiomyomatous stroma in tuberous sclerosis complex: a distinct entity. Virchows Arch 2021;478:793–9.
11. Hes O, Compérat EM, Rioux-Leclercq N. Clear cell papillary renal cell carcinoma, renal angiomyoadenomatous tumor, and renal cell carcinoma with leiomyomatous stroma relationship of 3 types of renal tumors: a review. Ann Diagn Pathol 2016; 21:59–64.
12. Shah RB, Stohr BA, Tu ZJ, et al. Renal cell carcinoma with leiomyomatous stroma" harbor somatic mutations of TSC1, TSC2, MTOR, and/or ELOC (TCEB1): clinicopathologic and molecular characterization of 18 sporadic tumors supports a distinct entity. Am J Surg Pathol 2020;44:571–81.
13. Ricketts CJ, De Cubas AA, Fan H, et al. The cancer genome atlas comprehensive molecular characterization of renal cell carcinoma. Cell Rep 2018;23: 313–26.e315.
14. Jonasch E, Walker CL, Rathmell WK. Clear cell renal cell carcinoma ontogeny and mechanisms of lethality. Nat Rev Nephrol 2021;17:245–61.
15. Clark DJ, Dhanasekaran SM, Petralia F, et al. Integrated proteogenomic characterization of clear cell renal cell carcinoma. Cell 2019;179:964–983 e931.
16. Latif F, Tory K, Gnarra J, et al. Identification of the von Hippel-Lindau disease tumor suppressor gene. Science 1993;260:1317–20.
17. Comprehensive molecular characterization of clear cell renal cell carcinoma. Nature 2013;499:43–9.
18. Gossage L, Eisen T, Maher ERVHL. the story of a tumour suppressor gene. Nat Rev Cancer 2015; 15:55–64.
19. Bui TO, Dao VT, Nguyen VT, et al. Genomics of clear-cell renal cell carcinoma: a systematic review and meta-analysis. Eur Urol 2022;81:349–61.
20. Maxwell PH, Dachs GU, Gleadle JM, et al. Hypoxia-inducible factor-1 modulates gene expression in solid tumors and influences both angiogenesis and tumor growth. Proc Natl Acad Sci U S A 1997;94: 8104–9.

21. Weidemann A, Johnson RS. Biology of HIF-1α. Cell Death Differ 2008;15:621–7.

22. Linehan WM, Ricketts CJ. The cancer genome atlas of renal cell carcinoma: findings and clinical implications. Nat Rev Urol 2019;16:539–52.

23. Turajlic S, Xu H, Litchfield K, et al. Deterministic evolutionary trajectories influence primary tumor growth: TRACERx renal. Cell 2018;173: 595–610.e511.

24. Gallan AJ, Parilla M, Segal J, et al. BAP1-mutated clear cell renal cell carcinoma. Am J Clin Pathol 2021;155:718–28.

25. Brunelli M, Eble JN, Zhang S, et al. Eosinophilic and classic chromophobe renal cell carcinomas have similar frequent losses of multiple chromosomes from among chromosomes 1, 2, 6, 10, and 17, and this pattern of genetic abnormality is not present in renal oncocytoma. Mod Pathol 2005; 18:161–9.

26. Michal M, Hes O, Svec A, et al. Pigmented microcystic chromophobe cell carcinoma: a unique variant of renal cell carcinoma. Ann Diagn Pathol 1998;2:149–53.

27. Michalova K, Tretiakova M, Pivovarcikova K, et al. Expanding the morphologic spectrum of chromophobe renal cell carcinoma: a study of 8 cases with papillary architecture. Ann Diagn Pathol 2020;44:151448.

28. Delahunt B, Cheville JC, Martignoni G, et al. The international society of urological pathology (ISUP) grading system for renal cell carcinoma and other prognostic parameters. Am J Surg Pathol 2013; 37:1490–504.

29. Delahunt B, Sika-Paotonu D, Bethwaite PB, et al. Fuhrman grading is not appropriate for chromophobe renal cell carcinoma. Am J Surg Pathol 2007;31:957–60.

30. Volpe A, Novara G, Antonelli A, et al. Chromophobe renal cell carcinoma (RCC): oncological outcomes and prognostic factors in a large multicentre series. BJU Int 2012;110:76–83.

31. Avulova S, Cheville JC, Lohse CM, et al. Grading Chromophobe Renal Cell Carcinoma: Evidence for a Four-tiered Classification Incorporating Coagulative Tumor Necrosis. Eur Urol 2021;79:225–31.

32. Paner GP, Amin MB, Alvarado-Cabrero I, et al. A novel tumor grading scheme for chromophobe renal cell carcinoma: prognostic utility and comparison with Fuhrman nuclear grade. Am J Surg Pathol 2010;34:1233–40.

33. Ohashi R, Martignoni G, Hartmann A, et al. Multi-institutional re-evaluation of prognostic factors in chromophobe renal cell carcinoma: proposal of a novel two-tiered grading scheme. Virchows Arch 2020;476:409–18.

34. Delahunt B, Samaratunga H, Egevad L. Re: Svetlana Avulova, John C. Cheville, Christine M.

Lohse, et al. Grading of chromophobe renal cell carcinoma: evidence for a four-tiered classification incorporating coagulative tumor necrosis. Eur Urol 2021;79:225-231: Should chromophobe renal cell carcinoma be graded? Eur Urol 2021; 79:e141–2.

35. Lopez-Beltran A, Montironi R, Cimadamore A, et al. Grading of chromophobe renal cell carcinoma: do we need it? Eur Urol 2021;79:232–3.

36. Wobker SE, Williamson SR. Modern pathologic diagnosis of renal oncocytoma. J Kidney Cancer VHL 2017;4:1–12.

37. Casuscelli J, Weinhold N, Gundem G, et al. Genomic landscape and evolution of metastatic chromophobe renal cell carcinoma. JCI Insight 2017;2.

38. Moch H, Cubilla AL, Humphrey PA, et al. The 2016 WHO classification of tumours of the urinary system and male genital organs-part A: renal, penile, and testicular tumours. Eur Urol 2016;70:93–105.

39. Tickoo SK, dePeralta-Venturina MN, Harik LR, et al. Spectrum of epithelial neoplasms in end-stage renal disease: an experience from 66 tumor-bearing kidneys with emphasis on histologic patterns distinct from those in sporadic adult renal neoplasia. Am J Surg Pathol 2006;30:141–53.

40. Williamson SR. Clear cell papillary renal cell carcinoma: an update after 15 years. Pathology 2021; 53:109–19.

41. Aron M, Chang E, Herrera L, et al. Clear cell-papillary renal cell carcinoma of the kidney not associated with end-stage renal disease: clinico-pathologic correlation with expanded immunophenotypic and molecular characterization of a large cohort with emphasis on relationship with renal angiomyoadenomatous tumor. Am J Surg Pathol 2015;39:873–88.

42. Zhao J, Eyzaguirre E. Clear cell papillary renal cell carcinoma. Arch Pathol Lab Med 2019;143: 1154–8.

43. Aydin H, Chen L, Cheng L, et al. Clear cell tubulo-papillary renal cell carcinoma: a study of 36 distinctive low-grade epithelial tumors of the kidney. Am J Surg Pathol 2010;34:1608–21.

44. Lawrie CH, Larrea E, Larrinaga G, et al. Targeted next-generation sequencing and non-coding RNA expression analysis of clear cell papillary renal cell carcinoma suggests distinct pathological mechanisms from other renal tumour subtypes. J Pathol 2014;232:32–42.

45. Massari F, Ciccarese C, Hes O, et al. The tumor entity denominated "clear cell-papillary renal cell carcinoma" according to the WHO 2016 new classification, have the clinical characters of a renal cell adenoma as does harbor a benign outcome. Pathol Oncol Res 2018;24:447–56.

46. Morlote DM, Harada S, Batista D, et al. Clear cell papillary renal cell carcinoma: molecular profile and virtual karyotype. Hum Pathol 2019;91:52–60.

47. Steward JE, Kern SQ, Cheng L, et al. Clear cell papillary renal cell carcinoma: Characteristics and survival outcomes from a large single institutional series. Urol Oncol 2021;39:370.e321–5.

48. Cheville J, Helenon O, Hes O, et al. WHO classification of tumours online: urinary and male genital tumours: clear cell papillary renal cell tumor. 2022. Available at: https://tumourclassification. iarc.who.int/welcome/. Accessed March 15, 2022.

49. Gandhi JS, Malik F, Amin MB, et al. MiT family translocation renal cell carcinomas: a 15th anniversary update. Histol Histopathol 2020;35:125–36.

50. de Jong B, Molenaar IM, Leeuw JA, et al. Cytogenetics of a renal adenocarcinoma in a 2-year-old child. Cancer Genet Cytogenet 1986;21:165–9.

51. Caliò A, Harada S, Brunelli M, et al. TFEB rearranged renal cell carcinoma. A clinicopathologic and molecular study of 13 cases. Tumors harboring MALAT1-TFEB, ACTB-TFEB, and the novel NEAT1-TFEB translocations constantly express PDL1. Mod Pathol 2021;34:842–50.

52. Xia QY, Wang XT, Ye SB, et al. Novel gene fusion of PRCC-MITF defines a new member of MiT family translocation renal cell carcinoma: clinicopathological analysis and detection of the gene fusion by RNA sequencing and FISH. Histopathology 2018;72:786–94.

53. Lang M, Vocke CD, Ricketts CJ, et al. Clinical and Molecular Characterization of Microphthalmia-associated Transcription Factor (MITF)-related Renal Cell Carcinoma. Urology 2021;149:89–97.

54. Bakouny Z, Sadagopan A, Ravi P, et al. Integrative clinical and molecular characterization of translocation renal cell carcinoma. Cell Rep 2022;38:110190.

55. Akgul M, Saeed O, Levy D, et al. Morphologic and immunohistochemical characteristics of fluorescent in situ hybridization confirmed TFE3-gene fusion associated renal cell carcinoma: a single institutional cohort. Am J Surg Pathol 2020;44:1450–8.

56. Skala SL, Xiao H, Udager AM, et al. Detection of 6 TFEB-amplified renal cell carcinomas and 25 renal cell carcinomas with MITF translocations: systematic morphologic analysis of 85 cases evaluated by clinical TFE3 and TFEB FISH assays. Mod Pathol 2018;31:179–97.

57. Kato I, Furuya M, Baba M, et al. RBM10-TFE3 renal cell carcinoma characterised by paracentric inversion with consistent closely split signals in break-apart fluorescence in-situ hybridisation: study of 10 cases and a literature review. Histopathology 2019;75:254–65.

58. Kuthi L, Somorácz Á, Micsik T, et al. Clinicopathological findings on 28 Cases with XP11.2 renal cell carcinoma. Pathol Oncol Res 2020;26:2123–33.

59. Argani P, Zhong M, Reuter VE, et al. TFE3-fusion variant analysis defines specific clinicopathologic associations among Xp11 translocation cancers. Am J Surg Pathol 2016;40:723–37.

60. Classe M, Malouf GG, Su X, et al. Incidence, clinicopathological features and fusion transcript landscape of translocation renal cell carcinomas. Histopathology 2017;70:1089–97.

61. Zhong M, De Angelo P, Osborne L, et al. Dual-color, break-apart FISH assay on paraffin-embedded tissues as an adjunct to diagnosis of Xp11 translocation renal cell carcinoma and alveolar soft part sarcoma. Am J Surg Pathol 2010;34:757–66.

62. Sidhar SK, Clark J, Gill S, et al. The t(X;1)(p11.2;q21.2) translocation in papillary renal cell carcinoma fuses a novel gene PRCC to the TFE3 transcription factor gene. Hum Mol Genet 1996;5:1333–8.

63. Argani P, Antonescu CR, Illei PB, et al. Primary renal neoplasms with the ASPL-TFE3 gene fusion of alveolar soft part sarcoma: a distinctive tumor entity previously included among renal cell carcinomas of children and adolescents. Am J Pathol 2001;159:179–92.

64. Clark J, Lu YJ, Sidhar SK, et al. Fusion of splicing factor genes PSF and NonO (p54nrb) to the TFE3 gene in papillary renal cell carcinoma. Oncogene 1997;15:2233–9.

65. Argani P, Zhang L, Reuter VE, et al. RBM10-TFE3 renal cell carcinoma: a potential diagnostic pitfall due to cryptic intrachromosomal Xp11.2 inversion resulting in false-negative TFE3 FISH. Am J Surg Pathol 2017;41:655–62.

66. Antic T, Taxy JB, Alikhan M, et al. Melanotic translocation renal cell carcinoma with a novel ARID1B-TFE3 gene fusion. Am J Surg Pathol 2017;41:1576–80.

67. Fukuda H, Kato I, Furuya M, et al. A novel partner of TFE3 in the Xp11 translocation renal cell carcinoma: clinicopathological analyses and detection of EWSR1-TFE3 fusion. Virchows Arch 2019;474:389–93.

68. Pei J, Cooper H, Flieder DB, et al. NEAT1-TFE3 and KAT6A-TFE3 renal cell carcinomas, new members of MiT family translocation renal cell carcinoma. Mod Pathol 2019;32:710–6.

69. Ye H, Qin S, Li N, et al. A Rare Partner of TFE3 in the Xp11 Translocation Renal Cell Carcinoma: Clinicopathological Analyses and Detection of MED15-TFE3 Fusion. Biomed Res Int 2019;2019:5974089.

70. Akgul M, Williamson SR, Ertoy D, et al. Diagnostic approach in TFE3-rearranged renal cell carcinoma: a multi-institutional international survey. J Clin Pathol 2021;74:291–9.

71. Sharain RF, Gown AM, Greipp PT, et al. Immunohistochemistry for TFE3 lacks specificity and sensitivity in the diagnosis of TFE3-rearranged neoplasms: a comparative, 2-laboratory study. Hum Pathol 2019;87:65–74.

72. Akgul M, Al-Obaidy KI, Cheng L, et al. Low-grade oncocytic tumour expands the spectrum of renal oncocytic tumours and deserves separate classification: a review of 23 cases from a single tertiary institute. J Clin Pathol 2021, online ahead of print.

73. Gupta S, Rowsey RA, Cheville JC, et al. Morphologic overlap between low-grade oncocytic tumor and eosinophilic variant of chromophobe renal cell carcinoma. Hum Pathol 2022;119:114–6.

74. Kravtsov O, Gupta S, Cheville JC, et al. Low-grade oncocytic tumor of kidney (CK7-Positive, CD117-Negative): incidence in a single institutional experience with clinicopathological and molecular characteristics. Hum Pathol 2021;114:9–18.

75. Morini A, Drossart T, Timsit MO, et al. Low-grade oncocytic renal tumor (LOT): mutations in mTOR pathway genes and low expression of FOXI1. Mod Pathol 2022;35:352–60.

76. Siadat F, Trpkov K. ESC, ALK, HOT and LOT: three letter acronyms of emerging renal entities knocking on the door of the WHO classification. Cancers (Basel) 2020;12:168.

77. Trpkov K, Williamson SR, Gao Y, et al. Low-grade oncocytic tumour of kidney (CD117-negative, cytokeratin 7-positive): a distinct entity? Histopathology 2019;75:174–84.

78. Trpkov K, Williamson SR, Gill AJ, et al. Novel, emerging and provisional renal entities: the genitourinary pathology society (GUPS) update on renal neoplasia. Mod Pathol 2021;34:1167–84.

79. Zhang HZ, Xia QY, Wang SY, et al. Low-grade oncocytic tumor of kidney harboring TSC/MTOR mutation: clinicopathologic, immunohistochemical and molecular characteristics support a distinct entity. Virchows Arch 2022;480:999–1008.

80. Farcas M, Gatalica Z, Trpkov K, et al. Eosinophilic vacuolated tumor (EVT) of kidney demonstrates sporadic TSC/MTOR mutations: next-generation sequencing multi-institutional study of 19 cases. Mod Pathol 2022;35:344–51.

81. He H, Trpkov K, Martinek P, et al. High-grade oncocytic renal tumor": morphologic, immunohistochemical, and molecular genetic study of 14 cases. Virchows Arch 2018;473:725–38.

82. Kapur P, Gao M, Zhong H, et al. Eosinophilic vacuolated tumor of the kidney: a review of evolving concepts in this novel subtype with additional insights from a case with MTOR Mutation and concomitant chromosome 1 loss. Adv Anat Pathol 2021;28:251–7.

83. Aldera AP, Hes O. Eosinophilic solid and cystic renal cell carcinoma with melanin pigment-expanding the morphological spectrum. Int J Surg Pathol 2022;30:295–9.

84. McKenney JK, Przybycin CG, Trpkov K, et al. Eosinophilic solid and cystic renal cell carcinomas have metastatic potential. Histopathology 2018;72:1066–7.

85. Mehra R, Vats P, Cao X, et al. Somatic Bi-allelic loss of TSC Genes in eosinophilic solid and cystic renal cell carcinoma. Eur Urol 2018;74:483–6.

86. Munari E, Settanni G, Caliò A, et al. TSC loss is a clonal event in eosinophilic solid and cystic renal cell carcinoma: a multiregional tumor sampling study. Mod Pathol 2022;35:376–85.

87. Tretiakova MS. Eosinophilic solid and cystic renal cell carcinoma mimicking epithelioid angiomyolipoma: series of 4 primary tumors and 2 metastases. Hum Pathol 2018;80:65–75.

88. Trpkov K, Abou-Ouf H, Hes O, et al. Eosinophilic solid and cystic renal cell carcinoma (ESC RCC): further morphologic and molecular characterization of ESC RCC as a distinct entity. Am J Surg Pathol 2017;41:1299–308.

89. Trpkov K, Hes O, Bonert M, et al. Eosinophilic, solid, and cystic renal cell carcinoma: clinicopathologic study of 16 unique, sporadic neoplasms occurring in women. Am J Surg Pathol 2016;40:60–71.

90. Amin MB, Crotty TB, Tickoo SK, et al. Renal oncocytoma: a reappraisal of morphologic features with clinicopathologic findings in 80 cases. Am J Surg Pathol 1997;21:1–12.

91. Al-Obaidy KI, Cheng L. Renal oncocytoma with adverse pathologic features: a clinical and pathologic study of 50 cases. Mod Pathol 2021;34:1947–54.

92. Williamson SR, Gadde R, Trpkov K, et al. Diagnostic criteria for oncocytic renal neoplasms: a survey of urologic pathologists. Hum Pathol 2017;63:149–56.

93. Hes O, Michal M, Boudova L, et al. Small cell variant of renal oncocytoma–a rare and misleading type of benign renal tumor. Int J Surg Pathol 2001;9:215–22.

94. Kuroda N, Yorita K, Naroda T, et al. Renal oncocytoma, small cell variant, with pseudorosettes, showing cyclin D1 expression and tubulovesicular cristae of mitochondria. Pathol Int 2016;66:409–10.

95. Li K, Wang C, Xiong X, et al. Small-cell variant renal oncocytoma: case report on its clinicopathological and genetic characteristics and literature review. Gene 2020;730:144266.

96. Magro G, Gardiman MP, Lopes MR, et al. Small-cell variant of renal oncocytoma with dominating solid growth pattern: a potential diagnostic pitfall. Virchows Arch 2006;448:379–80.

97. Williamson SR. Renal Oncocytoma With Perinephric Fat Invasion. Int J Surg Pathol 2016;24:625–6.

98. Wobker SE, Przybycin CG, Sircar K, et al. Renal oncocytoma with vascular invasion: a series of 22 cases. Hum Pathol 2016;58:1–6.

99. Sukov WR, Ketterling RP, Lager DJ, et al. CCND1 rearrangements and cyclin D1 overexpression in renal oncocytomas: frequency, clinicopathologic features, and utility in differentiation from chromophobe renal cell carcinoma. Hum Pathol 2009;40:1296–303.

100. Trpkov K, Hes O, Williamson SR, et al. New developments in existing WHO entities and evolving molecular concepts: the genitourinary pathology society (GUPS) update on renal neoplasia. Mod Pathol 2021;34:1392–424.

101. Ruiz-Cordero R, Rao P, Li L, et al. Hybrid oncocytic/chromophobe renal tumors are molecularly distinct from oncocytoma and chromophobe renal cell carcinoma. Mod Pathol 2019;32:1698–707.

102. Menko FH, van Steensel MA, Giraud S, et al. Birt-Hogg-Dubé syndrome: diagnosis and management. Lancet Oncol 2009;10:1199–206.

103. Schmidt LS, Linehan WM. FLCN: The causative gene for Birt-Hogg-Dubé syndrome. Gene 2018;640:28–42.

104. Furuya M, Hasumi H, Yao M, et al. Birt-Hogg-Dubé syndrome-associated renal cell carcinoma: Histopathological features and diagnostic conundrum. Cancer Sci 2020;111:15–22.

105. Pavlovich CP, Walther MM, Eyler RA, et al. Renal tumors in the Birt-Hogg-Dubé syndrome. Am J Surg Pathol 2002;26:1542–52.

106. Napolitano G, Di Malta C, Esposito A, et al. A substrate-specific mTORC1 pathway underlies Birt-Hogg-Dubé syndrome. Nature 2020;585:597–602.

107. Gupta S, Swanson AA, Chen YB, et al. Incidence of succinate dehydrogenase and fumarate hydratase-deficient renal cell carcinoma based on immunohistochemical screening with SDHA/SDHB and FH/2SC. Hum Pathol 2019;91:114–22.

108. Wang G, Rao P. Succinate dehydrogenase-deficient renal cell carcinoma: a short review. Arch Pathol Lab Med 2018;142:1284–8.

109. Fuchs TL, Maclean F, Turchini J, et al. Expanding the clinicopathological spectrum of succinate dehydrogenase-deficient renal cell carcinoma with a focus on variant morphologies: a study of 62 new tumors in 59 patients. Mod Pathol 2022;35:836–49.

110. Aggarwal RK, Luchtel RA, Machha V, et al. Functional succinate dehydrogenase deficiency is a common adverse feature of clear cell renal cancer. Proc Natl Acad Sci U S A 2021;118, e2106947118.

111. Williamson SR, Hornick JL, Eble JN, et al. Renal cell carcinoma with angioleiomyoma-like stroma and clear cell papillary renal cell carcinoma: exploring SDHB protein immunohistochemistry and the relationship to tuberous sclerosis complex. Hum Pathol 2018;75:10–5.

112. Mancilla-Jimenez R, Stanley RJ, Blath RA. Papillary renal cell carcinoma: a clinical, radiologic, and pathologic study of 34 cases. Cancer 1976;38:2469–80.

113. Li CX, Lu Q, Huang BJ, et al. Routine or enhanced imaging to differentiate between type 1 and type 2 papillary renal cell carcinoma. Clin Radiol 2021;76:135–42.

114. Magers MJ, Perrino CM, Cramer HM, et al. Cytomorphologic comparison of type 1 and type 2 papillary renal cell carcinoma: a retrospective analysis of 28 cases. Cancer Cytopathol 2019;127:370–6.

115. Motoshima T, Komohara Y, Ma C, et al. PD-L1 expression in papillary renal cell carcinoma. BMC Urol 2017;17:8.

116. Murugan P, Jia L, Dinatale RG, et al. Papillary renal cell carcinoma: a single institutional study of 199 cases addressing classification, clinicopathologic and molecular features, and treatment outcome. Mod Pathol 2022;35:825–35.

117. Ravaud A, Oudard S, De Fromont M, et al. First-line treatment with sunitinib for type 1 and type 2 locally advanced or metastatic papillary renal cell carcinoma: a phase II study (SUPAP) by the French Genitourinary Group (GETUG). Ann Oncol 2015;26:1123–8.

118. Ungari M, Trombatore M, Ferrero G, et al. Eosinophilic cytoplasmic inclusions in type 2 papillary renal cell carcinoma. Pathologica 2019;111:369–74.

119. Warrick JI, Tsodikov A, Kunju LP, et al. Papillary renal cell carcinoma revisited: a comprehensive histomorphologic study with outcome correlations. Hum Pathol 2014;45:1139–46.

120. Wong ECL, Di Lena R, Breau RH, et al. Morphologic subtyping as a prognostic predictor for survival in papillary renal cell carcinoma: Type 1 vs. type 2. Urol Oncol 2019;37:721–6.

121. Williamson SR, Gill AJ, Argani P, et al. Report from the international society of urological pathology (ISUP) consultation conference on molecular pathology of urogenital cancers: III: molecular pathology of kidney cancer. Am J Surg Pathol 2020;44:e47–65.

122. Linehan WM, Spellman PT, Ricketts CJ, et al. Comprehensive molecular characterization of papillary renal-cell carcinoma. N Engl J Med 2016;374:135–45.

123. Srigley JR, Delahunt B, Eble JN, et al. The international society of urological pathology (ISUP) vancouver classification of renal neoplasia. Am J Surg Pathol 2013;37:1469–89.

124. Al-Obaidy KI, Eble JN, Cheng L, et al. Papillary renal neoplasm with reverse polarity: a morphologic, immunohistochemical, and molecular study. Am J Surg Pathol 2019;43:1099–111.

125. Saleeb RM, Brimo F, Farag M, et al. Toward biological subtyping of papillary renal cell carcinoma with clinical implications through histologic, immunohistochemical, and molecular analysis. Am J Surg Pathol 2017;41:1618–29.

126. Kunju LP, Wojno K, Wolf JS Jr, et al. Papillary renal cell carcinoma with oncocytic cells and nonoverlapping low grade nuclei: expanding the morphologic spectrum with emphasis on clinicopathologic, immunohistochemical and molecular features. Hum Pathol 2008;39:96–101.

127. Al-Obaidy KI, Eble JN, Nassiri M, et al. Recurrent KRAS mutations in papillary renal neoplasm with reverse polarity. Mod Pathol 2020;33:1157–64.

128. Wei S, Kutikov A, Patchefsky AS, et al. Papillary renal neoplasm with reverse polarity is often cystic: report of 7 cases and review of 93 cases in the literature. Am J Surg Pathol 2022;46:336–43.

129. Zhou L, Xu J, Wang S, et al. Papillary renal neoplasm with reverse polarity: a clinicopathologic study of 7 cases. Int J Surg Pathol 2020;28:728–34.

130. Parwani AV, Husain AN, Epstein JI, et al. Low-grade myxoid renal epithelial neoplasms with distal nephron differentiation. Hum Pathol 2001;32:506–12.

131. Billis A. Phenotypic, molecular and ultrastructural studies of a novel low grade renal epithelial neoplasm possibly related to the loop of Henle. Int Braz J Urol 2002;28:477–8.

132. Fine SW, Argani P, DeMarzo AM, et al. Expanding the histologic spectrum of mucinous tubular and spindle cell carcinoma of the kidney. Am J Surg Pathol 2006;30:1554–60.

133. Yang C, Cimera RS, Aryeequaye R, et al. Adverse histology, homozygous loss of CDKN2A/B, and complex genomic alterations in locally advanced/metastatic renal mucinous tubular and

spindle cell carcinoma. Mod Pathol 2021;34:445–56.

134. Ren Q, Wang L, Al-Ahmadie HA, et al. Distinct genomic copy number alterations distinguish mucinous tubular and spindle cell carcinoma of the kidney from papillary renal cell carcinoma with overlapping histologic features. Am J Surg Pathol 2018;42:767–77.

135. Wang L, Zhang Y, Chen YB, et al. VSTM2A overexpression is a sensitive and specific biomarker for mucinous tubular and spindle cell carcinoma (MTSCC) of the kidney. Am J Surg Pathol 2018;42:1571–84.

136. Lau HD, Chan E, Fan AC, et al. A clinicopathologic and molecular analysis of fumarate hydratase-deficient renal cell carcinoma in 32 patients. Am J Surg Pathol 2020;44:98–110.

137. Buelow B, Cohen J, Nagymanyoki Z, et al. Immunohistochemistry for 2-succinocysteine (2SC) and fumarate hydratase (FH) in cutaneous leiomyomas may aid in identification of patients With HLRCC (Hereditary Leiomyomatosis and Renal Cell Carcinoma Syndrome). Am J Surg Pathol 2016;40:982–8.

138. Ezekian B, Englum B, Gilmore BF, et al. Renal medullary carcinoma: a national analysis of 159 patients. Pediatr Blood Cancer 2017;64:e26609.

139. Baniak N, Tsai H, Hirsch MS. The differential diagnosis of medullary-based renal masses. Arch Pathol Lab Med 2021;145:1148–70.

140. Calderaro J, Moroch J, Pierron G, et al. SMARCB1/INI1 inactivation in renal medullary carcinoma. Histopathology 2012;61:428–35.

141. Jia L, Carlo MI, Khan H, et al. Distinctive mechanisms underlie the loss of SMARCB1 protein expression in renal medullary carcinoma: morphologic and molecular analysis of 20 cases. Mod Pathol 2019;32:1329–43.

142. Bratslavsky G, Gleicher S, Jacob JM, et al. Comprehensive genomic profiling of metastatic collecting duct carcinoma, renal medullary carcinoma, and clear cell renal cell carcinoma. Urol Oncol 2021;39:367.e361–5.

Kidney Tumors
New and Emerging Kidney Tumor Entities

Farshid Siadat, MD, FRCPC[a], Mehdi Mansoor, MD, FRCPC[a],
Ondrej Hes, MD, PhD[b,1], Kiril Trpkov, MD, FRCPC[a,*]

KEYWORDS

- Kidney • Renal cell carcinoma • Unclassified renal tumor • Unclassified renal cell carcinoma
- Novel entities • Pathology • WHO • GUPS

Key points

- Several novel and emerging renal entities have been recently characterized, owing to the rapid acquisition of new evidence and knowledge.
- This review summarizes the current state of the art on several new and emerging renal entities, including eosinophilic solid and cystic renal cell carcinoma, renal cell carcinoma with fibromyomatous stroma, anaplastic lymphoma kinase-rearranged renal cell carcinoma, low-grade oncocytic renal tumor, eosinophilic vacuolated tumor, thyroid-like follicular renal cell carcinoma, and biphasic hyalinizing psammomatous renal cell carcinoma.
- Pathologists played a key role in characterizing these new and emerging tumors; importantly the diagnosis of most of them rests primarily on recognizing their morphologic features with the aid of immunohistochemistry.
- We hope that this updated review will promote awareness of these entities, and will stimulate additional studies for their further characterization, resulting in more accurate diagnosis and improved patient prognostication and management.

ABSTRACT

This review summarizes current knowledge on several novel and emerging renal entities, including eosinophilic solid and cystic renal cell carcinoma (RCC), RCC with fibromyomatous stroma, anaplastic lymphoma kinase-rearranged RCC, low-grade oncocytic renal tumor, eosinophilic vacuolated tumor, thyroidlike follicular RCC, and biphasic hyalinizing psammomatous RCC. Their clinical features, gross and microscopic morphology, immunohistochemistry, and molecular and genetic features are described. The diagnosis of most of them rests on recognizing their morphologic features using immunohistochemistry. Accurate diagnosis of these entitles will further reduce the category of "unclassifiable renal carcinomas/tumors" and will lead to better clinical management and improved patient prognostication.

EOSINOPHILIC SOLID AND CYSTIC RENAL CELL CARCINOMA

INTRODUCTION

Eosinophilic solid and cystic renal cell carcinoma (ESC RCC) is a recently characterized renal cell

[a] Department of Pathology and Laboratory Medicine, Cumming School of Medicine, University of Calgary, Rockyview General Hospital, 7007 14 Street, Calgary, Alberta T2V 1P9, Canada; [b] Department of Pathology, Charles University in Prague, Faculty of Medicine in Plzeň, University Hospital Plzen, Alej Svobody 80, 304 60 Pilsen, Czech Republic
[1] Deceased July 2, 2022
* Corresponding author.
E-mail address: kiril.trpkov@albertaprecisionlabs.ca
Twitter: @FSiadat (F.S.); Twitter: @Kiril_T_Can (K.T.)

Surgical Pathology 15 (2022) 713–728
https://doi.org/10.1016/j.path.2022.07.006

surgpath.theclinics.com

neoplasm demonstrating a unique set of clinical, microscopic, immunohistochemical, and molecular features.[1,2] Such tumors were likely designated previously as "unclassified RCC" or "unclassified renal neoplasm/RCC with oncocytic/eosinophilic features."

CLINICAL FEATURES

ESC RCC is typically sporadic and solitary tumor, found in patients of broad age range; most tumors are identified in females.[1–3] A subset has been documented in patients with tuberous sclerosis complex (TSC).[4,5] Although a great majority of ESC RCCs have indolent behavior, rare tumors with metastatic disease have also been reported, warranting the designation of "carcinoma" for this entity.[6–8]

GROSS

As the descriptive name implies, solid and cystic components are the main gross features of ESC RCC. The tumors are well delineated, but nonencapsulated, and show a variable mix of solid parts and macrocysts. The cysts range from few millimeters to few centimeters. Rare cases have predominantly solid growth, with only rare microcysts. Tumor cut section is yellow, gray, and tan. Reported size varied broadly, but most tumors are less than 5 cm in size.[1,2]

MICROSCOPY

The solid parts are composed of eosinophilic cells exhibiting diffuse, compact acinar, or nested growth (Fig. 1A–B).[1,2] Scattered foamy histiocytes and lymphocytes are also common, as are psammoma bodies. A characteristic feature is the presence of coarse, basophilic to purple, cytoplasmic granules (stippling). The nuclei are round to oval with focally prominent nucleoli. Focal papillary growth, clear cell areas, focal insular or tubular growth, and clusters of multinucleated cells can also be found.

IMMUNOHISTOCHEMISTRY

ESC RCC shows either diffuse or focal CK20 expression (see **Fig. 1**C), although rare cases may be CK20 negative.[1,2] CK7 is typically negative or very focally positive. At least focal cathepsin K expression has been documented in a great majority of cases. Other positive stains include PAX8, AE1/AE3, CK8/18, and vimentin. Negative stains include CD117 and CAIX; HMB45 and melan-A are also negative in a great majority of cases, although rare cases show focal reactivity.

MOLECULAR AND GENETIC FINDINGS

Most sporadic ESC RCCs have recurrent, somatic biallelic losses or mutations in *TSC2* and *TSC1*. A subset of tumors has been identified in patients with TSC. These genetic changes result in dysregulation of the mammalian target of rapamycin (mTOR) signaling pathway.[6,9,10]

DIFFERENTIAL DIAGNOSIS

1. Oncocytoma: Typically lacks large cysts; cells have homogeneous oncocytic cytoplasm, without coarse granules. Immunohistochemistry (IHC): CD117+/CK20−/vimentin− (vs ESC RCC: CD117−/CK20+/vimentin+).

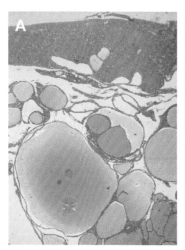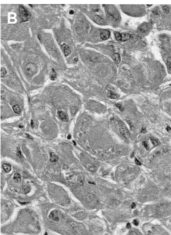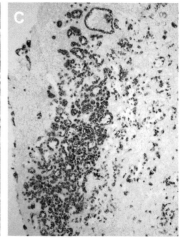

Fig. 1. ESC RCC. (*A*) At low power, it is an eosinophilic tumor that shows solid and cystic components; the cysts vary in size from macroscopic to microscopic. (*B*) The cells have voluminous eosinophilic cytoplasm with characteristic coarse cytoplasmic granules (stippling). (*C*) ESC RCC is typically CK20 positive (either diffuse or focal).

2. Chromophobe RCC, eosinophilic: Typically lacks large cysts, and cells lack coarse granules; irregular (raisinoid) nuclei with perinuclear halos are typical. IHC: CD117+/CK7+/CK20−/vimentin− (vs ESC RCC: CD117−/CK7−/CK20+/vimentin+).

3. SDH-deficient RCC: Cells have more flocculent cytoplasm and intracytoplasmic vacuoles. IHC: SDHB−/CK20−.

4. Epithelioid angiomyolipoma: Typically lacks large cysts (although smaller cysts can be present in some cases); cells lack coarse granules. IHC: PAX8−/CK20− (vs ESC RCC: PAX8+/CK20+).

RENAL CELL CARCINOMA WITH FIBROMYOMATOUS STROMA

INTRODUCTION

Renal cell carcinoma with fibromyomatous stroma (RCC FMS) was described by Canzonieri and colleagues[11] in 1993, named as *mixed renal tumor with carcinomatous and fibroleiomyomatous components*. Over the years, various names were used in the literature to describe this entity, including: *RCC with prominent smooth muscle stroma*, *mixed renal tumor with carcinomatous and fibroleiomyomatous components*, *RCC associated with prominent angioleiomyoma-like proliferation*, *clear cell RCC with smooth muscle stroma*, and *RCC with clear cells, smooth muscle stroma, and negativity for 3p deletion*.[12] The name renal cell carcinoma with fibromyomatous stroma was officially endorsed by the Genitourinary Pathology Society (GUPS) in 2021, based on a broad consensus.[14] Recently published fifth edition of World Health Organization (WHO) classification of genitourinary tumors refers to this tumor as "renal cell carcinoma with prominent leiomyomatous stroma."[13]

CLINICAL FEATURES

RCC FMS occurs more frequently in women (male:female [M:F] = 1:2) and is seen in adults of broad age range. The tumor is usually sporadic, but rare cases had familial association with TSC.[15] The prognosis is generally good and a great majority of cases had an indolent clinical course.[14,16,17] One case has been reported with lymph node metastasis in a patient with tuberous sclerosis and multifocal tumors.[18]

GROSS

RCC FMS is a well-circumscribed, solid tumor, usually of small size (mean: 2.7 cm). Cut surface has a tan-brown color, often with lobulated appearance due to fibromyomatous septae.[12,19,20]

MICROSCOPY

RCC FMS is typically composed of an epithelial neoplastic component, often forming nodules, separated by and admixed with a fibromuscular stromal component (Fig. 2A). The epithelial component consists of cells with voluminous clear cytoplasm, arranged in solid sheets, nests, branching tubules, and focal papillary structures (see Fig. 2B–C). The nuclei are WHO grade 2 or 3 (equivalent). The fibromyomatous stromal component can be variable and often appears more prominent at the periphery of the tumor.[12,14,19]

IMMUNOHISTOCHEMISTRY

The characteristic IHC profile for RCC FMS includes diffuse positivity for CK7 (see Fig. 2D), as well as CAIX and CD10.[14,16,21] CAIX staining is usually diffuse membranous, but focally it can be cup shaped. Other positive stains include vimentin and high-molecular-weight cytokeratin. AMACR is typically negative. CK20 has been found positive in an apical pattern in some cases.[22]

MOLECULAR AND GENETIC FINDINGS

Molecular studies have provided evidence of association of RCC FMS with mutations involving the TSC/MTOR pathway.[14,16,22] A subset of tumors has shown mutations of *ELOC* (previously known as *TCEB1*) and monosomy of chromosome 8.[23] Unlike conventional clear cell RCC, these tumors are not associated with loss of heterozygosity (LOH) in chromosome 3p or *VHL* mutations.[14,24] Fibromyomatous stroma has been shown to be polyclonal and nonneoplastic.[24]

DIFFERENTIAL DIAGNOSIS

1. Clear cell RCC: Typically lacks fibromyomatous stroma (although rare cases may show focally prominent stroma). Focal papillary structures are not usually present. IHC: CK7 is negative (or only focally positive); CD10 and AMACR are usually positive.

2. Clear cell papillary renal cell tumor: Cells have scant clear cytoplasm and form tubular and focal papillary structures. The nuclei are of lower grade (WHO/ISUP grade1 equivalent) and have a linear arrangement along the luminal surface. IHC: diffuse positivity for CAIX (cup shaped, not box shaped) and CK7, but CD10 is negative, as is AMACR.

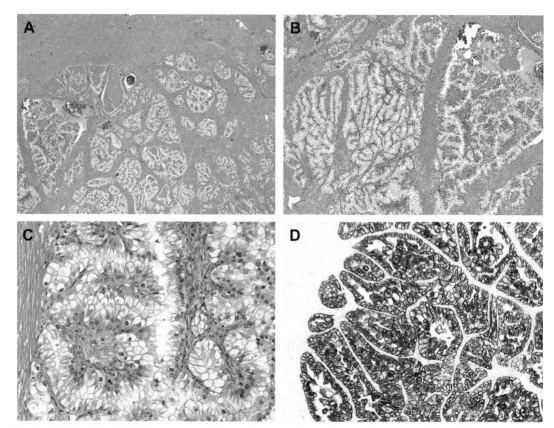

Fig. 2. RCC FMS. (A) RCC FMS has a clear cell morphology, with epithelial cells organized in lobules, separated by fibromuscular stroma. (B) The epithelial component often forms compact branching tubules (left) and focal papillary formations (right). (C) At high power, the nuclei are enlarged and may show more prominent nucleoli. (D) CK7 is typically diffusely positive.

ANAPLASTIC LYMPHOMA KINASE-REARRANGED RENAL CELL CARCINOMA

INTRODUCTION

Anaplastic lymphoma kinase-rearranged renal cell carcinoma (ALK RCC) is a renal entity first described in 2011.[25,26] ALK RCC is listed in the 2022 fifth edition of WHO classification of genitourinary tumors as a molecularly defined entity.[13] ALK RCC is characterized by an *ALK* gene fusion with various partner genes, leading to aberrant *ALK* activation. *ALK* rearrangement can be identified either by ALK protein expression on IHC, fluorescence in situ hybridization (FISH), or by sequencing methods. ALK RCC is a clinically important diagnosis because targeted therapies with ALK inhibitors are available and can be used as in other *ALK* rearrangement-associated neoplasms.[27,28]

CLINICAL FEATURES

ALK RCCs have been reported in patients of wide age range, including pediatric and adolescent patients with sickle cell trait, as well as adult patients who typically did not harbor a sickle cell trait.[29] ALK RCC is not associated with other extrarenal tumors harboring ALK rearrangement. ALK RCC is slightly more common in males (M:F = 1.5:1). Patients had a diverse racial background, including African American, Caucasian, and Asian. ALK RCCs are indolent in most cases, although some may show aggressive clinical course, including metastasis and death.

GROSS

ALK RCC usually presents as a solitary and circumscribed tumor, often less than 5 cm in size; it may be solid or solid-cystic, with tan-gray or variegated cut surface. Pseudocapsule of varying thickness can also be found.

MICROSCOPY

ALK RCC typically demonstrates variable and diverse morphology with no characteristic or specific morphologic features. The growth patterns may include papillary, solid, tubular, trabecular cystic, cribriform, signet-ring, single cells, "mucinous tubular and spindle cell RCC-like" and "metanephric adenoma-like" (Fig. 3A–C).[14,29] However, mucinous or myxoid component (intracellular or interstitial) has been commonly found. Thus, a diagnostic consideration of ALK RCC and screening for ALK should be done in all difficult-to-classify renal tumors with variable and admixed patterns, unusual morphologies, or containing a mucinous component. Psammoma bodies and tumor necrosis are also common.

IMMUNOHISTOCHEMISTRY

ALK protein expression by IHC, typically diffuse cytoplasmic and membranous, is a defining feature of ALK RCC (see Fig. 3D). Remaining immunoprofile is nonspecific and includes reactivity for PAX8, CK7, vimentin, INI1 (retained), 34βE12, and AMACR. Negative IHC stains include CK20, GATA3, melan-A, HMB45, S100, and cathepsin K.[14,29] TFE3 reactivity by IHC was

reported in some cases, but without evidence of TFE3 rearrangement by FISH.[30]

MOLECULAR AND GENETIC FINDINGS

Several ALK fusion partners were identified in ALK RCC, including VCL, HOOK1, STRN, TPM3, EML4, and PLEKHA7.[14] A recent multi-institutional study reported 3 additional fusion partners CLIP1, KIF5B, and KIAA1217.[29]

DIFFERENTIAL DIAGNOSIS

The differential diagnosis of ALK RCC is broad, because its heterogeneous morphology may mimic a wide spectrum of other renal tumors, including SMARCB1-deficient renal medullary carcinoma (in children and adolescents), papillary RCC, MiTF RCC (TFE3 and TFEB), rhabdoid RCC (or clear cell RCC with rhabdoid features), collecting duct carcinoma, metanephric adenoma, mucinous tubular and spindle cell RCC, or unclassifiable RCC/tumor. A negative ALK IHC along with

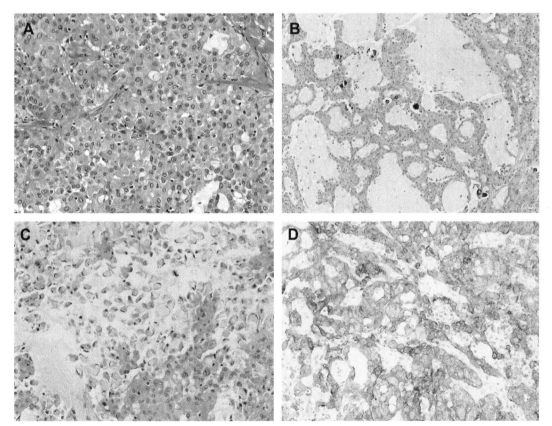

Fig. 3. ALK RCC. (A–C) ALK RCC shows mixed and variable patterns occurring in the same tumor, including, for example, solid areas (A); papillary, trabecular and tubulocystic areas, often with scattered psammomatous calcification (B); and focal single signet-ring cells (C). Note the extracellular mucinous background (B) and intracellular mucin in the signet-ring cells (C). (D) ALK expression is uniformly positive.

more specific immunomarkers for certain entities may help rule out ALK RCC.

EOSINOPHILIC VACUOLATED TUMOR

INTRODUCTION

Eosinophilic vacuolated tumor (EVT) is a recently described renal entity that emerged from the group of eosinophilic/oncocytic tumors with shared features between renal oncocytoma and chromophobe RCC.[31–33] EVT was described by He and colleagues[34] (as high-grade oncocytic tumor [HOT])[34] and by Chen and colleagues[35] (as sporadic RCC with eosinophilic and vacuolated cytoplasm). The recent GUPS consensus proposed the name *eosinophilic vacuolated tumor* for this entity.[14] EVT was also identified in some patients with TSC.[22,36–38] The 2022 fifth edition of WHO classification regards this tumor as one of the two emerging entities within the broader category of "other oncocytic tumors."[13]

CLINICAL FEATURES

EVT is found in patients of broad age range and occurs more frequently in women (M:F = 1:2.5).[14,34,35,39] All reported EVT cases had benign behavior, without evidence of recurrence or metastatic disease.[14,39,40]

GROSS

EVT is mostly a solitary and sporadic tumor of smaller size, about 3 to 4 cm in greatest dimension, although rare EVTs have been documented exceeding 10 cm.[34,35,38,39] EVT is typically solid, gray, or tan to brown tumor.[14,34,35,38,39]

MICROSCOPY

EVT has a diffuse and solid growth, often admixed with nested and tubulocystic foci. Thick-walled vessels are virtually always present at the periphery, but a well-formed capsule is lacking. The cells have an eosinophilic cytoplasm and prominent intracytoplasmic vacuoles (Fig. 4A). The nuclei are round to oval, with prominent nucleoli that focally can be quite large and resemble viral inclusion.[34,35]

IMMUNOHISTOCHEMISTRY AND ELECTRON MICROSCOPY

EVT is positive for CD117 (KIT), CD10, antimitochondrial antigen antibody, and cathepsin K, in some cases focally (see Fig. 4B); CK7 is typically expressed only in rare, scattered cells.[34,39] The immunoprofile "CD117+ and CK7+ only in rare cells" resembles that of an oncocytoma. EVT is negative for vimentin. Fumarate hydratase (FH) and succinate dehydrogenase B (SDHB) are retained. p-S6 and p-4EBP1, markers associated with mTOR pathway activation, have also been found to be expressed in EVT.[35]

On electron microscopy, EVT demonstrated numerous intracytoplasmic mitochondria, as well as dilated cisterns of rough endoplasmic reticulum.[38,40]

MOLECULAR AND GENETIC FINDINGS

Losses of chromosomes 1 and 19p were frequently found in EVT, along with loss of heterozygosity at 16p11 and 7q31.[34] However, complete losses or gains of other chromosomes, as in chromophobe RCC, have not been found. *TSC/mTOR* mutations seem to be consistent molecular findings in EVT.[35,38] In a recent study, Farcas and colleagues[39] demonstrated nonoverlapping mutations in *MTOR*, *TSC2*, and *TSC1* in all evaluated cases, associated with low mutational burden. Thus, EVT is associated with either germline or somatic mutations leading to mTORC1 activation.[38]

DIFFERENTIAL DIAGNOSIS

1. Hybrid oncocytic tumor (Birt-Hogg Dubé syndrome): Typically multiple/bilateral tumors with hybrid (oncocytoma/chromophobe RCC-like) look; no stromal areas; often scattered cells with clear cytoplasm (mosaic pattern); the nuclei are typically low-grade and without prominent nucleoli; may show perinuclear halos. IHC: CD117+, CK7+ only focally, cathepsin K+/− (limited data).
2. Oncocytoma: Can show tubulocystic growth; cells lack perinuclear halos; stromal archipelaginous areas are present containing larger cell aggregates. IHC: CD117+, CK7+ only in scattered cells, but cathepsin K− and often CD10−.
3. Chromophobe RCC, classic: Cells usually have more prominent membranes and show irregular (raisinoid) nuclei with uniform perinuclear halos. IHC: CD117+, CK7+, but cathepsin K− and often CD10−.
4. SDH-deficient RCC: Cells have more flocculent cytoplasm and intracytoplasmic vacuoles; lack perinuclear halos. Edematous stromal areas with individual cells (as in LOT) can be seen. IHC: SDHB−/CD117−/CK7−.

LOW-GRADE ONCOCYTIC TUMOR

INTRODUCTION

Low-grade oncocytic tumor (LOT) is another recently described renal tumor that emerged

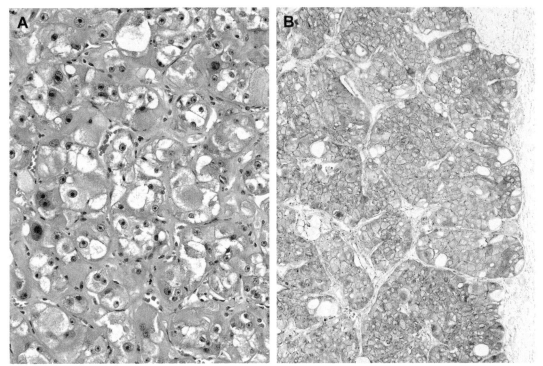

Fig. 4. EVT. (*A*) EVT is composed of eosinophilic cells with voluminous cytoplasm, typically showing prominent intracytoplasmic vacuoles, and enlarged, round to oval nuclei, often with very prominent nucleoli, imparting a "high-grade" appearance. (*B*) Cathepsin K is typically positive.

from the spectrum of eosinophilic/oncocytic tumors with shared features between renal oncocytoma and chromophobe RCC.[12,41] Rare examples have been found in patients with TSC.[42] LOT is another emerging entity included within the broader category of "other oncocytic tumors" in the fifth edition of the 2022 WHO classification.[13]

CLINICAL FEATURES

LOT is typically found as a single and incidental tumor, but multiple LOTs have also been documented, either in patients with end-stage kidney disease[43] or in patients with TSC.[42] Lerma and colleagues[37] recently reported four patients, in whom LOT was associated with other recently described renal tumors, typically found in patients with TSC, including eosinophilic solid and cystic ESC RCC, EVT, RCC FMS, as well as angiomyolipoma and papillary adenoma.[37]

LOT was identified in patients of broad age range, but usually older patients. Overall, LOT is slightly more frequent in females (M:F = 1:1.3). All reported LOTs with available follow-up have behaved in a benign fashion, without evidence of disease progression and metastatic disease.[41–46]

GROSS

LOT is usually a smaller tumor with median size between 3 and 4 cm, but similar to EVT; larger tumors have also been reported, exceeding 10 cm.[41,43,44] Grossly, LOT is a solid and compact tumor, without necrosis or cysts. Cut surface is tan-yellow to mahogany-brown, similar to oncocytoma.[41] Hemorrhagic areas may also be seen, usually more centrally.

MICROSCOPY

LOT has a diffuse and solid growth, typically showing compact nests, and focal tubular, tubuloreticular, or trabecular growth. LOT lacks a well-formed capsule, and entrapped tubules may be seen at the periphery.[14,41] The neoplastic cells are eosinophilic with round to oval nuclei, lacking significant irregularities, and may show focal perinuclear halos or clearings (Fig. 5A–B). An important finding is that of sharply delineated, edematous stromal areas with scattered individual cells that can be elongated, and may form cordlike formations ("boats in a bay"), or may have an irregular "tissue culture" arrangement.[14,41] Edematous areas often contain fresh hemorrhage. Small

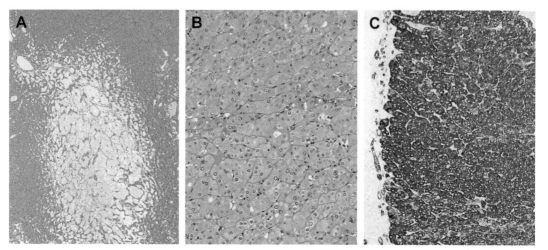

Fig. 5. LOT. (*A*) At low power, LOT is an eosinophilic solid tumor, often exhibiting sharply delineated, edematous areas with scattered individual cells ("boats in a bay"). (*B*). Higher magnification reveals eosinophilic cells with "low-grade" round to oval nuclei, and occasional perinuclear clearings. (*C*) EVT is diffusely positive for CK7 (shown) and negative for CD117 (not shown).

lymphocytic collections can also be often seen in the solid areas.[14,41] Adverse features, such as coagulative necrosis, nuclear pleomorphism, cell atypia, multinucleation, and mitotic activity are typically absent.

IMMUNOHISTOCHEMISTRY AND ELECTRON MICROSCOPY

LOT is diffusely positive for CK7 (see **Fig. 5C**) and is negative, or in rare cases, very focally and weakly positive for CD117. LOT is also positive for PAX8, e-cadherin, BerEP4, and MOC31.[41] Negative stains include CAIX, CK20, CK5/6, p63, CD15, HMB45, melan-A, cathepsin K, and vimentin. CD10 and AMACR can be either negative or focally positive. FH and SDHB are retained. LOT is consistently positive for GATA3. LOT also expresses, at least focally, p-S6 and p-4EBP1, both markers associated with mTOR pathway activation.[42,45] Another novel marker FOXI1, typically expressed in both oncocytoma and chromophobe RCC, has been recently found to be negative or with very low reactivity in LOT.[47,48] In the normal kidney, FOXI1 is positive in the intercalated cells.[48]

On electron microscopy, LOT exhibits abundant, closely packed cytoplasmic mitochondria, similar to oncocytoma.[40]

MOLECULAR AND GENETIC FEATURES

LOT shows frequent deletions at 19p13, 1p36, and 19q13, or may show a disomic chromosomal status.[41] No other complete chromosomal gains or losses were found. *CCND1* rearrangements are not found in LOT (unlike in oncocytoma, in which they are frequent).[43]

Recent studies demonstrated common involvement of the mTOR pathway genes in LOT. In one study, abnormalities in mTOR pathway genes were found in 80% (8 of 10) of evaluated LOTs, including *mTOR* (7 of 8) and *TSC1* (1 of 8).[45] Another study found somatic, likely activating, mutations in *mTOR* (4 of 6) and *RHEB* (1 of 6) in 6 evaluable LOTs; one additional patient with multiple bilateral LOTs had a pathogenic germline mutation in *TSC1* (1 of 6).[42] *TSC1* germline mutations were also found in 2 patients with *TSC* mutations who had multiple LOTs.[37]

DIFFERENTIAL DIAGNOSIS

1. Oncocytoma: Can show tubulocystic growth, cells lack perinuclear halos, and archipelaginous areas are present containing larger cell aggregates. IHC: CD117+, CK7+ only in scattered cells.
2. Chromophobe RCC, eosinophilic: Lacks hypocellular stromal areas, cells usually have irregular (raisinoid) nuclei with uniform perinuclear halos. IHC: CD117+, CK7+.
3. SDH-deficient RCC: Cells have more flocculent cytoplasm and intracytoplasmic vacuoles, lack perinuclear halos. Edematous stromal areas with individual cells (as in LOT) may be present. IHC: SDHB−, CD117−, CK7−.

THYROID-LIKE FOLLICULAR RENAL CELL CARCINOMA

INTRODUCTION

Thyroid-like follicular renal cell carcinoma (TLF RCC) is a rare tumor with less than 50 cases described in the literature, mostly published as individual case reports. TLF RCC has also been considered an emerging renal entity in the recent GUPS update[14] and is listed in the 2022 fifth edition of WHO as an "emerging entity."[13]

CLINICAL FEATURES

The sex distribution of TLF RCC has a slight female predominance (M:F = 1:1.8). Age range is broad (from 10 to 83 years).[49–51] No specific clinical features have been associated with TLF RCC. The clinical behavior was usually indolent in most reported cases, but lymph node and distant metastases were documented in about 10% of the patients.[52–55] Some reports have documented associations in individual patients with a family history of hereditary leiomyomatosis-associated RCC but without *FH* mutation, with mixed epithelial stromal tumor of the kidney, nephrolithiasis, and polycystic kidney disease.[14,54,56–59]

GROSS

TLF RCC is a solitary, solid, well-circumscribed, and nonencapsulated tumor. The reported size range was wide (from 0.8 to 16.5 cm).[14,49–51]

MICROSCOPY

TLF RCC resembles thyroid gland morphology (Fig. 6A–B). The tumors demonstrated follicular pattern, but focal branching and papillary structures were also reported. The size of the follicles was variable, and they were typically lined by a single layer of cuboidal or low columnar epithelial cells. The reported WHO grade was 2 or 3 (equivalent).[12,14,49–52,60–63] Sarcomatoid differentiation has been reported in one case.[64]

IMMUNOHISTOCHEMISTRY

TLF RCC is usually positive for CK7, vimentin, and PAX8, and less frequently for RCC, AMACR, CD10, and CK20. An important finding is the negative staining for TTF1 and thyroglobulin, in contrast to true metastatic carcinomas of the thyroid.[14,58]

MOLECULAR AND GENETIC FEATURES

An association of TLF RCC and *EWSR1* gene abnormality has been recently reported by Al-Obaidy and colleagues,[58] documenting a fusion of *EWSR1-PATZ1* genes in 3 cases. The reported copy number variations have been variable, but neither consistent copy number changes nor other recurrent gene alterations have been found in TLF RCC.[49,55,60,64–66]

DIFFERENTIAL DIAGNOSIS

1. Metastasis of thyroid gland carcinoma to the kidney: This is the most important differential diagnosis that can be easily ruled out by IHC, because TTF1+ and thyroglobulin+ are found in a thyroid metastasis, in contrast to TLF RCC, which is negative for both. Caution: metastatic thyroid carcinoma is PAX8+, which may be a pitfall, because PAX8+ is found in almost all thyroid gland tumors.
2. Atrophic kidney-like lesion: Rare, well-demarcated, brown, tumor-like mass; considered nonneoplastic and likely reactive. This lesion is composed of atrophic renal tubules admixed with rare collapsed glomeruli. The key morphologic findings are the atrophic tubules and the collapsed glomeruli, which are not found in TLF RCC.

BIPHASIC HYALINIZING PSAMMOMATOUS RENAL CELL CARCINOMA

INTRODUCTION

Biphasic hyalinizing psammomatous renal cell carcinoma (BHP RCC) is a recently proposed renal tumor entity, invariably demonstrating neurofibromin 2 (*NF2*) mutations.[67] However, it is unclear whether *NF2* abnormalities represent a specific feature or a genetic driver in a group of related tumors that may represent an entity, or if they are a nonspecific finding, because they have been found in other RCC subtypes with various morphologies.[67–69] For example, in one recent study, 2 tumors described as BHP RCC did not show *NF2* abnormality.[70] In contrast, *NF2* abnormalities have been identified in some advanced papillary RCCs.[69] Thus, further study is necessary to validate whether BHP RCC represents a distinct renal entity sharing *NF2* gene abnormalities.[14,68,71]

CLINICAL FEATURES

No specific clinical features were identified in the initial series of 8 cases,[67] and in a subsequent series of 6 cases.[72] There were 6 males and 1 female (1 unknown gender) in the study by Argani and colleagues,[67] and 3 males and 3 females in the study by Wang and colleagues.[72] Age range was broad

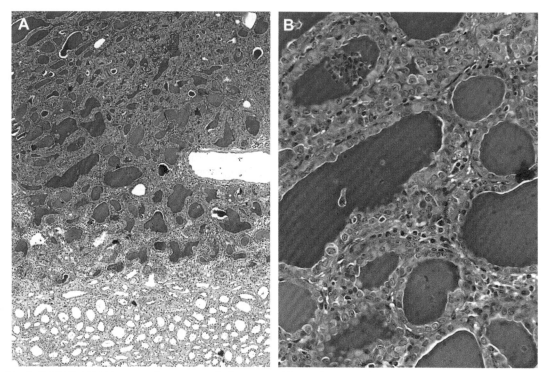

Fig. 6. TLF RCC. (*A*) This tumor shows a morphology resembling a thyroid gland, and is composed of back-to-back arranged, variable-sized follicles, with "colloid-like" luminal content. (*B*) At high power, the follicles are lined by a single layer of cuboidal to low columnar epithelial cells.

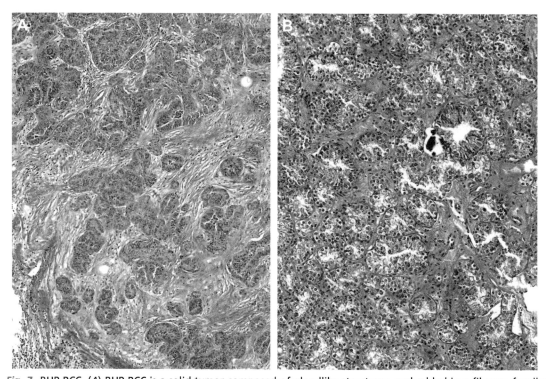

Fig. 7. BHP RCC. (*A*) BHP RCC is a solid tumor composed of glandlike structures, embedded in a fibrous, focally hyalinized stroma. These tumors typically show biphasic cell composition with smaller cells forming pseudoro-settes. (*B*) Some areas show tubular morphology, and scattered psammoma bodies are common.

Table 1
Features of novel and emerging renal entities

Type	Clinical Features	Morphology	Immunohistochemistry	Molecular Features
ESC RCC	Mostly in females, mostly sporadic and solitary, rare cases in patients with TSC, indolent (great majority)	Solid and cystic, voluminous eosinophilic cells, cytoplasmic stippling	CK20+ CK7– CD117–v imentin+c athepsin K+ (focal)	Somatic biallelic loss or mutations of *TSC1* and *TSC2*
RCC FMS	Mostly sporadic and solitary, rare cases in patients with TSC, indolent (great majority)	Solid, smaller tumor, tan to brown, frequent lobulated appearance; clear cells with voluminous cytoplasm forming nodules, separated and encircled by fibromuscular stroma	CK7+ CAIX+ (membranous) CD10+ AMACR–	Frequent mutations in *TSC/mTOR* pathway genes, *ELOC (TCEB1)* mutation in some cases; some lack *VHL* mutations, or LOH/deletion of chromosome 3
ALK RCC	Broad age range, solitary tumor, some in patients with sickle cell trait	Diverse (variable admixed patterns), often mucinous/myxoid background; medullary carcinoma-like morphology in children	ALK+ Other IHC nonspecific Rare cases TFE3+ (without translocation)	*ALK* rearrangement Fusion partners: *VCL, HOOK1, STRN, TPM3, EML4, PLEKHA7, CLIP1, KIF5B,* and *KIAA1217*
EVT	Broad age range, sporadic and solitary, rare cases in patients with TSC, indolent	Solid, smaller tumor, tan to brown or gray, large vessels often found at the periphery; eosinophilic cells with frequent and prominent intracytoplasmic vacuoles, large nucleoli	cathepsin K+ CD117+ CD10+ CK7– (only rare cells +) CK20–v imentin–	*TSC/mTOR* mutations virtually in all cases, deletions of chromosome 19 and 1 also found
LOT	Older patients, sporadic and solitary, rare cases in patients with TSC, indolent	Solid, smaller tumor, tan to mahogany brown; sharp transition to edematous areas with scattered individual cells; round to oval nuclei without irregularities and prominent nucleoli, often with perinuclear halos	CK7+ (diffuse) CD117– (rarely weak +) GATA3+ (limited data) FOXI1– CK20–v imentin–	Frequent *TSC/MTOR* mutations, lacks multiple chromosomal losses, deletions of chromosomes 19p, 19q and 1p also found, no *CCND1* rearrangements

(continued on next page)

Table 1
(continued)

Type	Clinical Features	Morphology	Immunohistochemistry	Molecular Features
TLF RCC	Broad age range including children, solitary, mostly indolent	Thyroid-like follicular arrangement, follicles of variable size with eosinophilic luminal content, lining cells cuboidal to cylindrical	CK7+ PAX8+ Vimentin− TTF1−t hyroglobulin−	Fusion of *EWSR1-PATZ1* found in 3 cases No other specific findings
BHP RCC	Adult patients, about half of tumors with aggressive clinical course	Tubulopapillary architecture, prominent fibrotic to hyalinized stroma, and microcalcifications Heterogeneous morphology	CK7+ PAX8+ CD10+ HMB45−m elan A−	*NF2* abnormalities , loss of chromosome 22 found in some cases

(39–82 years), and no hereditary/syndromic or other associations were reported. Approximately half of the cases reported in the literature demonstrated metastatic disease.[70,71]

GROSS

BHP RCC is a well-demarcated, solid, solitary tumor, occasionally demonstrating a peripheral capsule. Size ranged from 0.9 to 7.5 cm.[67,70–73]

MICROSCOPY

BHP RCC is a solid tumor, with variable architecture, often including papillary and tubular growth. The tumors were typically composed of biphasic neoplastic cells, with smaller cells clustering around basement membrane material forming pseudorosettes and resembling the classic morphology of TFEB RCC (Fig. 7A–B). The second cell population consisted of larger cells with pale cytoplasm. Some reported tumors resembled a gonadoblastoma and formed solid pseudotubules or pseudoresettes, composed of cuboidal to cylindrical cells with pale to eosinophilic cytoplasm. Another morphologic variation was the presence of focal tubulopapillary growth, associated with basement membrane material, resulting in a glomeruloid appearance. The stromal component was typically sclerotic and focally hyalinized and scattered psammoma bodies were common.[67,71–73]

IMMUNOHISTOCHEMISTRY

The neoplastic cells were usually reactive for PAX8, CD10, and CK7, but were negative for GATA3, cathepsin K, melan-A, inhibin, SF1, and WT1. All tested cases were also negative for TFE3 and TFEB rearrangements by break-apart FISH.

MOLECULAR AND GENETIC FEATURES

A typical molecular feature identified in all analyzable cases of BHP RCC was a mutations of the NF2 gene.[67,71,72] In a recent study, two tumors described as BHP RCC lacked NF2 abnormalities.[70] Additional mutations in PBMRT1, BAP1, ARID1A, DNMT3A, TERT, and SMARCB1 were also found in some cases. The copy number variation pattern was not uniform and showed multiple chromosomal gains and losses, most commonly a loss of chromosome 22. Coalteration of NF2 and PBMRT1 was found in some cases with aggressive clinical course.[71]

DIFFERENTIAL DIAGNOSIS

BHP RCC represents a heterogeneous group of renal tumors with a limited number of reported cases, usually demonstrating prominent fibrotic and hyalinized stroma, microcalcification, and tubulopapillary architecture. The differential diagnosis of BHP RCC is broad and may include papillary RCC, MiTF family RCC (often demonstrating cathepsin K or melanotic marker expression, as well as TFE3/TFEB rearrangements), ALK-rearranged RCC (typically showing ALK rearrangements), and metastatic sex core stromal tumor, such as gonadoblastoma (which can be ruled out by the absence of gonadal primary and inhibin and SF1 immunoreactivity). However, without genetic testing for NF2, the diagnosis of BHP RCC remains virtually impossible.

SUMMARY

This article provides an overview of several new and emerging renal entities. The summary of their key features is shown in Table 1. The awareness of these renal neoplasms is essential for practicing pathologists because the navigation through this evolving field is a challenging task, even in places with large volumes of renal tumors. Such cases can, however, be seen in practices of any scope, and their correct classification requires diagnostic awareness among general pathologists, because they can be often diagnosed, or at least suspected, on morphology in combination with IHC. The recognition of such novel renal entities will guide both pathologists and clinicians in translating these developments into more accurate diagnosis and better patient management.

DISCLOSURE

Authors have no conflicts of interest to declare that are relevant to the content of this article.

REFERENCES

1. Trpkov K, Hes O, Bonert M, et al. Eosinophilic, Solid, and Cystic Renal Cell Carcinoma: Clinicopathologic Study of 16 Unique, Sporadic Neoplasms Occurring in Women. Am J Surg Pathol 2016;40(1):60–71.
2. Trpkov K, Abou-Ouf H, Hes O, et al. Eosinophilic Solid and Cystic Renal Cell Carcinoma (ESC RCC): Further Morphologic and Molecular Characterization of ESC RCC as a Distinct Entity. Am J Surg Pathol 2017;41(10):1299–308.
3. Li Y, Reuter VE, Matoso A, et al. Re-evaluation of 33 'unclassified' eosinophilic renal cell carcinomas in young patients. Histopathology 2018;72(4):588–600.

4. Guo J, Tretiakova MS, Troxell ML, et al. Tuberous Sclerosis-associated Renal Cell Carcinoma: A Clinicopathologic Study of 57 Separate Carcinomas in 18 Patients. Am J Surg Pathol 2014;38(11): 1457–67.

5. Schreiner A, Daneshmand S, Bayne A, et al. Distinctive morphology of renal cell carcinomas in tuberous sclerosis. Int J Surg Pathol 2010;18(5):409–18.

6. Palsgrove DN, Li Y, Pratilas CA, et al. Eosinophilic Solid and Cystic (ESC) Renal Cell Carcinomas Harbor TSC Mutations: Molecular Analysis Supports an Expanding Clinicopathologic Spectrum. Am J Surg Pathol 2018;42(9):1166–81.

7. McKenney JK, Przybycin CG, Trpkov K, et al. Eosinophilic solid and cystic renal cell carcinomas have metastatic potential. Histopathology 2018;72(6): 1066–7.

8. Tretiakova MS. Eosinophilic solid and cystic renal cell carcinoma mimicking epithelioid angiomyolipoma: series of 4 primary tumors and 2 metastases. Hum Pathol 2018;80:65–75.

9. Mehra R, Vats P, Cao X, et al. Somatic Bi-allelic Loss of TSC Genes in Eosinophilic Solid and Cystic Renal Cell Carcinoma. Eur Urol 2018;74(4):483–6.

10. Tjota M, Chen H, Parilla M, et al. Eosinophilic Renal Cell Tumors With a TSC and MTOR Gene Mutations Are Morphologically and Immunohistochemically Heterogenous: Clinicopathologic and Molecular Study. Am J Surg Pathol 2020;44(7):943–54.

11. Canzonieri V, Volpe R, Gloghini A, et al. Mixed renal tumor with carcinomatous and fibroleiomyomatous components, associated with angiomyolipoma in the same kidney. Pathol Res Pract 1993;189(8): 951–6, [discussion: 957-959].

12. Trpkov K, Hes O. New and emerging renal entities: a perspective post-WHO 2016 classification. Histopathology 2019;74(1):31–59.

13. WHO Classification of Tumours. Edited by the WHO Classification of Tumours Editorial Board. Urinary and male genital tumours. 5th edition. WHO classification of tumours series, 8. Lyon (France): International Agency for Research on Cancer; 2022. https://publications.iarc.fr.

14. Trpkov K, Williamson SR, Gill AJ, et al. Novel, emerging and provisional renal entities: The Genitourinary Pathology Society (GUPS) update on renal neoplasia. Mod Pathol 2021;34(6):1167–84.

15. Gournay M, Dugay F, Belaud-Rotureau MA, et al. Renal cell carcinoma with leiomyomatous stroma in tuberous sclerosis complex: a distinct entity. Virchows Arch 2021;478(4):793–9.

16. Shah RB, Stohr BA, Tu ZJ, et al. Renal Cell Carcinoma With Leiomyomatous Stroma" Harbor Somatic Mutations of TSC1, TSC2, MTOR, and/or ELOC (TCEB1): Clinicopathologic and Molecular Characterization of 18 Sporadic Tumors Supports a Distinct Entity. Am J Surg Pathol 2020;44(5):571–81.

17. Williamson SR, Hornick JL, Eble JN, et al. Renal Cell Carcinoma with Angioleiomyoma-Like Stroma and Clear Cell Papillary Renal Cell Carcinoma: Exploring SDHB Protein Immunohistochemistry and the Relationship to Tuberous Sclerosis Complex. Hum Pathol 2018;75:10–5.

18. Gupta S, Lohse CM, Rowsey R, et al. Renal Neoplasia in Polycystic Kidney Disease: An Assessment of Tuberous Sclerosis Complex-associated Renal Neoplasia and PKD1/TSC2 Contiguous Gene Deletion Syndrome. Eur Urol 2021; S0302-2838(21):02161–8. https://doi.org/10.1016/j.eururo.2021.11.013. Online ahead of print.

19. Martignoni G, Brunelli M, Segala D, et al. Renal cell carcinoma with smooth muscle stroma lacks chromosome 3p and VHL alterations. Mod Pathol 2014; 27(5):765–74.

20. Parilla M, Alikhan M, Al-Kawaaz M, et al. Genetic Underpinnings of Renal Cell Carcinoma With Leiomyomatous Stroma. Am J Surg Pathol 2019;43(8): 1135–44.

21. Williamson SR, Cheng L, Eble JN, et al. Renal cell carcinoma with angioleiomyoma-like stroma: clinicopathological, immunohistochemical, and molecular features supporting classification as a distinct entity. Mod Pathol 2015;28(2):279–94.

22. Gupta S, Jimenez RE, Herrera-Hernandez L, et al. Renal Neoplasia in Tuberous Sclerosis: A Study of 41 Patients. Mayo Clin Proc 2021;96(6):1470–89.

23. Hakimi AA, Tickoo SK, Jacobsen A, et al. TCEB1-mutated renal cell carcinoma: a distinct genomic and morphological subtype. Mod Pathol 2015; 28(6):845–53.

24. Petersson F, Martinek P, Vanecek T, et al. Renal Cell Carcinoma With Leiomyomatous Stroma: A Group of Tumors With Indistinguishable Histopathologic Features, But 2 Distinct Genetic Profiles: Next-Generation Sequencing Analysis of 6 Cases Negative for Aberrations Related to the VHL gene. Appl Immunohistochem Mol Morphol 2018;26(3):192–7.

25. Marino-Enriquez A, Ou WB, Weldon CB, et al. ALK rearrangement in sickle cell trait-associated renal medullary carcinoma. Genes Chromosomes Cancer 2011;50(3):146–53.

26. Debelenko LV, Raimondi SC, Daw N, et al. Renal cell carcinoma with novel VCL-ALK fusion: new representative of ALK-associated tumor spectrum. Mod Pathol 2011;24(3):430–42.

27. Pal SK, Bergerot P, Dizman N, et al. Responses to Alectinib in ALK-rearranged Papillary Renal Cell Carcinoma. Eur Urol 2018;74(1):124–8.

28. Hallberg B, Palmer RH. Mechanistic insight into ALK receptor tyrosine kinase in human cancer biology. Nat Rev Cancer 2013;13(10):685–700.

29. Kuroda N, Trpkov K, Gao Y, et al. ALK rearranged renal cell carcinoma (ALK-RCC): a multi-institutional study of twelve cases with identification

of novel partner genes CLIP1, KIF5B and KIAA1217. Mod Pathol 2020;33(12):2564–79.

30. Thorner PS, Shago M, Marrano P, et al. TFE3-positive renal cell carcinomas are not always Xp11 translocation carcinomas: Report of a case with a TPM3-ALK translocation. Pathol Res Pract 2016; 212(10):937–42.

31. Trpkov K, Hes O, Williamson SR, et al. New developments in existing WHO entities and evolving molecular concepts: The Genitourinary Pathology Society (GUPS) update on renal neoplasia. Mod Pathol 2021;34(7):1392–424.

32. Williamson SR, Gadde R, Trpkov K, et al. Diagnostic criteria for oncocytic renal neoplasms: a survey of urologic pathologists. Hum Pathol 2017;63:149–56.

33. Hes O, Petersson F, Kuroda N, et al. Renal hybrid oncocytic/chromophobe tumors - a review. Histol Histopathol 2013;28(10):1257–64.

34. He H, Trpkov K, Martinek P, et al. High-grade oncocytic renal tumor": morphologic, immunohistochemical, and molecular genetic study of 14 cases. Virchows Arch 2018;473(6):725–38.

35. Chen YB, Mirsadraei L, Jayakumaran G, et al. Somatic Mutations of TSC2 or MTOR Characterize a Morphologically Distinct Subset of Sporadic Renal Cell Carcinoma With Eosinophilic and Vacuolated Cytoplasm. Am J Surg Pathol 2019;43(1): 121–31.

36. Trpkov K, Bonert M, Gao Y, et al. High-grade oncocytic tumour (HOT) of kidney in a patient with tuberous sclerosis complex. Histopathology 2019;75(3): 440–2.

37. Lerma LA, Schade GR, Tretiakova MS. Co-existence of ESC-RCC, EVT, and LOT as synchronous and metachronous tumors in six patients with multifocal neoplasia but without clinical features of tuberous sclerosis complex. Hum Pathol 2021;116:1–11.

38. Kapur P, Gao M, Zhong H, et al. Eosinophilic Vacuolated Tumor of the Kidney: A Review of Evolving Concepts in This Novel Subtype With Additional Insights From a Case With MTOR Mutation and Concomitant Chromosome 1 Loss. Adv Anat Pathol 2021;28(4):251–7.

39. Farcas M, Gatalica Z, Trpkov K, et al. Eosinophilic vacuolated tumor (EVT) of kidney demonstrates sporadic TSC/MTOR mutations: next-generation sequencing multi-institutional study of 19 cases. Mod Pathol 2021. https://doi.org/10.1038/s41379-021-00923-6.

40. Siadat F, Trpkov K. ESC, ALK, HOT and LOT: Three Letter Acronyms of Emerging Renal Entities Knocking on the Door of the WHO Classification. Cancers (Basel) 2020;12(1).

41. Trpkov K, Williamson SR, Gao Y, et al. Low-grade Oncocytic Tumor of Kidney (CD117 Negative, Cytokeratin 7 Positive): A Distinct Entity? Histopathology 2019;75(2):174–84.

42. Kapur P, Gao M, Zhong H, et al. Germline and sporadic mTOR pathway mutations in low-grade oncocytic tumor of the kidney. Mod Pathol 2021. https://doi.org/10.1038/s41379-021-00896-6.

43. Kravtsov O, Gupta S, Cheville JC, et al. Low-Grade Oncocytic Tumor of Kidney (CK7-Positive, CD117-Negative): Incidence in a Single Institutional Experience with Clinicopathological and Molecular Characteristics. Hum Pathol 2021;114:9–18.

44. Akgul M, Al-Obaidy KI, Cheng L, et al. Low-grade oncocytic tumour expands the spectrum of renal oncocytic tumours and deserves separate classification: a review of 23 cases from a single tertiary institute. J Clin Pathol 2021. https://doi.org/10.1136/jclinpath-2021-207478, jclinpath-2021-207478.

45. Morini A, Drossart T, Timsit MO, et al. Low-grade oncocytic renal tumor (LOT): mutations in mTOR pathway genes and low expression of FOXI1. Mod Pathol 2021. https://doi.org/10.1038/s41379-021-00906-7.

46. Guo Q, Liu N, Wang F, et al. Characterization of a distinct low-grade oncocytic renal tumor (CD117-negative and cytokeratin 7-positive) based on a tertiary oncology center experience: the new evidence from China. Virchows Arch 2020;449–58.

47. Tong K, Hu Z. FOXI1 expression in chromophobe renal cell carcinoma and renal oncocytoma: a study of The Cancer Genome Atlas transcriptome-based outlier mining and immunohistochemistry. Virchows Arch 2021;478(4):647–58.

48. Skala SL, Wang X, Zhang Y, et al. Next-generation RNA Sequencing-based Biomarker Characterization of Chromophobe Renal Cell Carcinoma and Related Oncocytic Neoplasms. Eur Urol 2020;78(1):63–74.

49. Amin MB, Gupta R, Ondrej H, et al. Primary thyroid-like follicular carcinoma of the kidney: report of 6 cases of a histologically distinctive adult renal epithelial neoplasm. Am J Surg Pathol 2009;33(3): 393–400.

50. Alessandrini L, Fassan M, Gardiman MP, et al. Thyroid-like follicular carcinoma of the kidney: report of two cases with detailed immunohistochemical profile and literature review. Virchows Arch 2012; 461(3):345–50.

51. Chen F, Wang Y, Wu X, et al. Clinical characteristics and pathology of thyroid-like follicular carcinoma of the kidney: Report of 3 cases and a literature review. Mol Clin Oncol 2016;4(2):143–50.

52. Dhillon J, Tannir NM, Matin SF, et al. Thyroid-like follicular carcinoma of the kidney with metastases to the lungs and retroperitoneal lymph nodes. Hum Pathol 2011;42(1):146–50.

53. Vicens RA, Balachandran A, Guo CC, et al. Multimodality imaging of thyroid-like follicular renal cell carcinoma with lung metastases, a new emerging tumor entity. Abdom Imaging 2014; 39(2):388–93.

54. Rao V, Menon S, Bakshi G, et al. Thyroid-Like Follicular Carcinoma of the Kidney With Low-Grade Sarcomatoid Component: A Hitherto Undescribed Case. Int J Surg Pathol 2021;29(3):327–33.

55. Ko JJ, Grewal JK, Ng T, et al. Whole-genome and transcriptome profiling of a metastatic thyroid-like follicular renal cell carcinoma. Cold Spring Harb Mol Case Stud 2018;4(6):a003137.

56. Wu WW, Chu JT, Nael A, et al. Thyroid-like follicular carcinoma of the kidney in a young patient with history of pediatric acute lymphoblastic leukemia. Case Rep Pathol 2014;2014:313974.

57. Volavsek M, Strojan-Flezar M, Mikuz G. Thyroid-like follicular carcinoma of the kidney in a patient with nephrolithiasis and polycystic kidney disease: a case report. Diagn Pathol 2013;8:108.

58. Al-Obaidy KI, Bridge JA, Cheng L, et al. EWSR1-PATZ1 fusion renal cell carcinoma: a recurrent gene fusion characterizing thyroid-like follicular renal cell carcinoma. Mod Pathol 2021;34: 1921–34.

59. Tretiakova MS, Kehr EL, Gore JL, et al. Thyroid-Like Follicular Renal Cell Carcinoma Arising Within Benign Mixed Epithelial and Stromal Tumor. Int J Surg Pathol 2020;28(1):80–6.

60. Ohe C, Kuroda N, Pan CC, et al. A unique renal cell carcinoma with features of papillary renal cell carcinoma and thyroid-like carcinoma: a morphological, immunohistochemical and genetic study. Histopathology 2010;57(3):494–7.

61. Dhillon J, Mohanty SK, Krishnamurthy S. Cytologic diagnosis of thyroid-like follicular carcinoma of the kidney: a case report. Diagn Cytopathol 2014; 42(3):273–7.

62. Dong L, Huang J, Huang L, et al. Thyroid-Like Follicular Carcinoma of the Kidney in a Patient with Skull and Meningeal Metastasis: A Unique Case Report and Review of the Literature. Medicine (Baltimore) 2016;95(15):e3314.

63. de Jesus LE, Fulgencio C, Leve T, et al. Thyroid-like follicular carcinoma of the kidney presenting on a 10 year-old prepubertal girl. Int Braz J Urol 2019;45(4): 834–42.

64. Jenkins TM, Rosenbaum J, Zhang PJ, et al. Thyroid-Like Follicular Carcinoma of the Kidney With Extensive Sarcomatoid Differentiation: A Case Report and Review of the Literature. Int J Surg Pathol 2019;27(6):678–83.

65. Jung SJ, Chung JI, Park SH, et al. Thyroid follicular carcinoma-like tumor of kidney: a case report with morphologic, immunohistochemical, and genetic analysis. Am J Surg Pathol 2006;30(3):411–5.

66. Fanelli GN, Fassan M, Dal Moro F, et al. Thyroid-like follicular carcinoma of the kidney: The mutational profiling reveals a BRAF wild type status. Pathol Res Pract 2019;215(9):152532.

67. Argani P, Reuter VE, Eble JN, et al. Biphasic Hyalinizing Psammomatous Renal Cell Carcinoma (BHP RCC): A Distinctive Neoplasm Associated With Somatic NF2 Mutations. Am J Surg Pathol 2020;44(7): 901–16.

68. Chen YB, Xu J, Skanderup AJ, et al. Molecular analysis of aggressive renal cell carcinoma with unclassified histology reveals distinct subsets. Nat Commun 2016;7:13131.

69. Yakirevich E, Pavlick DC, Perrino CM, et al. NF2 Tumor Suppressor Gene Inactivation in Advanced Papillary Renal Cell Carcinoma. Am J Surg Pathol 2021;45(5):716–8.

70. Chumbalkar V, Wang P, Paner GP. Spectrum of biphasic renal cell carcinomas with hyalinized stroma and psammoma bodies associated and not associated with NF2 alteration. Hum Pathol 2021. https://doi.org/10.1016/j.humpath.2021.12.001. S0046-8177(21)00199-4.

71. Paintal A, Tjota MY, Wang P, et al. NF2-mutated Renal Carcinomas Have Common Morphologic Features Which Overlap With Biphasic Hyalinizing Psammomatous Renal Cell Carcinoma: A Comprehensive Study of 14 Cases. Am J Surg Pathol 2022. https://doi.org/10.1097/PAS.0000000000001846.

72. Wang G, Amin MB, Grossmann P, et al. Renal cell tumor with sex-cord/gonadoblastoma-like features: analysis of 6 cases. Virchows Arch 2021. https://doi.org/10.1007/s00428-021-03235-x.

73. Gopinath A, Mubeen A, Jamal M, et al. Biphasic Hyalinizing Psammomatous Renal Cell Carcinoma: Another Provisional Entity Emerging From the Papillary Renal Cell Carcinoma Pandora's Box. Int J Surg Pathol 2021;29(7):783–7.

Testicular Tumors
New Developments in Germ Cell and Sex Cord Stromal Tumors

Abhishek Dashora, MD, FRCPath[a], Thomas Wagner, MD[b,c],
Daniel M. Berney, FRCPath[a,d],*

KEYWORDS

• Testis • Germ cell tumor • Sex cord stromal tumor • Recent developments

---

Key points

- GCNIS is the standard terminology for preinvasive TGCTs.
- Amplification on chromosome 12p (isochromosome 12p) by molecular analysis is a useful test for confirming GCNIS-derived GCTs in challenging cases.
- Seminoma is the most common TGCT having an excellent prognosis. They can exhibit diverse histologic patterns and may lead to a potential diagnostic pitfall.
- Testicular teratomas are classified into postpubertal and prepubertal types and have entirely different derivations and behavior.
- Teratoma with somatic type malignancy occurs in a small subset of postpubertal-type teratoma either within the testis or more commonly in metastatic sites and is characterized by an expansile mass of a pure tumor type.

ABSTRACT

This article reviews the recent advances and potential future changes in the classification of testicular germ cell and sex cord stromal tumors, highlighting changes in the classification system and terminology with description on newer entities. A discussion on approaching difficult areas and diagnostic pitfalls is also included along with the utility of ancillary investigations. Areas with limited knowledge are highlighted to providing direction for future studies and a bulleted summary in the form of critical care points is provided.

INTRODUCTION

Testicular tumors, although being the most common solid neoplasm of young men, are rare accounting for only 1% to 2% of all neoplasms in men.[1] They exhibit a diverse morphologic spectrum and can be diagnostically challenging due to their relative unfamiliarity. They are also one of the most curable solid neoplasms with 5-year survival rates of up to 99% in some tumor types, which makes stratification of pathologic risk factors difficult and raises concerns on overtreatment that in turn may lead to increased morbidity.[2] This is particularly worrisome considering long-term survival in this era of modern chemotherapy and imaging which comes with increased risk of secondary malignancies. There is constant evolution in our understanding of testicular neoplasia reflected by successive revisions of World Health Organization (WHO) classification of the Urinary System and Male Genital Organs with the fifth edition just released.[3] The scope of this review article

---

[a] Department of Cellular Pathology, Barts Health NHS Trust, London, United Kingdom; [b] Department of Pathology, Copenhagen University Hospital, Rigshospitalet, Copenhagen, Denmark; [c] Department of Oncology, Copenhagen University Hospital, Rigshospitalet, Copenhagen, Denmark; [d] Department of Molecular Oncology, Barts Health Cancer and Barts Health NHS Trust, London, United Kingdom
* Corresponding author. Department of Molecular Oncology, Barts Cancer Institute, Queen Mary University of London, London EC1A 7BE, United Kingdom.
E-mail address: Daniel.Berney@nhs.net

Surgical Pathology 15 (2022) 729–743
https://doi.org/10.1016/j.path.2022.07.007

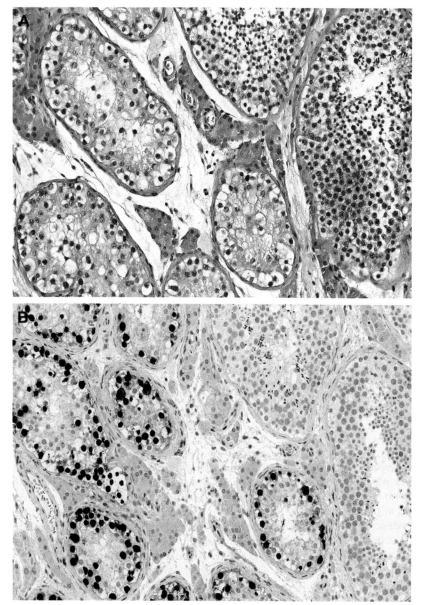

Fig. 1. GCNIS with characteristic ring-like arrangement of vacuolated neoplastic cells (*A*) with strong nuclear positivity for OCT3/4 (*B*).

will cover new advances in the knowledge of testicular germ cell and sex cord tumors with emphasis on updates in classification and terminology, profiles on recently described entities and discussion of approach in some difficult areas as well as diagnostic pitfalls, which could be of significant clinical relevance.

GERM CELL TUMORS

The WHO 2016 fourth edition introduced the term germ cell neoplasia in situ (GCNIS) and standardized the terminology of preinvasive testicular germ cell tumors (TGCTs) after unanimous agreement of the WHO editors.[4] This term provides multitude of benefits such as avoiding the epithelial connotations of carcinoma in situ/testicular intraepithelial neoplasia, dropping the unclassified letter U from previously used term intratubular germ cell neoplasia unclassified type and aligning this preneoplastic entity with the nomenclature of preinvasive conditions in general. The lesion arises in the spermatogonial niche located between the basement membrane and the tight junctions of Sertoli cells characterized by large vacuolated cells with prominent nucleoli arranged in a ring like fashion in the seminiferous tubules uniformly expressing OCT3/4 (**Fig. 1**).[5]

Normal spermatogonia may have similar appearance and absence of spermatogenesis is a good diagnostic clue for the presence of GCNIS particularly in small testicular biopsies.

GCNIS forms the basis of classification into 2 broad categories: GCNIS-derived and non–GCNIS-derived germ cell tumors (GCTs).

GERM CELL NEOPLASIA IN SITU-DERIVED GERM CELL TUMORS

These are malignant tumors usually presenting in young men or adolescents.[6,7] They are further subclassified histologically as seminoma and nonseminomatous GCTs (NSGCTs); with the latter presenting either as pure or mixed forms of embryonal carcinoma (EC), yolk sac tumors (YST), choriocarcinoma (CC), and postpubertal-type teratomas. Large-scale whole genome sequencing studies have confirmed pathognomonic amplification of 12p (isochromosome 12p) occurring in about 90% of these cases and its detection is very helpful in challenging cases to ascertain germ cell nature of the tumor especially in the metastatic setting and in somatically transformed tumors.[8]

Seminomas

Seminoma is the most common testicular tumor accounting for 50% of TGCTs presenting at a mean age of 40 years.[9] Some have expressed their disagreement regarding the different nomenclature being used for this tumor based purely on the site such as seminoma in testis, dysgerminoma in ovary, and germinoma in other sites. The tumor shows identical morphologic, immunohistochemical (IHC) and molecular characteristic with similar clinical management and therefore a single unifying name or being categorized as germinoma is suggested which would lead to better consistency and avoid confusion for the treating physicians.[10]

Histologic features of classic seminoma are well described with diagnosis usually straightforward. However, a wide variety of patterns exists leading to potential pitfalls. Tubular/pseudoglandular, signet ring, rhabdoid, and pure intertubular (Fig. 2) are a few of such subtypes, which can mimic carcinoma or sarcoma.[11] In addition to expressing PLAP, OCT3/4, and CD117, these subtypes may have areas elsewhere with more typical appearance of seminoma and a careful search with generous sampling of tumor may prevent this misdiagnosis.[12] Syncytiotrophoblast-rich seminomas (see Fig. 2) may be associated with modestly raised levels of serum human chorionic gonadotrophin and should be differentiated from CC by an absence of a biphasic population of cells. Very rarely florid inflammation, granulomatous

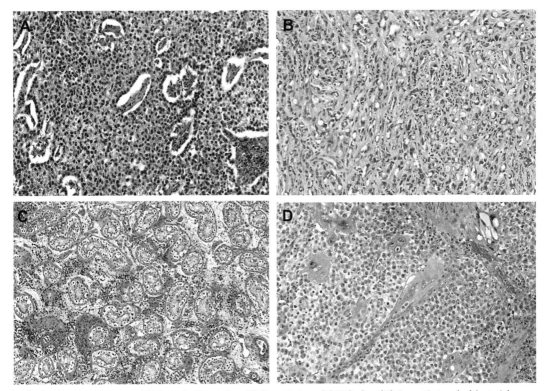

Fig. 2. Seminoma patterns. (*A*) Pseudoglandular. (*B*) Signet ring. (*C*) Tubular. (*D*) Syncytiotrophoblast rich.

response, or infarct type necrosis may almost completely overgrow the seminoma. To avoid this, extensive sampling of various areas, correlation with tumor markers is mandatory, and immunohistochemistry and discussion at multidisciplinary team meeting may be useful. There are no known prognostic or treatment differences within these histologic subtypes. Seminomas have an excellent prognosis with 5-year survival of greater than 95%. There is no conclusive evidence on anaplastic features or degree of differentiation in seminomas that can affect prognosis or alter management decisions and hence are not required in a routine pathology reports.[13]

Nonseminomatous Germ Cell tumors

NSGCTs tend to arise a decade earlier than seminomas presenting as enlarging testicular mass having variegated appearance with occult metastasis in up to one-third of cases.[14,15] An estimate on the percentage of different tumor elements in mixed NSGCT by a basic "eye-balling" should always be given in a pathology report because it is predictive of the relapse risk, particularly proportion of EC.[16,17]

Embryonal carcinoma

Embryonal carcinoma presents challenges in posttherapy and metastatic settings. Although it may show typical morphologic appearance, there is often widespread necrosis. Atypical patterns encountered include intratubular EC, micropapillary, blastocyst-like, anastomosing glandular, and sieve-like glandular patterns (Fig. 3).[18] Loss of CD30 expression is reported in some metastatic cases and therefore reliance on a combination of markers such as OCT3/4 and CD117 should be undertaken in such scenarios.[19,20]

Postpubertal-type teratoma

Testicular teratomas, in contrast to their ovarian counterparts, are classified based on their derivation from GCNIS and categorized into postpubertal and prepubertal-types, the former being GCNIS-derived and the latter not. The presence or absence of immature elements or neuroepithelium has no known prognostic significance,[13] and hence, the use of terms such as mature and immature teratoma should be avoided.

Postpubertal-type teratomas are malignant GCTs irrespective of maturity or cytologic atypia in its constituents with metastasis at presentation in 22% to 37% of cases.[4] A description on "immature" elements is relevant only in 2 settings: first, when they form an expansile mass overgrowing other GCT elements suggesting a transformation into somatic malignancy, and second, its presence excludes possibility of prepubertal-type teratoma.[10]

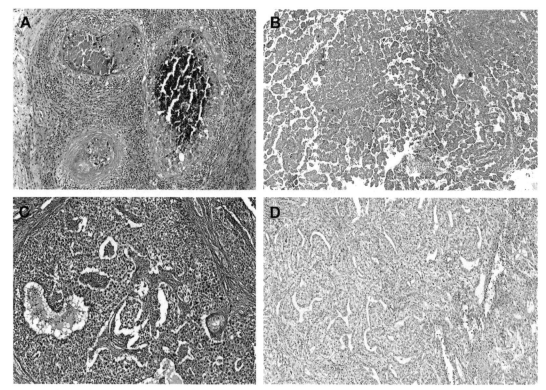

Fig. 3. Embryonal carcinoma patterns. (*A*) Intratubular. (*B*) Micropapillary. (*C*) Solid and glandular. (*D*) Glandular.

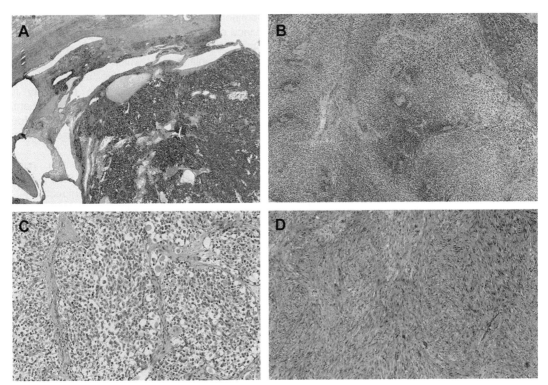

Fig. 4. Somatic-type malignancies in GCTs. (*A*) Nephroblastoma. (*B*) ENET. (*C*) Rhabdomyosarcoma. (*D*) Leiomyosarcoma.

Teratoma with somatic type malignancy

Criteria defining somatic transformation in teratomas are challenging and definitions are somewhat crude. The new WHO classification is likely to eschew the use of field diameters to measure the size of the transformation and suggest using an expansile nodule size of at least 5 mm instead of "a nodule of malignant cells equivalent to area seen by 4X objective and overgrowing other GCT elements."[4] The neoplasm should consist of pure population of atypical epithelial or mesenchymal elements giving rise to carcinomas, sarcomas, nephroblastomas, hematological, or other malignancies (Fig. 4).

Primitive neuroepithelium is one such commonly encountered element that could give rise to somatic malignancy currently called primitive neuroectodermal tumor (PNET).[4,21] The term PNET was historically taken from central nervous system (CNS) tumors and applied to various anatomic sites. PNETs in testis are akin to pediatric type CNS PNETs and lack the translocations (*EWSR1* gene on chromosome 22) of Ewing sarcoma or peripheral PNETs.[22–24] The WHO 2016 revision of CNS tumors changed the name of PNET to "Embryonal tumor with multi-layered rosettes, C19mc altered or not otherwise specified (NOS)".[25] In light of these changes, and that misdiagnosis as a Ewing sarcoma might lead to inappropriate therapy, it is suggested the term "Embryonic-type neuroectodermal tumor" (ENET) instead of PNET and "ENET areas of differentiation" where somatic malignancy has not yet occurred.[26] Teratoma with somatic malignancy is more common in metastatic sites after chemotherapy and has a poor prognosis due to insensitivity to chemotherapy as compared with when confined within the testis, which could be treated with orchidectomy and surveillance.[20,27–29]

Yolk sac tumors

The diverse and complex histologic patterns seen in YST can be a diagnostic challenge. Small areas of YST are often missed in NSGCTs, and we find correlation with levels of serum alpha-fetoprotein and application of Glypican3 immunostaining very helpful. Solid YST may be mistaken for seminoma leading to inappropriate therapy.[30] A recent study on somatic malignancies in teratomas suggests a proportion of them are actually variants of YSTs. In one study, a proportion of sarcomas showed immunoreactivity to Glypican 3 and SALL4 with some morphologic features of parietal YST differentiation suggesting a sarcomatoid variant of YST.[31] Similarly, some of the adenocarcinomas showed immunoprofile in keeping with YST with the absence of EMA/CK7 supporting their reclassification as glandular variant of YST. Hepatoid YST is another such pattern common in late relapses, which could be mistaken for hepatocellular carcinoma.[20,32,33] Late recurrences of yolks sac tumor may be insensitive to chemotherapy, and their identification is, therefore, important. The more unusual variants may also be more common in patients with disorders of sexual development.[34,35]

Trophoblastic tumors
Trophoblastic tumors of the testis include CC, the most aggressive form of GCT and other very rare nonchoriocarcinomatous trophoblastic tumors, which are more indolent in the limited data that has become available in recent times.[36–38] The latter group includes cystic trophoblastic tumor (CTT), epithelioid trophoblastic tumors, and placental site trophoblastic tumor, which are usually seen either as a part of mixed GCT or as residual disease at metastatic site after chemotherapy.[4] Cystic change with prominent cytoplasmic lacunae is seen in CTT, which usually occurs after chemotherapy.[4]

Regressed germ cell tumors
Also referred to as "burnt out" GCTs, they are categorized under GCTs of unknown type in WHO 2022 classification and usually present as retroperitoneal lymph node masses with an occult or regressed primary testicular tumor. A high index of clinical suspicion with thorough sampling and correlation with serum markers is essential in identifying them because they may mimic testicular torsion.[39] An active and meticulous search for certain specific features that includes GCNIS in the background testicular parenchyma, hemosiderin-laden macrophages, and coarse calcification in tubules of scarred area should be undertaken (**Fig. 5**).[40] A completely regressed tumor may only show scar tissue in the testis with no evidence of any residual tumor, GCNIS or calcification. In such cases, it is almost impossible to distinguish them from nonneoplastic scarring and a close follow-up is the only viable option. Identifying a testicular primary is important because without an orchidectomy, the disease may relapse and also present at higher stage.[13,41]

NON-GERM CELL NEOPLASIA IN SITU-DERIVED GERM CELL TUMORS

This group of tumors shows no evidence of derivation from GCNIS with an absence of isochromosome 12p and includes spermatocytic tumor, prepubertal-type teratomas, and prepubertal YST with some mixed forms.[4]

Spermatocytic Tumor

Spermatocytic tumor (ST) was renamed in the 2016 WHO revision (from spermatocytic seminoma) reflecting its benign behavior.[42,43] Incidence of ST peaks at a relatively older age than other TGCTs and presents usually with painless testicular enlargement which is reported bilateral in 9% of cases.[4] There is a typical polymorphous population of tumor cells with negativity for OCT3/4 immunoreactivity (**Fig. 6**). More recently described features include edema, granulomatous inflammation, intratubular spread, vessel invasion, and necrosis.[44]

Although c-kit is frequently positive, newer immunochemical markers such as SSX proteins may be helpful.[45] Although orchidectomy is considered curative due to its indolent nature, a handful of aggressive types have been described in the literature with metastasis. This is reported in relation to sarcomatous transformation and very recently identification of STs with hybrid genetics characterized by chromosome 12p amplification, a highly unusual and intriguing finding. Authors have found lymphovascular invasion in these cases and speculated that gain of 12p might be linked to metastatic potential in STs analogous to this phenomenon in GCNIS-derived GCTs.[43,46–49] Further research is needed to define possible biomarkers of aggressive clinical behavior in this otherwise benign tumor.[50]

Prepubertal-Type Teratoma

These are essentially benign tumors resembling somatic tissue of all 3 lineages (ectoderm, endoderm, and mesoderm) with significant difference in prognosis and management from postpubertal-type teratomas. Distinguishing these 2 entities is not entirely based on attaining puberty as they can both be seen postpubertally and prepubertally and depends on examination of the background testis for atrophic changes, microlithiasis, GCNIS which are not seen in prepubertal type. Significant immaturity and embryonic areas are not seen within these tumors. In challenging cases, absence of chromosome 12p amplifications by molecular analyses can aid conformation of prepubertal-type teratoma.[13,51] Various specialized subtypes such as dermoid cyst, epidermoid cyst, and monodermal teratoma are described, with a higher incidence of well differentiated neuroendocrine tumor (NET) in association with prepubertal type teratomas (**Fig. 7**).[51,52] Recent consensus papers have recommended discarding the term "carcinoid" and using NET in line with WHO guidance of other anatomic sites.[53] Although mostly indolent,[54,55] further study assessing Ki67 proliferation index and mitotic index is suggested to better prognosticate testicular NETs.

CLINICS CARE POINTS

- GCNIS is the standard terminology for preinvasive TGCTs.

- Amplification on chromosome 12p (isochromosome 12p) by molecular analysis is a useful test for confirming GCNIS-derived GCTs in challenging cases.

- Seminoma is the most common TGCT having an excellent prognosis. They can exhibit diverse histologic patterns and may lead to a potential diagnostic pitfall.

- Testicular teratomas are classified into postpubertal and prepubertal types and have entirely different derivations and behavior.

- Teratoma with somatic type malignancy occurs in a small subset of postpubertal-type teratoma either within the testis or more commonly in metastatic sites and is characterized by an expansile mass of a pure tumor type.

- Criteria for teratoma with somatic type malignancy needs further refinement with the current recommendation to use 5 mm as minimum size of expansile nodule rather than 4X objective.

- The term PNET is outdated and should be replaced by the term ENET.

- Neuroendocrine tumor should be used in place of carcinoid.

- YSTs show diverse and complex histologic patterns with recently described patterns, which could mimic sarcoma and carcinoma.

- STs are non–GCNIS-derived indolent neoplasms with rare reported cases of sarcomatous transformation and metastasis. Recent studies have found rare chromosome 12 amplification and introduced a novel concept of hybrid genetics in these tumors.

SEX CORD STROMAL TUMORS

Sex cord stromal tumors (SCSTs) are relatively rare and account for 4% to 8% of all testicular tumors, with a higher proportion of cases in pediatric population.[56] SCSTs can be a diagnostic challenge due to their relative unfamiliarity, wide heterogeneity in morphology, and inconsistent IHC expression. Newer markers such as SOX9, FOXL2, and SF-1 are helpful in this regard.[57] Association with rare genetic alterations and the potential for malignancy causes further challenges in some subtypes.[58–60]

SCSTs usually present as a nodule or painless swelling of testicle with occasional hormonal manifestations. The incidence is apparently increasing secondary to the increase in detection and later excision of ultrasound-detected masses of uncertain clinical significance.[61] Grossly, they are usually well-circumscribed, lobulated tan white to yellow in appearance.[56] Most behave indolently, particularly the tumors in the fibroma-thecoma group but a minority of SCSTs may metastasize. However, the data for malignant behavior are challenging due to referral practice bias, lack of follow-up of supposed benign lesions and inconsistent recording of data.[62] High-risk features are described correlating with malignant potential, which should be documented in a pathology report. These include tumor size greater than 50 mm, infiltrative borders, cytologic atypia, 3 or more mitotic figures per 10 high power fields (HPF), lymphovascular invasion, extratesticular growth, and necrosis.[63,64] To achieve more uniformity and comparability in assessing mitotic counts, it has been now recommended to use square millimeter rather than number high or low power fields in all SCSTs.[59]

Sertoli cell tumors (SCTs) demonstrate a huge range of morphologic complexity and a definitive diagnosis may be difficult especially in solid/undifferentiated forms with minimal identifiable tubulopapillary pattern. Nuclear expression of SF1 on immunohistochemistry is a consistent marker to ascertain such tumors as sex-cord stromal.[65] In addition, CTNNB1 gene mutation with nuclear expression of β-catenin on immunohistochemistry (Fig. 8) is seen in 60% to 70% of SCTs NOS and is a robust diagnostic tool in differentiating them from GCTs in challenging cases.[66] Malignant SCTs may mimic seminoma and can be misdiagnosed as such leading to inappropriate therapy.[67] Similar to the prior edition, the WHO 2022 revision did not separately classify sclerosing SCT but noted SCTs with this rare morphologic pattern seem to have a better prognosis than other SCTs.[3,59] It is recommended to indicate percentage of sclerosing pattern in these tumors because the metastatic potential was less in tumors with abundant sclerosis, compared with their cellular counterparts.[3,59]

In terms of treatment, most SCSTS are benign and orchidectomy (total or partial) remains the most effective therapeutic approach. However, in cases with high-risk features, management, and follow-up remains controversial. Systemic chemotherapy/radiation have limited efficacy in unresectable metastatic disease.[64,68] Further genomic profiling studies and clinical trials are required to explore targeted therapies and guide management.[69]

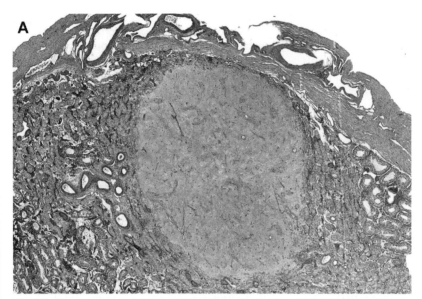

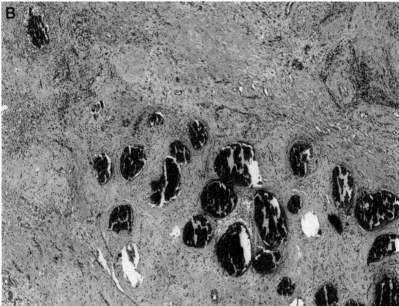

Fig. 5. Regressed germ cell tumor showing (*A*) a well-circumscribed scar tissue with surrounding GCNIS and (*B*) background testicular atrophy, coarse calcification, and hemosiderin-laden macrophages.

NEWLY DESCRIBED TYPES OF SEX CORD STROMAL TUMORS

One of the recently described patterns in SCTs is of a striking signet ring appearance, which seems to have an indolent behavior and demonstrates nuclear expression of β-catenin. These tumors can mimic and be misclassified as metastatic adenocarcinoma; however, they are entirely benign.[70] Recent studies have showed its similar morphologic, IHC, and molecular alterations with pancreatic solid pseudopapillary neoplasm suggesting a common pathogenesis while others thought this may represent just a pattern of

SCT.[71,72] It is important to be aware of this tumor due to the significantly different clinical course and potentially should be classified as a separate entity "signet ring stromal tumor."[3]

Myoid gonadal stromal tumor is another rare indolent testicular neoplasm characterized by a spindle cell proliferation with features of gonadal stroma and smooth muscle in a background containing collagen and tubules (Fig. 9). These tumors have a low mitotic activity and coexpress S100 and smooth muscle actin in addition to SCST markers such as SF1 and inhibin, which may show focal positivity. This was considered as

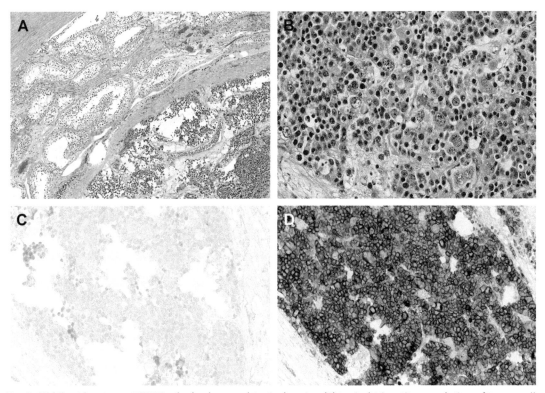

Fig. 6. ST (*A*) without any GCNIS in the background testis showing (*B*) typical tripartite population of tumor cells. (*C*) Tunour cells are negative for OCT3/4 with (*D*) diffuse expression of CD117.

emerging entity in WHO 2016 and is recognized as a distinct entity in the 2022 edition.[3,73]

Large cell calcifying SCT (LCCSCT) and intratubular large cell hyalinizing Sertoli cell neoplasia (ILCHSCT) are distinct neoplasms of Sertoli cells having genetic associations. LCCSCT (Fig. 10) may either occur sporadically or in association with Carney complex with germline mutation in

Fig. 7. Prepubertal-type teratoma with well-differentiated NET.

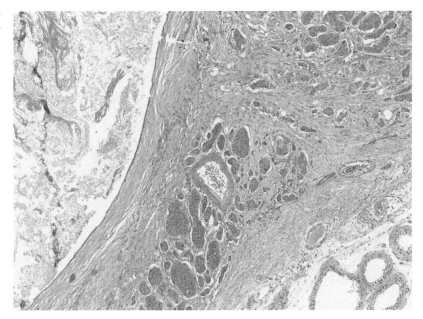

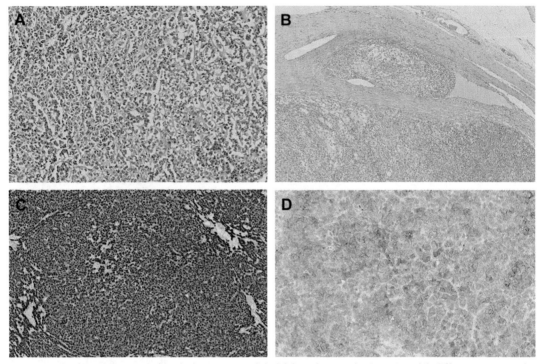

Fig. 8. SCT showing (*A*) a vaguely tubular pattern with (*B*) lymphovascular invasion, (*C*) diffuse strong nuclear expression of β-catenin, and (*D*) patchy positivity for CD99.

PRKAR1A gene on chromosome 17q22 to 24. ILCHSCT almost exclusively occurs in patients with Peutz-Jeghers syndrome characterized by germline mutation in *STK11* gene and shows histologic features overlapping with LCCSCT but with prominent intratubular growth accompanied by thick basement membrane and are usually benign.[74,75]

Furthermore, Leydig cell tumors may rarely also show genetic predisposition and be associated with Klinefelter syndrome, hereditary leiomyomatosis, and hereditary renal cell cancer

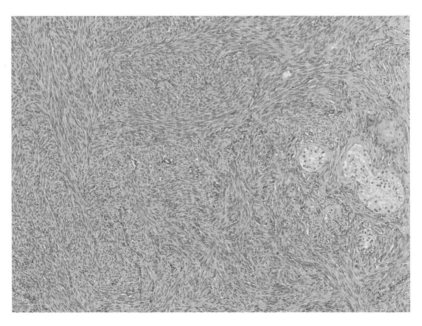

Fig. 9. Myoid gonadal stromal tumor composed of spindle cells and tubules in a collagenous background.

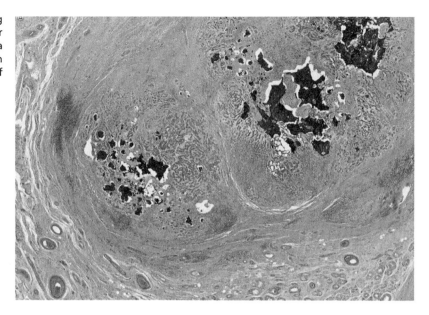

Fig. 10. LCCSCT showing nests and cords of tumor cells embedded in a collagenous stroma with prominent foci of calcification.

syndromes with germline fumarate hydratase mutation.[76] Genetic counseling should be offered in men with such tumors if clinically indicated.[59,77]

TUMORS CONTAINING BOTH GERM CELL AND SEX CORD-STROMAL ELEMENTS

WHO 2022 includes gonadoblastoma (GB) as an in situ form of malignant GCT consisting of GCNIS, seminoma, or dysgerminoma cells, and incompletely differentiated sex cord cells reminiscent of Sertoli or granulosa cells. This tumor occurs solely in individuals with a disorder of sex development.[3] Most people with this abnormality are phenotypically female, although a minority are phenotypic men with undescended gonads.[78] All karyotypically possess a Y chromosome. The dysgenetic gonads are composed of germ cells and sex cord stromal derivatives resembling immature sex cord cells. However, in fact, the immature sex cord cells are not neoplastic, and it merely represents a very unusual form of in situ germ cell malignancy. Pure GB is therefore considered as noninvasive neoplasm having excellent prognosis with local excision of bilateral dysgenetic gonads.[78] However, if left in place, progression into seminoma is seen in 80% of cases and into nonseminoma in around 20%. Moreover, an associated malignant GCT is seen in around 60% of classic GB at presentation.[59,79]

A recent study has argued in favor of existence of true testicular mixed germ cell-sex cord tumor (MGSCT) and proposed its recognition in line with the ovarian counterpart.[80] In this study with a relatively small but unique series, authors found extratesticular invasion by a germ cell component with some features of ST along with the presence of atypical mitoses and multiple chromosomal aberrations. In the past, this has been regarded as SCST with entrapped nonneoplastic germ cells and therefore further research is required to ascertain its existence. We would contend that this is likely to be a collision tumor rather than a neoplasm differentiating along such widely divergent lines.

CLINICS CARE POINTS

- Most SCSTs are indolent in behavior.

- High-risk features include tumor size greater than 50 mm, infiltrative borders, cytologic atypia, 3 or more mitotic figures per 10 HPF, lymphovascular invasion, extratesticular growth and necrosis. It is now recommended that mitotic activity be represented in square millimeter rather than HPF.

- Nuclear expression of β-catenin and SF1 are robust IHC markers for SCT. SOX 9 and FOXL2 are also helpful.

- Signet ring stromal tumor and myoid gonadal stromal tumor are both indolent tumors and may potentially be classified as separate entities.

- LCCSCT and ILCHSCT are distinct neoplasms of Sertoli cells having genetic associations.

- Diagnosis of a pure GB is straightforward but a cautious approach should be taken in distinguishing GB, especially dissecting GB, a morphologic variant of GB, and undifferentiated gonadal tissue from germinomas as the management and prognosis are significantly different.

- Evidence in favor of true testicular MGSCT is being published and is potentially another emerging entity.

SUMMARY

In summary, recent advances has led to refinement and stabilization of the classification of testicular tumors and is aligned toward achieving uniformity by minimizing interobserver variation and incorporating updates in tumors of other organ systems. Evolving knowledge has led us to understand the disease biology better enabling an improved patient management but at the same time posed us with some challenges and confounding facts to fuel further research and development.

CONFLICTS OF INTEREST

The authors state that they have no conflicts of interest. D.M. Berney is supported by Orchid.

REFERENCES

1. Park JS, Kim J, Elghiaty A, et al. Recent global trends in testicular cancer incidence and mortality. Medicine (Baltimore) 2018;97(37):e12390.
2. Oldenburg J, Berney DM, Bokemeyer C, et al. Testicular seminoma and non-seminoma: ESMO-EURACAN Clinical Practice Guideline for diagnosis, treatment and follow-up. Ann Oncol Off J Eur Soc Med Oncol 2022;S0923-7534(22):00007–12.
3. WHO Classification of Tumours Editorial Board. Urinary and male genital tumours [Internet], [cited YYYY Mmm D]. 5th edition.. WHO classification of tumours series, 8 Lyon (France): International Agency for Research on Cancer; 2022. Available from: https://tumourclassification.iarc.who.int/chapters/36.
4. Ulbright TM, Amin MB, Balzer B, et al. Tumors of the testis and paratesticular tissue. In: Moch H, Humphrey PA, Ulbright TM, et al, editors. World Health Organization classification of tumours of the urinary system and male genital organs. 4th edition. Lyon (France): IARC Press; 2016. p. 185–258.
5. Berney DM, Looijenga LHJ, Idrees M, et al. Germ cell neoplasia in situ (GCNIS): evolution of the current nomenclature for testicular pre-invasive germ cell malignancy. Histopathology 2016;69(1):7–10.
6. Cheng L, Albers P, Berney DM, et al. Testicular cancer. Nat Rev Dis Primer 2018;4(1):29.
7. Oosterhuis JW, Looijenga LHJ. Human germ cell tumours from a developmental perspective. Nat Rev Cancer 2019;19(9):522–37.
8. Fichtner A, Richter A, Filmar S, et al. The detection of isochromosome i(12p) in malignant germ cell tumours and tumours with somatic malignant transformation by the use of quantitative real-time polymerase chain reaction. Histopathology 2021;78(4):593–606.
9. Howitt BE, Berney DM. Tumors of the Testis: Morphologic Features and Molecular Alterations. Surg Pathol Clin 2015;8(4):687–716.
10. Berney DM, Stoneham S, Arora R, et al. Ovarian germ cell tumour classification: views from the testis. Histopathology 2020;76(1):25–36.
11. Ulbright TM, Young RH. Seminoma with conspicuous signet ring cells: a rare, previously uncharacterized morphologic variant. Am J Surg Pathol 2008;32(8):1175–81.
12. Ulbright TM. Pitfalls in the interpretation of specimens from patients with testicular tumours, with an emphasis on variant morphologies. Pathology (Phila) 2018;50(1):88–99.
13. Williamson SR, Delahunt B, Magi-Galluzzi C, et al. The world health organization 2016 classification of testicular germ cell tumours: a review and update from the international society of urological pathology testis consultation panel. Histopathology 2017;70(3):335–46.
14. Daugaard G, Gundgaard MG, Mortensen MS, et al. Surveillance for stage I nonseminoma testicular cancer: outcomes and long-term follow-up in a population-based cohort. J Clin Oncol Off J Am Soc Clin Oncol 2014;32(34):3817–23.
15. Nayan M, Jewett MAS, Hosni A, et al. Conditional Risk of relapse in surveillance for clinical stage i testicular cancer. Eur Urol 2017;71(1):120–7.
16. Berney DM, Comperat E, Feldman DR, et al. Datasets for the reporting of neoplasia of the testis: recommendations from the International Collaboration on Cancer Reporting. Histopathology 2019;74(1):171–83.
17. Blok JM, Pluim I, Daugaard G, et al. Lymphovascular invasion and presence of embryonal carcinoma as risk factors for occult metastatic disease in clinical stage I nonseminomatous germ cell tumour: a systematic review and meta-analysis. BJU Int 2020;125(3):355–68.
18. Kao CS, Ulbright TM, Young RH, et al. Testicular embryonal carcinoma: a morphologic study of 180 cases highlighting unusual and unemphasized aspects. Am J Surg Pathol 2014;38(5):689–97.
19. Berney DM, Shamash J, Pieroni K, et al. Loss of CD30 expression in metastatic embryonal carcinoma: the effects of chemotherapy? Histopathology 2001;39(4):382–5.
20. Berney DM, Lu YJ, Shamash J, et al. Postchemotherapy changes in testicular germ cell tumours: biology and morphology. Histopathology 2017;70(1):26–39.

21. Michael H, Hull MT, Ulbright TM, et al. Primitive neuroectodermal tumors arising in testicular germ cell neoplasms. Am J Surg Pathol 1997;21(8):896–904.

22. Ulbright TM, Hattab EM, Zhang S, et al. Primitive neuroectodermal tumors in patients with testicular germ cell tumors usually resemble pediatric-type central nervous system embryonal neoplasms and lack chromosome 22 rearrangements. Mod Pathol Off J U S Can Acad Pathol Inc 2010;23(7):972–80.

23. Matoso A, Idrees MT, Rodriguez FJ, et al. Neuroglial differentiation and neoplasms in testicular germ cell tumors lack immunohistochemical evidence of alterations characteristic of their cns counterparts: a study of 13 cases. Am J Surg Pathol 2019;43(3):422–31.

24. Kilpatrick SE, Reith JD, Rubin B. Ewing sarcoma and the history of similar and possibly related small round cell tumors: from whence have we come and where are we going? Adv Anat Pathol 2018;25(5):314–26.

25. Louis DN, Perry A, Reifenberger G, et al. The 2016 world health organization classification of tumors of the central nervous system: a summary. Acta Neuropathol (Berl) 2016;131(6):803–20.

26. Flood TA, Ulbright TM, Hirsch MS. Embryonic-type Neuroectodermal Tumor" should replace "primitive neuroectodermal tumor" of the testis and gynecologic tract: a rationale for new nomenclature. Am J Surg Pathol 2021;45(10):1299–302.

27. Necchi A, Colecchia M, Nicolai N, et al. Towards the definition of the best management and prognostic factors of teratoma with malignant transformation: a single-institution case series and new proposal. BJU Int 2011;107(7):1088–94.

28. Scheckel CJ, Kosiorek HE, Butterfield R, et al. Germ cell tumors with malignant somatic transformation: a mayo clinic experience. Oncol Res Treat 2019;42(3):95–100.

29. Motzer RJ, Amsterdam A, Prieto V, et al. Teratoma with malignant transformation: diverse malignant histologies arising in men with germ cell tumors. J Urol 1998;159(1):133–8.

30. Kao CS, Idrees MT, Young RH, et al. Solid pattern yolk sac tumor: a morphologic and immunohistochemical study of 52 cases. Am J Surg Pathol 2012;36(3):360–7.

31. Howitt BE, Magers MJ, Rice KR, et al. Many post-chemotherapy sarcomatous tumors in patients with testicular germ cell tumors are sarcomatoid yolk sac tumors: a study of 33 cases. Am J Surg Pathol 2015;39(2):251–9.

32. Michael H, Lucia J, Foster RS, et al. The pathology of late recurrence of testicular germ cell tumors. Am J Surg Pathol 2000;24(2):257–73.

33. Al-Obaidy KI, Williamson SR, Shelman N, et al. Hepatoid teratoma, hepatoid yolk sac tumor, and hepatocellular carcinoma: a morphologic and immunohistochemical study of 30 cases. Am J Surg Pathol 2021;45(1):127–36.

34. Magers MJ, Kao CS, Cole CD, et al. Somatic-type" malignancies arising from testicular germ cell tumors: a clinicopathologic study of 124 cases with emphasis on glandular tumors supporting frequent yolk sac tumor origin. Am J Surg Pathol 2014;38(10):1396–409.

35. Segura SE, Young RH, Oliva E, et al. Malignant Gonadal Germ Cell Tumors (Other Than Pure Germinoma) in Patients With Disorders of Sex Development: A Report of 21 Cases Based Largely on the Collection of Dr Robert E. Scully, Illustrating a High Frequency of Yolk Sac Tumor With Prominent Hepatoid and Glandular Features. Am J Surg Pathol Published online September 23, 2021. doi:10.1097/PAS.0000000000001815.

36. Petersson F, Grossmann P, Vanecek T, et al. Testicular germ cell tumor composed of placental site trophoblastic tumor and teratoma. Hum Pathol 2010;41(7):1046–50.

37. Ulbright TM, Henley JD, Cummings OW, et al. Cystic trophoblastic tumor: a nonaggressive lesion in postchemotherapy resections of patients with testicular germ cell tumors. Am J Surg Pathol 2004;28(9):1212–6.

38. Idrees MT, Kao CS, Epstein JI, et al. Nonchoriocarcinomatous trophoblastic tumors of the testis: the widening spectrum of trophoblastic neoplasia. Am J Surg Pathol 2015;39(11):1468–78.

39. Kao CS, Zhang C, Ulbright TM. Testicular hemorrhage, necrosis, and vasculopathy: likely manifestations of intermittent torsion that clinically mimic a neoplasm. Am J Surg Pathol 2014;38(1):34–44. https://doi.org/10.1097/PAS.0b013e31829c0206.

40. Miller JS, Lee TK, Epstein JI, et al. The utility of microscopic findings and immunohistochemistry in the classification of necrotic testicular tumors: a study of 11 cases. Am J Surg Pathol 2009;33(9):1293–8.

41. Balzer BL, Ulbright TM. Spontaneous regression of testicular germ cell tumors: an analysis of 42 cases. Am J Surg Pathol 2006;30(7):858–65.

42. Lombardi M, Valli M, Brisigotti M, et al. Spermatocytic seminoma: review of the literature and description of a new case of the anaplastic variant. Int J Surg Pathol 2011;19(1):5–10.

43. Moch H, Cubilla AL, Humphrey PA, et al. The 2016 WHO classification of tumours of the urinary system and male genital organs-part a: renal, penile, and testicular tumours. Eur Urol 2016;70(1):93–105.

44. Hu R, Ulbright TM, Young RH. Spermatocytic seminoma: a report of 85 cases emphasizing its morphologic spectrum including some aspects not widely known. Am J Surg Pathol 2019;43(1):1–11.

45. Anderson WJ, Maclean FM, Acosta AM, et al. Expression of the C-terminal region of the SSX protein is a useful diagnostic biomarker for spermatocytic tumour. Histopathology 2021;79(5):700–7.

46. Horn T, Schulz S, Maurer T, et al. Poor efficacy of BEP polychemotherapy in metastatic spermatocytic seminoma. Med Oncol Northwood Lond Engl 2011; 28(Suppl 1):S423–5.

47. Mikuz G, Böhm GW, Behrend M, et al. Therapy-resistant metastasizing anaplastic spermatocytic seminoma: a cytogenetic hybrid: a case report. Anal Quant Cytopathol Histopathol 2014;36(3):177–82.

48. Steiner H, Gozzi C, Verdorfer I, et al. Metastatic spermatocytic seminoma–an extremely rare disease. Eur Urol 2006;49(1):183–6.

49. Wagner T, Grantham M, Berney D. Metastatic spermatocytic tumour with hybrid genetics: breaking the rules in germ cell tumours. Pathology (Phila) 2018;50(5):562–5.

50. Grogg JB, Schneider K, Bode PK, et al. A systematic review of treatment outcomes in localised and metastatic spermatocytic tumors of the testis. J Cancer Res Clin Oncol 2019;145(12):3037–45.

51. Wagner T, Scandura G, Roe A, et al. Prospective molecular and morphological assessment of testicular prepubertal-type teratomas in postpubertal men. Mod Pathol Off J U S Can Acad Pathol Inc 2020;33(4):713–21.

52. Zhang C, Berney DM, Hirsch MS, et al. Evidence supporting the existence of benign teratomas of the postpubertal testis: a clinical, histopathologic, and molecular genetic analysis of 25 cases. Am J Surg Pathol 2013;37(6):827–35.

53. Rindi G, Klimstra DS, Abedi-Ardekani B, et al. A common classification framework for neuroendocrine neoplasms: an International Agency for Research on Cancer (IARC) and World Health Organization (WHO) expert consensus proposal. Mod Pathol Off J U S Can Acad Pathol Inc 2018;31(12):1770–86.

54. Wang WP, Guo C, Berney DM, et al. Primary carcinoid tumors of the testis: a clinicopathologic study of 29 cases. Am J Surg Pathol 2010;34(4):519–24.

55. Amine MM, Mohamed B, Mourad H, et al. Neuroendocrine Testicular Tumors: A Systematic Review and Meta-Analysis. Curr Urol 2017;10(1):15–25.

56. Dilworth JP, Farrow GM, Oesterling JE. Non-germ cell tumors of testis. Urology 1991;37(5):399–417.

57. Lau HD, Kao CS, Williamson SR, et al. Immunohistochemical characterization of 120 testicular sex cord-stromal tumors with an emphasis on the diagnostic utility of SOX9, FOXL2, and SF-1. Am J Surg Pathol 2021;45(10):1303–13.

58. Young RH. Sex cord-stromal tumors of the ovary and testis: their similarities and differences with consideration of selected problems. Mod Pathol Off J U S Can Acad Pathol Inc 2005;18(Suppl 2):S81–98.

59. Idrees MT, Ulbright TM, Oliva E, et al. The World Health Organization 2016 classification of testicular non-germ cell tumours: a review and update from the International Society of Urological Pathology Testis Consultation Panel. Histopathology 2017;70(4):513–21.

60. Mosharafa AA, Foster RS, Bihrle R, et al. Does retroperitoneal lymph node dissection have a curative role for patients with sex cord-stromal testicular tumors? Cancer 2003;98(4):753–7.

61. Scandura G, Verrill C, Protheroe A, et al. Incidentally detected testicular lesions <10 mm in diameter: can orchidectomy be avoided? BJU Int 2018;121(4): 575–82.

62. Fankhauser CD, Grogg JB, Rothermundt C, et al. Treatment and follow-up of rare testis tumours. J Cancer Res Clin Oncol 2022;20. https://doi.org/ 10.1007/s00432-021-03890-2.

63. Grogg JB, Schneider K, Bode PK, et al. Risk factors and treatment outcomes of 239 patients with testicular granulosa cell tumors: a systematic review of published case series data. J Cancer Res Clin Oncol 2020;146(11):2829–41.

64. Grogg J, Schneider K, Bode PK, et al. Sertoli cell tumors of the testes: systematic literature review and meta-analysis of outcomes in 435 patients. Oncologist 2020;25(7):585–90.

65. Sangoi AR, McKenney JK, Brooks JD, et al. Evaluation of SF-1 expression in testicular germ cell tumors: a tissue microarray study of 127 cases. Appl Immunohistochem Mol Morphol AIMM 2013;21(4):318–21.

66. Zhang C, Ulbright TM. Nuclear localization of β-catenin in sertoli cell tumors and other sex cord-stromal tumors of the testis: an immunohistochemical study of 87 cases. Am J Surg Pathol 2015;39(10):1390–4.

67. Henley JD, Young RH, Ulbright TM. Malignant Sertoli cell tumors of the testis: a study of 13 examples of a neoplasm frequently misinterpreted as seminoma. Am J Surg Pathol 2002;26(5):541–50.

68. Fankhauser CD, Grogg JB, Hayoz S, et al. Risk factors and treatment outcomes of 1,375 patients with testicular leydig cell tumors: analysis of published case series data. J Urol 2020;203(5):949–56.

69. Necchi A, Bratslavsky G, Shapiro O, et al. Genomic features of metastatic testicular sex cord stromal tumors. Eur Urol Focus 2019;5(5):748–55.

70. Kao CS, Ulbright TM. A morphologic and immunohistochemical comparison of nuclear β-catenin expressing testicular sertoli cell tumors and pancreatic solid pseudopapillary neoplasms supporting their continued separate classification. Am J Surg Pathol 2020;44(8):1082–91.

71. Michalova K, Michal M, Kazakov DV, et al. Primary signet ring stromal tumor of the testis: a study of 13 cases indicating their phenotypic and genotypic analogy to pancreatic solid pseudopapillary neoplasm. Hum Pathol 2017;67:85–93.

72. Ulbright TM, Young RH. Pseudo-"solid pseudopapillary neoplasms" of the testis: in reality Sertoli cell tumors. Hum Pathol 2019;83:228–30.

73. Renne SL, Valeri M, Tosoni A, et al. Myoid gonadal tumor. case series, systematic review, and Bayesian analysis. Virchows Arch Int J Pathol 2021;478(4):727–34.

74. Anderson WJ, Gordetsky JB, Idrees MT, et al. Large cell calcifying sertoli cell tumour: a contemporary multi-institutional case series highlighting the diagnostic utility of PRKAR1A immunohistochemistry. *Histopathology.* Published online November 15, 2021. doi:10.1111/his.14599.

75. Ulbright TM, Amin MB, Young RH. Intratubular large cell hyalinizing sertoli cell neoplasia of the testis: a report of 8 cases of a distinctive lesion of the Peutz-Jeghers syndrome. Am J Surg Pathol 2007; 31(6):827–35.

76. Carvajal-Carmona LG, Alam NA, Pollard PJ, et al. Adult leydig cell tumors of the testis caused by germline fumarate hydratase mutations. J Clin Endocrinol Metab 2006;91(8):3071–5.

77. Mooney KL, Kao CS. A contemporary review of common adult non-germ cell tumors of the testis and paratestis. Surg Pathol Clin 2018;11(4):739–58.

78. Roth LM, Cheng L. Gonadoblastoma: origin and outcome. Hum Pathol 2020;100:47–53.

79. Kao CS, Idrees MT, Young RH, et al. Dissecting Gonadoblastoma" of scully: a morphologic variant that often mimics germinoma. Am J Surg Pathol 2016; 40(10):1417–23.

80. Michalova K, McKenney JK, Kristiansen G, et al. Novel insights into the mixed germ cell-sex cord stromal tumor of the testis: detection of chromosomal aneuploidy and further morphological evidence supporting the neoplastic nature of the germ cell component. Virchows Arch Int J Pathol 2020;477(5):615–23.

Testicular Cancer
Contemporary Updates in Staging

Khaleel I. Al-Obaidy, MD[a], Martin J. Magers, MD[b], Muhammad T. Idrees, MD[c],*

KEYWORDS

• Testis staging • Germ cell tumor • American Joint Commission on Cancer • Testicular tumors

Key points

• In pure seminoma, T1 is subclassified as T1a and T1b according to tumor's size using a 3 cm cutoff.

• Epididymal amd hilar soft tissue invasions are considered T2.

• Discontinuous spermatic cord involvement by vascular-lymphatic invasion represents M1 disease.

ABSTRACT

Testicular tumors are the most common solid tumors in young men, the vast majority of which are of germ cell origin. The staging of human cancers is paramount to correct patient management. Staging systems have passed through several developments leading to the release of the most recent 8th edition of the American Joint Committee for Cancer (AJCC) staging manual, which is based on the current understanding of tumor behavior and spread. In this review, the authors summarize the current AJCC staging of the germ cell tumors, highlight essential concepts, and provide insight into the most important parameters of testicular tumors.

OVERVIEW

The fundamentals of the malignant tumor staging, TNM (primary *t*umor, lymph *n*ode, and *m*etastasis), were developed by Professor Pierre Denoix in the mid-twentieth century.[1] Thereafter, the Union for International Cancer Control (UICC), in collaboration with Dr Denoix, chaired the UICC TNM Prognostic Factors Project committee to refine the TNM staging system, which eventually led to the publication of a pocketbook "Livre de Poche" in 1968. In the meantime, the American Joint Committee for Cancer (AJCC) started developing other but related definitions of the TNM categories, with the first AJCC cancer staging manual published in 1977. Subsequently, the UICC and the AJCC classifications were unified in 1987 to provide objective parameters to guide management decisions.[2]

Testicular tumors are the most common solid cancers in young men, of which germ cell tumors (GCTs) account for the vast majority.[3] The GCTs are divided into seminomatous and non-seminomatous tumors, with increasing risk around puberty and peaking at the ages of 25 and 35 years for non-seminomatous and seminomatous, respectively, exhibiting a bell-shaped curve of distribution. The first testicular AJCC staging system followed the same guidelines of the TNM stage categories. The T0 indicated no evidence of primary tumor, whereas T1 indicated a primary tumor limited to the testis, T2 indicated a tumor extending beyond the tunica albuginea, T3 indicated a tumor involving the rete testis or the epididymis, and T4 was divided into T4a or T4b, which indicated invasion of the spermatic cord or scrotum, respectively. Similarly, the N stage category was divided into N0-4, where N0 indicated no regional lymph node involvement; N1 indicated the involvement of a single (and mobile, if inguinal) ipsilateral regional

a Department of Pathology and Laboratory Medicine, Henry Ford Health, Detroit, MI 48202, USA; b IHA Pathology and Laboratory Medicine, Ann Arbor, MI 48106, USA; c Department of Pathology, Indiana University School of Medicine, Indianapolis, IN 46202, USA
* Corresponding author. Department of Pathology and Laboratory Medicine, School of Medicine, Indiana University, 350 West 11th Street, Suite 4014, Indianapolis, IN 46202.
E-mail address: midrees@iupui.edu

Surgical Pathology 15 (2022) 745–757
https://doi.org/10.1016/j.path.2022.07.010

lymph node; N2 indicated the involvement of contralateral, bilateral, or multiple (mobile, if inguinal) lymph nodes; N3 indicated the presence of fixed inguinal lymph nodes or palpable abdominal mass; and N4 indicated the involvement of juxtaregional lymph nodes. Distant metastasis was staged as M0 (no known distant metastases) or M1 (distant metastasis present). All TNM stage categories had an X classifier used when that component could not be assessed. Since the 1st edition, several advancements have developed leading to the release of the current 8th edition of the AJCC classification system.[4,5] In this article, the authors review the current classification system, highlight the major changes to the previous staging criteria, and provide insights into the current and contemporary staging of testicular cancer, focusing mainly on GCTs.

ANATOMY AND HISTOLOGY OF THE TESTIS

The testis is a paired oval-shaped organ located within the scrotum and suspended by the spermatic cord. The spermatic cord is covered by three layers derived from the abdominal wall coverings as they pass through the inguinal canal during the testicular descent into the scrotum. These layers are the internal spermatic fascia, the cremasteric muscle and fascia, and the external spermatic fascia. The spermatic cord comprises six structures: the vas deferens, arteries, veins (pampiniform plexus), lymphatics, nerves, and the processus vaginalis. The vas deferens arises from the lower pole of the epididymis, located at the posterolateral aspect of the testis. The testis is covered by the fibrous tissue (tunica albuginea) within the scrotum, with the anterior and medial aspects lying freely in the tunica vaginalis space. All these structures (testis, epididymis, and tunica vaginalis) are in turn covered by the three layers (internal spermsatic, cremaster muscle, and external spermatic fascia) surrounding the spermatic cord.

Histologically, the upper end of the epididymis is attached to the testis, where a fibrous tissue mass, the mediastinum testis, is present. It sends out multiple radiating septae reaching into the surrounding tunica albuginea and dividing the testis into nearly 250 lobules containing the highly compacted seminiferous tubules. The seminiferous tubules open into the rete testis at the mediastinum testis, which in turn open into the efferent ductules that communicate with the epididymis. Underneath the tunica albuginea is a vascular-rich fibrous tissue called the tunica vasculosa.

On cross section, the seminiferous tubules are lined by multiple layers of cells surrounded by a fibrous membrane. The outermost layer is formed by the spermatogonia, which divide to produce primary spermatocytes, further dividing to give rise to secondary spermatocytes. These almost immediately divide to produce spermatids that undergo metamorphosis and give rise to mature spermatozoa. In addition, the seminiferous tubules contain supporting cells, Sertoli cells, and Leydig cells, which lie in the fibrous septae outside the seminiferous tubules and secrete the testosterone hormone.

TESTICULAR GROSSING

The first step in accurate pathologic assessment is the gross examination and selection of the appropriate tissue sample for microscopic evaluation (Fig. 1A–F). This is especially true for testicular tumors. Grossing of testicular tumors is prone to multiple difficulties, including the presence of highly compacted seminiferous tubules, the friable nature of GCTs, and the mobility of the tunica vaginalis and tunica albuginea; therefore, careful assessment of the outer surface is an essential first step to the correct staging and for selection of which sections to submit for microscopic examination for diagnostic/staging confirmation. The extreme friability of tumorous tissue necessitates sectioning of the spermatic cord first, where an en face section of the surgical margin is to be taken before sectioning through the testicular parenchyma to avoid artifactual tumor displacement in the margin. In addition, GCTs can be assessed grossly to discern if there is direct extension into the epididymis and/or hilar soft tissue (pT2) or spermatic cord (pT3), or has discontinuously spread into the spermatic cord (pM1). Therefore, grossing of testicular tumors should address the following questions based on gross examination to appropriately get tissue sections for microscopic examination:

- Is there any tumor at the spermatic cord margin? (Section is taken before opening/bivalving the testis).
- Is there any gross tumor extension/metastasis in the spermatic cord outside the margin? (Ideally, sections are taken before opening/bivalving the testis).

Following these initial steps, the testis is ideally bivalved and left to fix overnight in formalin to minimize the amount of floating tissue before addressing the following additional questions with representative sections for microscopic examination:

- What is the size, color, consistency, and focality of the tumor?
- Are there any heterogeneous areas potentially indicating different histologic components (eg, cystic or rubbery [cartilaginous] areas

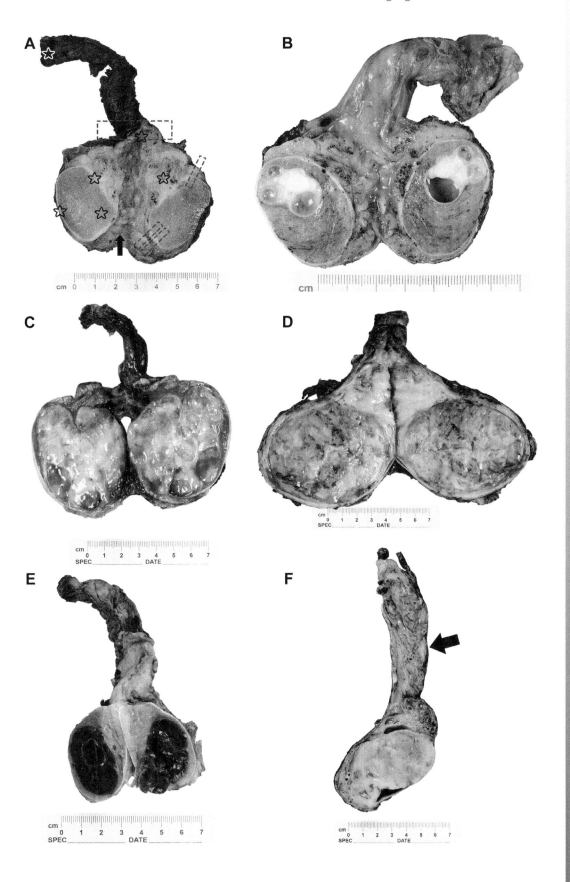

of teratoma or areas of hemorrhage in choriocarcinoma)?

- What is the relationship between the tumor and the adjacent tissues? (ie, the adjacent normal parenchyma, the tunica albuginea, the tunica vaginalis, the rete testis, the hilar fat/soft tissue, the epididymis, the spermatic cord, and scrotum, if present)?
- Are there any areas of fibrous scar indicating possible tumor regression?

TUMOR, NODES, METASTASIS STAGING AND DISCUSSION

Like any other organ system, the TNM staging is critical in the evaluation of the testicular tumors which dictates the clinical management and prognosis. The testis is unique because of its location and structural relationships to the paratesticular soft tissue and adnexal structures. Gross anatomy evaluation is critical for staging as different and distinct tumor involvement patterns of the paratesticular and adnexal structures make the staging of testicular tumors quite complex and demands attention to detail. It is unique that the AJCC developed this classification on GCTs; however, similar concepts may be applied for other malignant types of tumors, as discussed in the following section.

PRIMARY TUMOR: pT

The size, location, and extent of tumor into adjacent structure(s), including testicular tunics, adnexal structure, and paratesticular soft tissue, are important parameters for the AJCC staging. The current classification included several new criteria based on accumulating evidence, yet some areas still need further studies to fine-tune the classification.

pTx: PRIMARY TUMOR CANNOT BE ASSESSED

This category should only be used when tissue is unavailable or insufficient for the diagnosis. As orchidectomy is the most common specimen, the classification is developed based on the assumption that the testis, tunics, appendages, and paratesticular soft tissue including the spermatic cord, are procured and available for examination. Understandably, pTx could only be used in rare, unique circumstances, if ever required. To avoid confusion and impracticality, it is best to avoid this designation.

pT0: NO EVIDENCE OF PRIMARY TUMOR

In certain circumstances, no tumor may be identified after careful and thorough evaluation. One prime example is complete tumor regression with no tumor identified on the gross and microscopic evaluation of the testis when lymph node metastasis is present. Often a typical scar is present (Fig. 2A) along with germ cell neoplasia in situ (GCNIS) in the adjacent seminiferous tubules.[6] Sometimes, GCNIS is not identified despite thorough evaluation (ie, additional sectioning and immunohistochemical staining for OCT4).[7] If there is a scar and GCNIS, the pTis category should be used. Other possible scenarios with this designation include previous tumor resection or testicular infarction. In the latter, OCT4 immunohistochemistry (IHC) may help as infarcted tumor cells may show nuclear expression.

pTis: GERM CELL NEOPLASIA IN SITU

If no invasive tumor is present despite adequate sampling and only GCNIS is identified, it is prudent to designate it as pTis (Fig. 2B). As mentioned previously, sequelae of a regressed GCT in the form of scar are often present. Of course, IHC (eg, OCT4, CD117) may help in difficult cases.

pT1: TUMORS LIMITED TO THE TESTIS WITHOUT LYMPHOVASCULAR INVASION

Invasive tumors limited to the testis in the absence of lymphovascular invasion (LVI) are classified as pT1. Seminomas are subclassified into pT1a and pT1b based on a size cutoff of 3 cm (ie, <3 cm = pT1a, ≥3 cm = pT1b).[5,8–11] Adjuvant radiation or carboplatin-based chemotherapy decision-making depends on the size of the seminoma. In addition, it has been shown that seminoma size is an independent factor for

---

Fig. 1. Gross photographs of radical orchiectomy specimens. (A) Bivalved testis with asterixis indicating sections required for appropriate histologic evaluation, red rectangles showing the plane of sections including the epididymis, tunica albuginea, and proximal spermatic cord, black arrow indicating the start of the spermatic cord. (B) Intratesticular mixed germ cell tumor (pT1). (C) Seminoma involving the entire testis. The tumor was 4.5 cm and staged as pT1b. (D) Mixed germ cell tumor with hilar soft tissue invasion. (E) Well circumscribed intratesticular tumor with brownish tan cut surface. Microscopic assessment reveals a Leydig cell tumor. (F) Seminoma with discontinuous spread to the spermatic cord (arrow), staged as M1.

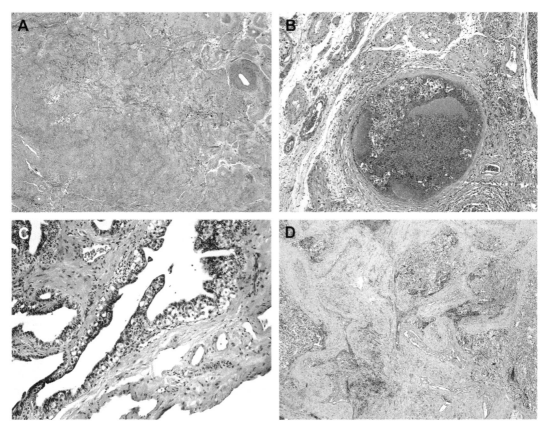

Fig. 2. Representative photographs showing (*A*) regressed germ cell tumor that is replaced by scar tissue with ghost tubules and hemosiderin pigment, (*B*) intratubular germ cell neoplasia (intratubular embryonal carcinoma), (*C*) rete testis with pagetoid spread, (*D*) invasion of the rete testis stroma by embryonal carcinoma, and also note rete testis hyperplasia usually associated with invasion.

disease progression.[8–12] There is no subdivision based on size for non-seminomatous GCTs, including mixed GCTs containing a seminoma component. Gross assessment is critical in this regard as macroscopic dimensions are usually incorporated into the template report. The utility of the 3 cm size cutoff to substage pure seminoma is debatable, and a cutoff closer to 4 cm is likely a better benchmark as supported by the larger studies.[8–11] This rather conservative approach adopted by the AJCC is contentious as more patients could receive unnecessary chemotherapy using the lower threshold for stage pT1b. It has been suggested in a few recent publications that rete testis stromal invasion may be associated with a higher clinical stage; however, AJCC thought that additional evidence is required to justify upstaging.[8,11–15] It is perplexing that a significant number of pathologists (21%) do not distinguish between stromal invasion and pagetoid extension of GCNIS in the rete testes (Fig. 2C, D).[15–18] This is partly due to nonuniformity concerning the definition and reporting of rete testis invasion.[16]

pT2: TUMOR INVADES EPIDIDYMIS AND/OR HILAR SOFT TISSUE AND/OR LYMPHOVASCULAR INVASION

GCTs commonly invade through the testicular hilum. The rete testis opens into the efferent ductules, and hilar soft tissue is contiguous with the base of the spermatic cord next to the head of the epididymis. Staging of hilar soft tissue invasion is problematic and lacks consensus among experts. For all practical purposes, the rete testis is considered part of the testis and invasion of rete testis is not considered an extension of the tumor out of the testis. The AJCC 8th edition stages the rete testis stromal invasion as pT1 (see Fig. 2D). However, there are limited data that suggest that the rete testis invasion does correlate with adverse prognosis, and it should be given a higher stage (pT2).[13,14,19] The pagetoid extension of GCNIS has not been shown as an independent factor for adverse outcome. In this area, there is a need for further larger multi-institutional studies to strengthen these observations, which are based on limited data. The hilar soft tissue invasion is defined as the adipose and loose fibrous connective tissue invasion. Owing to the relative sparsity of data and to elude the possibility of understaging, invasion of hilar soft tissue is staged as pT2. Therefore, the grosser should be mindful that for the confirmation, a section of the spermatic cord should be taken at the level of the head of the epididymis and designated as the proximal spermatic cord because hilar soft tissue cannot be morphologically distinguished from the soft tissue of the spermatic cord. This is critical and is addressed further in the discussion of pT3 staging.

In addition, invasion of the epididymis and other appendageal structures in the hilar soft tissue, including efferent ductules, is also staged as pT2 in the current staging scheme (Fig. 3C, D).[19] These were not addressed in the previous AJCC classifications. It is logical to think that epididymal invasion can only occur through invasion of hilar soft tissue; however, very rarely, a direct extension of tumor through tunica vaginalis can be seen. The perforation of tunica vaginalis by tumor is an infrequent event, and there is not much evidence to support a higher staging for this scenario; hence, it is kept in the pT2 category.

LVI is staged as pT2 regardless of the site of LVI (ie, intratesticular or extratesticular including spermatic cord) (Fig. 3A, E).[16–18] Documenting vascular invasion is more critical for nonseminomatous GCTs than pure seminomas.[8,11,17] Artifactual displacement of tumor cells into vessels is extremely common, especially in seminoma, so LVI should only be reported if there is unequivocal morphologic evidence (Fig. 3A, B).[20]

pT3: TUMOR INVADES SPERMATIC CORD WITH OR WITHOUT LYMPHOVASCULAR INVASION

A tumor that spreads into the spermatic cord via hilar soft tissue is staged as pT3. The start of the spermatic cord is arbitrarily defined at the level above the head of the epididymis. As previously mentioned, it is mandatory to evaluate the proximal spermatic cord to document the direct contiguous extension of the tumor through hilar soft tissue. It is also essential to grossly evaluate the entire spermatic cord and take sections from the center, and from any other area suspicious for tumor in addition to the distal cord margin. Several recent studies have suggested that spermatic cord LVI (see Fig. 3E) may be related to higher clinical stage and recurrence and should be classified

as pT3; however, it is still premature to adopt this based on limited data.[21,22] The discontinuous spread of the tumor in the spermatic cord outside of lymphovascular spaces is considered metastasis (Fig. 3F) and is further discussed in the metastasis (M) section.

pT4: INVASION OF SCROTUM WITH OR WITHOUT VASCULAR INVASION

Invasion of the scrotum is staged as pT4 and is extremely rare in developed countries. The definition of scrotal invasion is not clear as it is not thoroughly discussed in the AJCC staging manual. However, it should be clear that the parietal layer of tunica vaginalis should not be considered part of the scrotum. Only invasion beyond tunica vaginalis and spermatic fascia (into soft tissue or skin of the scrotum) is acceptable for pT4 consideration.

REGIONAL LYMPH NODES: pN

The GCTs from the testes typically metastasize to the retroperitoneal lymph nodes along the aorta and vena cava. These include interaortocaval, paraaortic (or periaortic), paracaval, preaortic, precaval, retroaortic, retrocaval, and lymph nodes along the spermatic vein. The tumor from the left side generally metastasizes to the left-sided retroperitoneal lymph nodes and seldom crosses over to the right side. Right-sided tumors predominantly metastasize to the right-sided retroperitoneal lymph nodes, but concurrent left-sided involvement can be seen as well compared with the left-sided tumors. The lymph node groups mentioned above are considered regional lymph nodes, and a pN stage is assigned. When patients have a previous inguinal or scrotal surgery, lymph nodes including intrapelvic, external iliac, and inguinal are also considered regional lymph nodes. Other abdominal lymph nodes and supradiaphragmatic nodes are considered nonregional, and an M stage is assigned to these nodes. The pN stage is divided based on the number of lymph nodes involved by the metastatic tumor, the size of the largest lymph node involved by the tumor, and the presence of extranodal extension. The size cutoffs remain unchanged in the AJCC 8th edition, but the criteria for numbers of involved lymph nodes and extranodal extension are modified and are introduced in this classification. It is important to carefully determine the number of lymph nodes and size of individual lymph nodes at grossing for the appropriate staging. Radiographic correlation is recommended to evaluate lymph node metastasis in the retroperitoneum or other sites.[23]

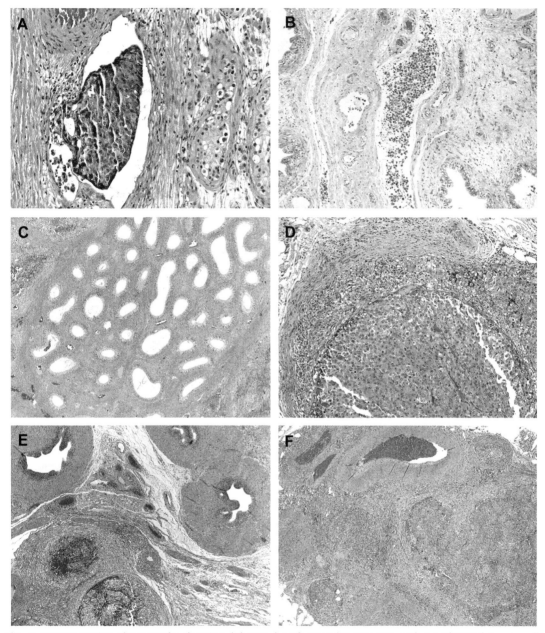

Fig. 3. Representative photographs showing (*A*) true lymphovascular invasion with intraluminal tumor cells adherent to the wall and (*B*) false lymphovascular invasion with intraluminal floating tumor cells, (*C*) epididymal invasion, (*D*) hilar soft tissue invasion, (*E*) lymphovascular invasion of the spermatic cord vessels, and (*F*) invasion of the spermatic cord stromal tissue.

It should be noted that the AJCC 8th edition emphasizes that the size cutoffs refer to the size of the involved lymph node and not the size of the metastatic deposit.

In addition, the metastatic deposit includes viable, nonviable tumor, hemorrhage, scarring, and chemotherapy-related changes. The percentage of the viable tumor should be included based on macroscopic and microscopic assessment.

Matted lymph nodes should be considered as one mass and reported as such.

pNx: REGIONAL LYMPH NODES CANNOT BE ASSESSED

If retroperitoneal lymph node dissection (RPLND) is not performed along with the radical orchiectomy and lymph nodes are not assessed, a pNx stage should be designated. RPLND performed on radiographically uninvolved lymph nodes or without evidence of metastatic disease is called virgin RPLND and is more commonly opted in North America than in European countries.

pN0: NO REGIONAL LYMPH NODE METASTASIS

A pN0 stage is assigned to regional lymph nodes if there is no evidence of metastatic disease on gross and microscopic examination. Necrosis, fibrosis, hemorrhage, scarring, and postchemotherapy changes involving the lymph nodes without viable tumor should be documented and quantified for facilitation of clinical and radiographical correlation. However, the nodal status remains pN0, and the prefix "y" is added if the patient is status post-chemotherapy (eg, ypN0).

pN1: LESS THAN FIVE POSITIVE LYMPH NODES, WITH NO SINGLE LYMPH NODE LARGER THAN 2 CM AND NO EXTRANODAL EXTENSION

The cumulative size of the tumor, including all the metastatic deposits in different lymph nodes, may be larger than 2 cm, but as long as the individual lymph nodes are less than 2 cm, it is staged as pN1. The AJCC did not discuss the determination of extranodal extension in matted lymph nodes; however, logically, the tumor cannot involve multiple matted lymph nodes without extranodal tumor extension, and the pN2 stage should be assigned in such a situation.

pN2: MORE THAN FIVE POSITIVE LYMPH NODES WITH NODAL SIZE RANGED BETWEEN 2 AND 5 CM AND/OR PRESENCE OF EXTRANODAL EXTENSION

The cumulative size of the metastatic foci may be larger than 5 cm, but only individual lymph nodes are accounted for the size. For example, if there are seven lymph nodes ranging in size from 2 to 4.5 cm, the assigned stage remains as pN2.

pN3: LYMPH NODE MEASURING LARGER THAN 5 CM IN GREATEST DIMENSION

pN3 staging should be assigned if any involved lymph node size is larger than 5 cm. The number of lymph nodes does not factor in this determination.

DISTANT METASTASIS: pM

Testicular GCTs typically spread to retroperitoneal lymph nodes. Spread to nonregional lymph nodes, lung, liver, bone, and other visceral sites can be sequential to or concurrent with regional lymph node metastasis. Rarely metastasis occurs in nonregional lymph nodes or other visceral sites without involving the retroperitoneal lymph nodes.

M0: NO DISTANT METASTASIS IDENTIFIED

If nonregional lymph nodes are histologically evaluated, the M stage is assigned. Like the N stage, if there is no viable tumor identified, an M0 stage is assigned; however, other findings, that is, such as necrosis, hemorrhage, scarring, and so forth, should be reported. Usually, the nonregional lymph nodes are not examined by the pathologists along with orchidectomy ± RPLND, and metastatic status is unknown; therefore, it is best not to comment on the M stage or report as "M stage-not applicable."

M1: DISTANT METASTASIS PRESENT

A tumor involving nonregional lymph nodes or visceral sites is reported as M1. In the AJCC 8th edition, M1 is further classified into M1a (nonretroperitoneal nodal or pulmonary metastases) and M1b (nonpulmonary visceral metastasis) in a slightly different manner from AJCC 7th edition, in which the M1a category included only the nonregional lymph nodes. However, pulmonary metastasis is lumped into M1a in the current edition. All other nonpulmonary visceral metastases are considered as M1b. Of course, the radiologic correlation is beneficial for adequate assessment.[23,24] Discontinuous spread of the tumor to the spermatic cord is staged as M1 without further subclassification, and it is unclear whether to classify it as M1a or M1b (discussed later).

SERUM TUMOR MARKERS: S

Serum tumor markers have great utility in testicular GCTs.[25,26] Reflecting this, the TNM staging system incorporates a fourth category for serum tumor markers (S). They aid in the diagnosis, prognosis, and therapeutic decision-making and should be measured before orchiectomy, after orchiectomy, during treatment to assess response, and during surveillance to monitor for recurrence.

However, as with any serum tumor marker, they are imperfect, and their interpretation must always be in conjunction with histologic, clinical, and radiographic findings.[27]

Alpha-fetoprotein (AFP), human chorionic gonadotropin (hCG), and lactate dehydrogenase (LDH) are the three serum tumor markers most associated with testicular GCTs and are included in the S category of the AJCC 8th edition TNM staging. AFP is synthesized in the yolk sac, liver, and intestine of fetuses, predominantly functioning as a serum binding protein. Serum AFP peaks at 12th to 14th week of gestation and subsequently decreases to less than 15 ng/mL during the first year after birth.

In germ cell neoplasia, AFP is primarily produced by yolk sac tumor, but it may also be produced, to a lesser extent, by embryonal carcinoma and teratoma. Pure choriocarcinoma and seminoma, however, do not produce AFP.[28] Because of this, a patient with an elevated AFP should be regarded as having a non-seminomatous GCT, even if seminoma is the only tumor type histologically identified. Owing to its half-life, serum levels of AFP should normalize in 20 to 28 days following therapy.

Placental syncytiotrophoblasts normally produce hCG, and increased levels in the setting of germ cell neoplasia are typically associated with trophoblastic tumors, primarily choriocarcinoma. Pure and predominant choriocarcinomas have markedly elevated serum hCG (above 55,000 with a median 199,000 IU/L).[29] Mixed GCTs with a minor ($\leq$0.5%) choriocarcinoma still have significantly elevated hCG (mean ~5000 IU/L).[30] However, elevated serum hCG may also occur in embryonal carcinoma and seminoma to a lesser extent.[28,31] Serum levels of hCG should normalize within 4 to 6 days following treatment.

Compared with AFP and hCG, LDH is more ubiquitously produced by many nonneoplastic tissue types, including muscle, liver, kidney, and brain. Because of this, it is not surprising that LDH is relatively nonspecific compared with AFP and hCG. Regardless, LDH is elevated in approximately half of the men with testicular GCTs.[32] Elevations of greater than 2000 U/L are consistent with the bulky seminomatous disease. LDH level is also related to tumor burden in non-seminomatous disease, and it may be the sole biochemical abnormality in ~10% of patients with persistent/recurrent non-seminomatous GCTs.[33]

The AJCC 8th edition S category is based on the pre-orchiectomy measurement of serum tumor markers. The category Sx is assigned when serum tumor markers have not been performed or are unavailable. The category of S0 is assigned when all serum tumor markers are within normal limits. If serum tumor markers are known to be elevated above normal limits, one of the categories of S1, S2, or S3 is applicable. S1 is assigned when at least one serum tumor marker is elevated above normal, and all the following criteria are met: LDH less than 1.5 times the upper limit of normal, hCG (mIU/mL) less than 5,000, and AFP (ng/mL) less than 1,000. S2 is assigned when one of the following criteria is present: LDH 1.5 to 10 times the upper limit of normal, hCG is between 5,000 and 50,000, or AFP is between 1,000 and 10,000. S3 is then assigned when LDH, hCG, or AFP are greater than their respective limit for the S2 category.

CHALLENGING ISSUES THAT NEED FURTHER STUDIES

- Subclassification of pT1 in pure seminoma is proposed in AJCC 8th edition based on a size cutoff of 3 cm (pT1a <3 cm and pT1b $\geq$ 3 cm). It is well known that the size of pure seminoma is an independent predictor of disease recurrence based on few credible studies.[8,10,11,15] There is some debate that AJCC has taken a very conservative approach by using a lower threshold of 3 cm for this subcategorization, as several larger studies suggested a higher cutoff close to 4 cm.[9,11,34,35] Substaging using 3 cm as the cutoff may lead to overtreatment of a subset of patients. On a positive note, this provides an opportunity to further look at comprehensive data to refine these criteria. There is pT1 substaging for the non-seminomatous GCTs, creating confusion for pathologists and the treating physicians.
- The contiguous tumor spread from hilar soft tissue to the spermatic cord is staged at pT3. As the distinction between the spermatic cord and hilar soft tissue is arbitrary and needs careful documentation of anatomical landmarks along with additional sections from the area, it is recommended to submit the entire hilar soft tissue and take a section of the proximal spermatic cord at the level above the head of the epididymis. Microscopic identification of the spermatic cord in the section ensures the appropriate documentation of the proximal spermatic cord.
- Noncontiguous spread of tumor in the soft tissue of spermatic cord is staged as M1. The

Table 1
The current 8th edition of the American Joint Committee for Cancer staging of testicular tumors

Pathologic Stage Category

Tumor (pT)	Criteria
pTX	Tumor cannot be assessed
pT0	No evidence of primary tumor
pTis	GCNIS
pT1	Tumor limited to the testis without LVI
pT1a	Tumor <3 cm in pure seminoma
pT1b	Tumor ≥3 cm in pure seminoma
pT2	Tumor extends to epididymis OR hilar soft tissue OR penetrates visceral mesothelial layer of the tunica albuginea with or without LVI OR Tumor limited to the testis with LVI
pT3	Direct invasion of the spermatic cord soft tissue
pT4	Invasion of the scrotum
Regional lymph node (pN)	
pNX	Lymph nodes cannot be assessed
pN0	No lymph nodes metastasis
pN1	A lymph node mass ≤2 cm OR metastasis to ≤5 lymph nodes, all are ≤2 cm
pN2	A lymph node mass >2 to 5 cm OR metastasis to >5 lymph nodes, all are ≤5 cm OR Presence of extranodal extension
pN3	A lymph node mass >5 cm
Metastasis (M)	
M0	No distant metastasis
M1	Distant metastasis
M1a	Pulmonary or non-RPLN metastasis
M1b	Nonpulmonary visceral metastasis

spermatic cord soft tissue invasion in this fashion is considered tumor spread secondary to vascular wall destruction leading to soft tissue extension. Extensive evaluation of the spermatic cord is required to identify any soft tissue extension of the tumor; additional routine sections and any suspicious area should therefore be sampled appropriately. The AJCC did not discuss whether this needs to be subclassified as M1a or M1b, and further clarification is required. One suggestion would be to classify it as M1sc (spermatic cord). Further comparative studies within the different cohorts of metastases (M1a vs. M1b vs. M1sc) are needed to clarify the prognostic significance of M1sc as an independent prognostic factor.

- Rete testes invasion is another contentious area where additional data are needed to refine the classification further. Currently, only limited data are available to suggest a classification of stromal invasion into higher stage (ie, pT2).

Table 2
A summary of the changes in the current 8th edition of the American Joint Committee for Cancer tumor, nodes, metastasis staging of testicular tumors

Stage Category	Summary of the Change
pT	T1 is subclassified into T1a and T1b according to the tumor size using a 3 cm cutoff in pure seminoma
pT	Epididymal invasion is considered T2
pT	Hilar soft tissue invasion is considered T2
pM	Discontinuous involvement of the spermatic cord by vascular-lymphatic invasion is M1 disease

Table 3
Differences in American Joint Committee for Cancer 8th edition and Union of International Cancer Control

Changes in AJCC 8th Edition	UICC Agreement with AJCC 8th Edition
In pure seminoma, T1 is subclassified as T1a and T1b according to tumor's size using a 3 cm cutoff.	NO
Epididymal invasion is considered T2 rather than T1.	NO
Hilar soft tissue invasion is considered T2.	NO
Discontinuous involvement of the spermatic cord by vascular-lymphatic invasion represents M1 disease	NO
For pTis, UICC uses term "intraepithelial germ cell neoplasia (carcinoma in situ)." Current terminology (WHO 2016) is "germ cell neoplasia in situ."	NO
Germ cell neoplasia in situ	*NO, still "intraepithelial germ cell neoplasia" or "carcinoma in situ"*

- Invasion of the scrotum (pT4) needs clarification as to what constitutes an actual invasion of the scrotum. This phenomenon is extremely rare but may be a more common finding in underdeveloped countries. The reasonable approach would be to consider invasion when the tumor permeates beyond the parietal layer of tunica vaginalis and spermatic cord fascia.
- Serum markers documentation is currently part of pathologic classification and is included in the College of American Pathologists cancer protocol template and is a reporting requirement. However, the serum markers are often not available to pathologists at the time of evaluation and consequently often are not added in the report. Emphasis on documentation and communication among interdisciplinary teams may improve this reporting requirement.
- The AJCC classification is more commonly used in North America; however, the rest of the world mostly follows UICC classification, and significant differences exist between the two classifications (Tables 1–3). Standardization and harmonization of these two different staging systems are essential to set aligning standards of care at the global level.
- The staging classifications for pediatric GCTs, sex cord stromal tumors, adnexal tumors, and paratesticular neoplasm do not exist and should be developed. Alternatively, current classifications for GCTs may be used with adequate modifications.
- International Germ Cell Consensus Classification Grouping has proposed guidelines for patient stratification into three risk categories (good, intermediate, and poor) considering serum markers and visceral metastasis including mediastinal location, which AJCC also endorsed. AJCC also provided its own guidelines to analyze established statistical prediction models for clinical purposes continuously. However, awareness of these guidelines is generally lacking for pathologists, and additional education or training is required to use these tools effectively.[36,37]

SUMMARY

Most of the tumors arising in the testis are GCTs. Owing to their relative rarity, extreme morphological diversity, unique presentations including young age at presentation, the diagnosis of these tumors is often challenging. However, these tumors have highly favorable prognosis as highly potent chemotherapy is available. It demands extraordinary attention and expertise in handling these tumors, which often present with complicated case histories and complex clinical scenarios. The current AJCC (8th edition) staging manual has provided refined classification criteria based on sound clinical and pathologic data relevant to overall survival and prognosis. Many abundantly beneficial modifications are provided compared with the previous edition; however, additional challenges exist that AJCC has identified and will continue to improve by incorporating the emerging data.

CLINICS CARE POINTS

- Spermatic cord margin should be taken before handing handling/ bivalving the orchiectomy specimens to avoid artifactual tumor displacement in the margin.

- Orchiectomy specimens should be bivalved before placing in formalin to avoid autolysis.

- Sections should be submitted to show the tumor's relation to adjacent structures are important for accurate staging the tumor.

- Contiguous tumor involvement of the spermatic cord is pT3, while discontinuous involvement through the vascular-lymphatic invasion is a metastatic deposit (M1).

- Lymph nodes with no residual viable tumor and only treatment effect should be reported and assigned pN0.

REFERENCES

1. Magers MJ, Idrees MT. Updates in staging and reporting of testicular cancer. Surg Pathol Clin 2018; 11(4):813–24.

2. Carr DT. The manual for the staging of cancer. Ann Intern Med 1977;87(4):491–2.

3. Al-Obaidy KI, Chovanec M, Cheng L. Molecular characteristics of testicular germ cell tumors: pathogenesis and mechanisms of therapy resistance. Expert Rev Anticancer Ther 2020;20(2):75–9.

4. Delahunt B, Egevad L, Samaratunga H, et al. UICC drops the ball in the 8th edition TNM staging of urological cancers. Histopathology 2017;71(1):5–11.

5. Amin MB, Greene FL, Edge SB, et al. The Eighth Edition AJCC Cancer Staging Manual: Continuing to build a bridge from a population-based to a more "personalized" approach to cancer staging. CA Cancer J Clin 2017;67(2):93–9.

6. Balzer BL, Ulbright TM. Spontaneous regression of testicular germ cell tumors: an analysis of 42 cases. Am J Surg Pathol 2006;30(7):858–65.

7. Emerson RE, Ulbright TM. Intratubular germ cell neoplasia of the testis and its associated cancers: the use of novel biomarkers. Pathology 2010;42(4): 344–55.

8. Chung P, Daugaard G, Tyldesley S, et al. Evaluation of a prognostic model for risk of relapse in stage I seminoma surveillance. Cancer Med 2015;4(1):155–60.

9. Mortensen MS, Lauritsen J, Gundgaard MG, et al. A nationwide cohort study of stage I seminoma patients followed on a surveillance program. Eur Urol 2014;66(6):1172–8.

10. Aparicio J, Maroto P, Garcia Del Muro X, et al. Prognostic factors for relapse in stage I seminoma: a new nomogram derived from three consecutive, risk-adapted studies from the Spanish Germ Cell Cancer Group (SGCCG). Ann Oncol 2014;25(11): 2173–8.

11. Warde P, Specht L, Horwich A, et al. Prognostic factors for relapse in stage I seminoma managed by surveillance: a pooled analysis. J Clin Oncol 2002; 20(22):4448–52.

12. Kamba T, Kamoto T, Okubo K, et al. Outcome of different post-orchiectomy management for stage I seminoma: Japanese multi-institutional study including 425 patients. Int J Urol 2010;17(12): 980–7.

13. Yilmaz A, Cheng T, Zhang J, et al. Testicular hilum and vascular invasion predict advanced clinical stage in nonseminomatous germ cell tumors. Mod Pathol 2013;26(4):579–86.

14. Vogt AP, Chen Z, Osunkoya AO. Rete testis invasion by malignant germ cell tumor and/or intratubular germ cell neoplasia: what is the significance of this finding? Hum Pathol 2010; 41(9):1339–44.

15. Berney DM, Algaba F, Amin M, et al. Handling and reporting of orchidectomy specimens with testicular cancer: areas of consensus and variation among 25 experts and 225 European pathologists. Histopathology 2015;67(3):313–24.

16. Alexandre J, Fizazi K, Mahé C, et al. Stage I nonseminomatous germ-cell tumours of the testis: identification of a subgroup of patients with a very low risk of relapse. Eur J Cancer 2001; 37(5):576–82.

17. Daugaard G, Gundgaard MG, Mortensen MS, et al. Surveillance for stage I nonseminoma testicular cancer: outcomes and long-term follow-up in a population-based cohort. J Clin Oncol 2014;32(34): 3817–23.

18. Lu K. Surveillance for stage I nonseminoma testicular cancer: outcomes and long-term follow-up in a population-based cohort. J Clin Oncol 2015;33(20): 2322.

19. Verrill C, Yilmaz A, Srigley JR, et al. Reporting and staging of testicular germ cell tumors: the international society of urological pathology (ISUP) testicular cancer consultation conference recommendations. Am J Surg Pathol 2017;41(6): e22–32.

20. Nazeer T, Ro JY, Kee KH, et al. Spermatic cord contamination in testicular cancer. Mod Pathol 1996;9(7):762–6.

21. McCleskey BC, Epstein JI, Albany C, et al. the significance of lymphovascular invasion of the spermatic cord in the absence of cord soft tissue invasion. Arch Pathol Lab Med 2017;141(6): 824–9.

22. Sanfrancesco JM, Trevino KE, Xu H, et al. The significance of spermatic cord involvement by testicular germ cell tumors: should we be staging discontinuous invasion from involved lymphovascular spaces differently from direct extension? Am J Surg Pathol 2018;42(3):306–11.

23. Coursey Moreno C, Small WC, Camacho JC, et al. Testicular tumors: what radiologists need to know– differential diagnosis, staging, and management. Radiographics 2015;35(2):400–15.

24. Hedgire SS, Pargaonkar VK, Elmi A, et al. Pelvic nodal imaging. Radiol Clin North Am 2012;50(6): 1111–25.

25. Ehrlich Y, Beck SD, Foster RS, et al. Serum tumor markers in testicular cancer. Urol Oncol 2013; 31(1):17–23.

26. Masterson TA, Rice KR, Beck SD. Current and future biologic markers for disease progression and relapse in testicular germ cell tumors: a review. Urol Oncol 2014;32(3):261–71.

27. Chakiryan NH, Dahmen A, Cucchiara V, et al. Reliability of serum tumor marker measurement to diagnose recurrence in patients with clinical stage I nonseminomatous germ cell tumors undergoing active surveillance: a systematic review. J Urol 2021;205(6):1569–76.

28. Bosl GJ, Motzer RJ. Testicular germ-cell cancer. N Engl J Med 1997;337(4):242–53.

29. Alvarado-Cabrero I, Hernandez-Toriz N, Paner GP. Clinicopathologic analysis of choriocarcinoma as a pure or predominant component of germ cell tumor of the testis. Am J Surg Pathol 2014;38(1): 111–8.

30. Hassan O, Epstein JI. The clinical significance of a small component of choriocarcinoma in testicular mixed germ cell tumor (MGCT). Am J Surg Pathol 2018;42(8):1113–20.

31. Gilbert SM, Daignault S, Weizer AZ, et al. The use of tumor markers in testis cancer in the United States: a potential quality issue. Urol Oncol 2008;26(2):153–7.

32. Gilligan TD, Seidenfeld J, Basch EM, et al. American society of clinical oncology clinical practice guideline on uses of serum tumor markers in adult males with germ cell tumors. J Clin Oncol 2010;28(20): 3388–404.

33. Skinner DG, Scardino PT. Relevance of biochemical tumor markers and lymphadenectomy in management of non-seminomatous testis tumors: current perspective. J Urol 1980;123(3):378–82.

34. Albers P, Albrecht W, Algaba F, et al. EAU guidelines on testicular cancer: 2011 update. Eur Urol 2011; 60(2):304–19.

35. Albers P, Albrecht W, Algaba F, et al. [EAU guidelines on testicular cancer: 2011 update. European Association of Urology]. Actas Urol Esp 2012; 36(3):127–45. Guía clínica sobre el cáncer de testículo de la EAU: actualización de 2011.

36. IGCCC G. A prognostic factor based staging system for metastatic germ-cell cancers. J Clin Oncol 1997;15(2):594–603.

37. Kattan MW, Hess KR, Amin MB, et al. American Joint Committee on Cancer acceptance criteria for inclusion of risk models for individualized prognosis in the practice of precision medicine. CA: A Cancer J Clinicians 2016;66(5):370–4.

Applications of Digital and Computational Pathology and Artificial Intelligence in Genitourinary Pathology Diagnostics

Ankush Uresh Patel, MBBCh, BAO, LRCP & SI[a],
Sambit K. Mohanty, MD[b,1],
Anil V. Parwani, MD, PhD, MBA[c,*]

KEYWORDS

- Genitourinary • Digital pathology • Computational pathology • Artificial intelligence • Quality control
- Whole-slide imaging • Generalizability • FDA

Key points

- Computational tools for pathology leverage AI algorithms for primary diagnostics and second-read applications, enhancing image analysis, quality control, and laboratory efficiency when implemented in clinical and anatomic pathology laboratory settings as adjuncts for pathologist diagnosis.

- Prostate pathology has been the primary focus of algorithmic development for genitourinary (GU) applications, however most studies pertaining to the algorithmic development of other GU systems are still relegated to academia and in need of further clinical exploration.

- Many limitations stymying the clinical implementation of ML algorithms stem from data concerns including data transparency, quality, standardization, availability, cost, and security.

- Population-wide generalizability has emerged as the pillar of clinical-grade AI, with FDA authorization of De Novo marketing status to the first clinical-grade AI solution for GU pathology followed extensive verification of the solution's generalizability.

- Multiple instance learning has been proposed as a viable method for developing clinical-grade AI, with the technique yielding achievement of an unprecedented degree of ML-model standardization applicable throughout a global patient population.

ABSTRACT

As machine learning (ML) solutions for genitourinary pathology image analysis are fostered by a progressively digitized laboratory landscape, these integrable modalities usher in a revolution in histopathological diagnosis. As technology advances, limitations stymying clinical artificial intelligence (AI) will not be extinguished without thorough validation and interrogation of ML tools by pathologists and regulatory bodies alike. ML solutions deployed in clinical settings for applications in prostate pathology yield promising results. Recent breakthroughs in clinical artificial intelligence for genitourinary pathology demonstrate unprecedented generalizability, heralding prospects for a future in which AI-driven assistive solutions may be seen as laboratory faculty, rather than novelty.

[a] Department of Laboratory Medicine and Pathology, Mayo Clinic, 200 First Street Southwest, Rochester, MN 55905, USA; [b] Surgical and Molecular Pathology, Advanced Medical Research Institute, Plot No. 1, Near Jayadev Vatika Park, Khandagiri, Bhubaneswar, Odisha 751019; [c] Department of Pathology, The Ohio State University, Cooperative Human Tissue Network (CHTN) Midwestern Division Polaris Innovation Centre, 2001 Polaris Parkway Suite 1000, Columbus, OH 43240, USA
[1]Present address: CORE Diagnostics (India), 406, Phase III, Udyog Vihar, Sector 19, Gurugram, Haryana 122016, India.
* Corresponding author.
E-mail address: anil.parwani@osumc.edu
Twitter: @SAMBITKMohanty1 (S.K.M.); @Aparwani_dpath (A.V.P.)

Surgical Pathology 15 (2022) 759–786
https://doi.org/10.1016/j.path.2022.08.001
1875-9181/22/© 2022 Elsevier Inc. All rights reserved.

OVERVIEW

Digital pathology (DP), machine learning (ML), and artificial intelligence (AI) are terms increasingly being used in pathology practice and are occasionally indistinguishable, though always traceable to a singular glass slide origin. Clinical implementation of DP is now orbits past its semicentennial anniversary, denoted by the 1972 implementation of the Spear CLAS-300, an early computer laboratory information system (LIS) at Cape Cod Hospital, Massachusetts.[1]

Two decades later, nascent satellite data technology for earth science applications was reshaped into primordial virtual microscopy software for whole slide image (WSI) viewing, predating the arrival of WSI scanners themselves.[2] Digital pathology today is synonymous with WSI, a medium now used for a litany of use-cases including primary diagnosis, consultation, telepathology, and quality assurance (QA). The rapid emergence of WSI systems has been met with adjunctive innovations in computational image analysis (IA) for the quantification of histologic features.

BASIC PRINCIPLES: COMPUTATIONAL PATHOLOGY AND ARTIFICIAL INTELLIGENCE

Computational tools for pathology have leveraged AI-algorithms to alleviate limitations commonly marring manual quantitative histopathological analysis, while enabling predictions and prognosis directly from the hematoxylin and eosin (H&E) stained WSIs (Box 1).[3]

Such limitations are exacerbated within the realm of genitourinary (GU) pathology, a forum plagued by high rates of specialist discordance, global urologic pathologist shortage, increasing prostate cancer cases, and biopsy volumes commanding navigation of increasingly intricate reporting complexity, all of which contribute to increased burdens for pathology departments. AI models using computer-based algorithms to advance the decision-making processes of pathologists now appear perched, primed, and prepared to advance the baton brought forth by laboratory digitization into the future of clinical medicine (Box 2).

DEVELOPMENT OF ARTIFICIAL INTELLIGENCE ALGORITHMS FOR PATHOLOGY

Machine learning measurement, quantification, and categorization of a WSI, for example, quantitative image analysis (QIA) is typically executed through pixel-, object-, and architecture-based methods (Table 1).

Systems for computer-aided diagnosis ("CAD") may apply image processing algorithms for staining standardization, tissue segmentation, histopathological feature extraction (Fig. 1), and morphologic classification (Fig. 2).[5] Many open-source and commercial vendors today offer platforms for image analysis (Table 2), several of which include solutions for GU-specific applications (Box 3).

DEEP LEARNING AND CONVOLUTIONAL NEURAL NETWORKS

Modeled after the human brain, the base components of artificial neural networks, for example, "nodes," bear structural and functional similarities to biological neurons of the central nervous system (CNS) (Fig. 3). Evolutionary advances have forged a cerebral network homed for pattern recognition vis a vis iterative information processing from a litany of past events, experiences, and emotions that may be used to navigate new challenges of a similar nature, yet never previously experienced. The "weight," that is, the importance of a particular experience in the context of a new setting gains relevance through mining a conglomerate of past experiences that are then triaged for pertinency to a present problem. Such understanding is used most effectively when not clouded by biases precluding an objective solution.

In a similar fashion, deep learning (DL) has emerged as an evolutionary progression of machine learning (Fig. 4) by which programmable neural networks may interpret or predict outcomes from WSI

Box 1
Limitations of manual quantitative histopathological image analysis

- Human interpretation factors, for example, biases, fatigue from pedantic and effort-intensive calculations, inconsistent application of scoring rules, suboptimal reproducibility, variations in experience

- Intra- and inter-observer variability

- Limited spatial coverage (only small areas can be realistically quantified with visual evaluation)

- Variations in field of view and microscope configuration

- Unscalable

> **Box 2**
> **Advantages of computer-aided image analysis**
>
> Enables the standardization of histopathology by reproducible, computer-driven quantitation conferring superior reliability to visual assessment.
> - Reduction of biased interpretations
>
> - Spatial coverage allowing for the quantification of a large ROI or an entire WSI
>
> - Fast speed of analysis
>
> - User friendly, open-source options available
>
> - Adjustment of cutoffs in real-time for clinically relevant algorithm development
>
> - Increased precision and accuracy in quantitative measurements
>
> - Recognition of morphologic patterns currently unrecognized for greater understanding of disease classification and prognosis
>
> - Ties morphologic features to molecular biology
>
> - Automated functionality reduces pathologist burden
>
> - Enhanced efficiency, for example, triaging of cases/screening
>
> - Digital prognostic signatures and biomarker discovery data utilizable for pharmaceutical breakthrough
>
> - May be further augmented with the application of deep learning algorithms

data inputs without the assistance of a predefined output set. CNNs have demonstrated efficacy in varying WSI analysis applications, including primary diagnosis of H&E images, through efficient and highly effective "end-to-end" training by which a model may use entire WSIs given single target labels, for example, Gleason grade, or up to millions of unlabeled regional WSI image-patches to autodidactically identify and extract features of importance in the processes between the WSI input and final output (**Fig. 5**).[6,7] Such techniques reduce effort-intensive human training while performing superiorly to algorithms developed using fully supervised pattern-recognition techniques dependent on manually annotated pixel-level feature extraction. DL for prostate histopathology has demonstrated great potential due to the vast swaths of pixels within a single WSI from which hundreds of examples of cancerous glands may be extracted (**Fig. 6**).[6,7]

DEVELOPMENT OF CLINICAL GRADE ARTIFICIAL INTELLIGENCE ALGORITHMS

Newer derivatives of CNN structure are customizable per user need, accessible via public domain, and are enabled for data-augmentation via temperature-based colorization, elasticity, for example, expansion and compression of images, and geometric flipping of images, for example, horizontally, and vertically (**Table 3**).

Such facilities for augmentation are not inherently dissimilar to those of light microscopy, in which a

pathologist may use controls to manipulate fine focus, illumination, for example, via condensers, and fine-tune a litany of other modules to enable the complete control of an environment personally crafted for his/her needs. Digital augmentation tools, however, possess the potential to offer greater faculties than the buttons and knobs ensconcing a microscope, as their merits are not limited to the practical application but extend toward the prospect of achieving global inter- and intra-laboratory standardization. Traditional laboratory peer-review practices predispose to substantial variability, as those who perform secondary evaluations on slides assessed by primary pathologists use microscopes they have never used before or are not as familiar with as those which they use on a regular basis. Validated AI systems offer the potential for mitigated discrepancies in this regard.

A systematic, pathologist-directed approach to the evaluation of an AI model must entail validation and verification processes for clinical implementation and continued utilization of computational tools (**Box 4**).

GENERALIZABILITY: THE PILLAR OF CLINICAL-GRADE ARTIFICIAL INTELLIGENCE

Clinical translation of algorithms requires generalizability throughout a wide breadth of patient populations and clinical institutions. QIA has advanced toward reproducibility of IHC results; however,

Table 1		
Machine learning approaches to IA and commonly used QIA algorithms[4]		
Approaches	**Description of Approaches**	**Example(s) of QIA Algorithm**
Pixel-based analysis	Most basic approach to IA in which filters are applied to separate red, green, and blue channels, producing a binary image format (with positive pixels above a threshold of inclusion and negative pixels below) that may then be analyzed for particles of interest	May be used to represent an output as an intensity heatmap or averaging pixel values over a ROI[A]. Positive pixel count algorithms are often included in vendor base packages. Not useful for clinical applications, though may be used as a foundation for which clinically useful algorithms are developed, for example, pixel-wise classification, that is, segmentation.
Object-based analysis	Categorizes pixels into an object, for example, nucleus, nucleolus, membrane, or an entire cell, for example, cell/area-based detection, acting similar to pathologist scoring of IHC within a clinical setting	May be used for scoring applications, for example, quantification of nuclear staining intensity based on average nuclear pixel intensity, scoring of predictive markers for breast tumors (% of positive cells), cell count and stain density/intensity, noncellular staining, for example, congo red/amyloid, cell morphology, for example, H. pylori detection, eosinophil count Area-based cell detection for the detection of all the cells present in an area based on the segmentation of nuclei; primarily based on nuclear detection Tumor-cell detection: *Non-Deep learning approach*: properties such as nuclear size can be used to separate tumor cells from other cells *Deep learning approach*: algorithms detect tumor cells based on training a dataset that provides ground truth Positive tumor cell detection is based on nuclear dab properties (DAB mean or DAB max); quantifies the number of positive cells within a specific area Hot Spot Identification: Positive and negative labels may be creation by the user for pathologist ground-truth analysis, followed by the selection of large image area for the application of fast cell count used for the creation of density maps, for example, % of positive cells for which the "hottest" areas consisting of the highest positive cell counts are colorized
Architecture-based analysis	Analyzes relationships of objects, similar to pathologist interpretation histopathological patterns	May be used to detect fibrosis, invasive tumor, epithelial surfaces, major tissue type, for example, bone and adipose, as well as architectural disruptions, for example, node effacement. Useful in pattern recognition/classification.

Key: "A" – Region of Interest.

Fig. 1. AI-based histologic feature extraction. Automated intelligent segmentation demonstrating the detection of digitized histologic patterns in a region of tissue classified as Gleason pattern 3 where blue = epithelial nuclei, red = epithelial cell cytoplasm, and brown = lumen.

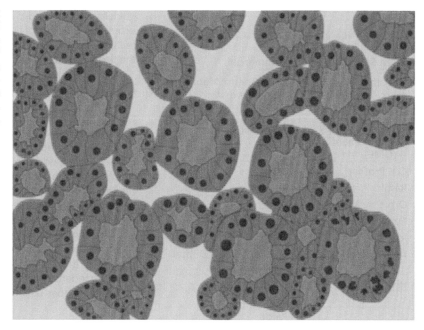

attention to variations within preanalytical factors compiled for training data is of importance (**Box 5**).

QC must be applied to every aspect of algorithm development (**Table 4**).

Quality and volume of data used to train CAD systems are tantamount to the relevancy, accuracy, and precision of the "decisions," that is, outputs, of such devices, and their capacity to aid clinical practice. An algorithmic model fit for clinical implementation must not fall susceptible to outlier data and remain robust, for example, generalizable to variability. Generalizability; that is, the applicability of an AI model output to the broader population of it has been designed to address, has emerged as the pillar of clinical grade AI (**Box 6**).

FDA authorization of De Novo marketing status to the first clinical-grade AI solution for GU pathology, Paige Prostate, followed extensive verification of the solution's generalizability. The AI-solution was deployed in conditions of significant preanalytical and analytical variability, elements of high importance for the FDA when determining performance

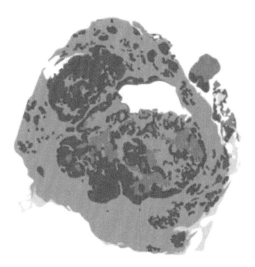 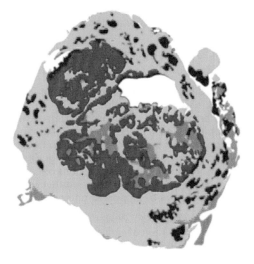

Fig. 2. AI-based segmentation/classification. Computational multi-class segmentation (*right*) applied to WSI specimen (*left*), colorized per pixel-wise tissue classification where red = carcinomatous region, blue = benign epithelium, green = stroma, orange = adipose, gray = necrotic area.

Table 2
Vendors offering image analysis platforms

Open Source	Commercial
QuPath	Leica Aperio Algorithm Framework
ImageJ/Fiji	HALO
Open Microscopy Environment (OME)	Visiopharm
Cell Profiler	Definiens
Ilastik	ImagePro
Orbit	inForm
Cytomine	Techyte
Icy	Tribvn
Augmentiqs	Hologic Genius Digital Diagnostics
HistoQC[A]	Ibex
	OptraScan
	Paige
	Deep Bio
	ContextVision (INIFY)
	AIRA Matrix

Key: "A" - automated Convolutional Neural Network (CNN)-based tool for WSI quality control (QC).

guidelines for the study.[8] A testing dataset marked by prominent inclusion of challenging histopathological features was crafted for its distinction compared with the training dataset used for the AI model (Box 7).

MULTIPLE INSTANCE LEARNING

Multiple instance learning (MIL), a highly unsupervised form of model training, circumvents the pixel-level, manual annotations required by more limited supervised learning techniques, to use data from entire WSIs and their corresponding pathology reports. MIL has been proposed as a viable method for developing clinical-grade AI,[9] as demonstrated recently during the development of the Paige Prostate solution.32,300 slides from 6700 patients and data sourced from multiple laboratories were involved in the training of Paige Prostate to achieve an unprecedented degree of model standardization applicable across a global population.[9]

COMPUTATIONAL PATHOLOGY IN GENITOURINARY PATHOLOGY: PROSTATE CANCER AS THE CASE OF STUDY

Paige Prostate Alpha, predecessor to the Paige Prostate solution, was validated for diagnostic

Box 3
Image analysis platforms with solutions for GU pathology

- Ibex (Image Analysis) – Galen Platform including Galen Prostate solution, granted breakthrough FDA device designation, first AI-based cancer detection platform deployed for routine clinical use in pathology laboratories. Algorithms are used to analyze images, detect, and grade cancer in biopsies and identify other findings with high clinical importance for reduced diagnostic error rates and efficient workflow.

- OptraScan OpptoraASSAYS image analysis solution contains algorithms for biomarker quantification using nuclear, membrane, and cytoplasmic stains, including turnkey PD-L1/Prostate/Breast Biomarker analysis.

- Pagie AI offers Paige Prostate, a clinical solution given De Novo marketing status by the FDA for the detection of areas suspicious of cancer.

- Deep Bio offers several solutions for prostate cancer including: 1. DeepDx-Prostate Basic (Slide viewer and binary screening solution); 2. DeepDx-Prostate Pro (distinguishes cancer severity via coloring tissue regions based on Gleason pattern classification results, then suggests a Gleason score using deep neural networks. Users may consult AI on hand-picked regions to obtain quick feedback on slides with large areas of tissue. Pre-filled pathology reports are generated once slides are analyzed using the AI from DeepDX-Prostate. Clinically significant information included in the pathology report includes Gleason score, relative proportions of each Gleason pattern, percentage involvement of cancer in tissue, and image samples representative of cancer found in the slide; 3) DeepDx Connect (DeepDx prostate for the web, supported on portable devices).

- Context Vision INIFY Prostate Screening solution implements deep learning algorithms for the automated annotation of cancer tissue using the patented "MasterAnnotation" method for CNN training (US 10,572,996). AI-solution assists pathologists with identifying cancer in prostate biopsies and is robust across different laboratories and scanners, adaptable to different workflows and user needs with seamless, customizable integration including optional, built-in case manager.

- AIRA Matrix offers clinical solutions for Gleason grading and radical prostatectomy reporting.

Fig. 3. Neuron versus node. The human neuron (*A*) consisting of a series of dendrites that receive information (input) then fed into a central soma/nucleus (node) from which signals are passed through an axon highway (output) and into multiple synapses which transmit the information along to other neurons in the network, very similar to the structure of the artificial neuron (*B*) which receives and transmits signals within an artificial neural network (ANN).

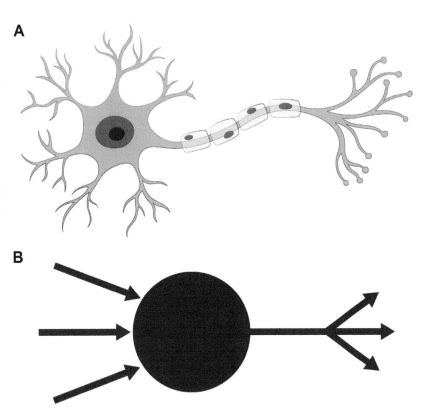

accuracy and efficiency to determine if the AI-model, when used as an assistive-tool during sign-out, could aid pathologists in improving diagnostic accuracy.[10] 254 prostate-biopsy slides enriched with small, well-differentiated foci of cancer, were selected for their high level of complexity, for example, inclusive of histopathological features reported as challenging, time-consuming, effort-intensive, yet frequently missed resulting in false negatives. Results demonstrated marked improvement (**Box 8**).

Fig. 4. AI Hierarchy. Machine learning (ML) is a subset of artificial intelligence (AI) that is capable of self-learning from training data, though is limited in the capacity to do so. Deep learning (DL) is a subset of machine learning (ML) using layered networks of machine-learning algorithms modeled after the neural structure of the human brain.

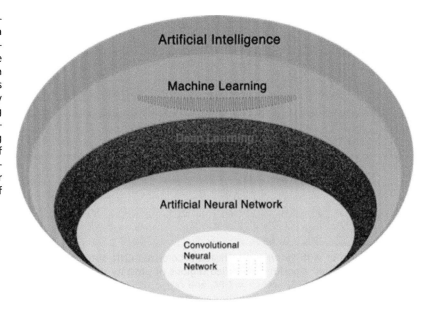

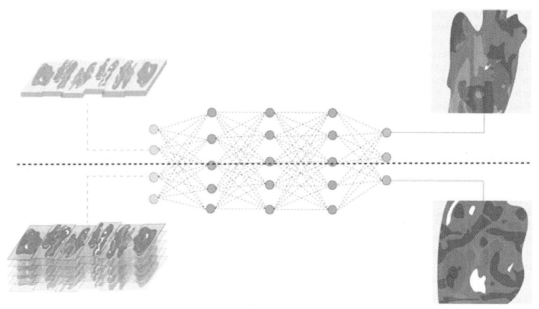

Fig. 5. CNN Structure and Function. A scaffolding of artificial nodes (blue – input; gray – hidden; green – output) supports network layers within a CNN that respond to different pattern-forming features in input data used for training (depicted below segmented *line*) or testing (depicted above segmented *line*). Output results from the interaction between the connection strength, that is, "weight," of node connection that adjusts with each input image, and bias, both of which are learnable parameters that represent the correlation of a prediction to ground truth and may be adjusted accordingly. A convolutional ("hidden") layer between input and output nodes uses complex feature maps to extract and classify patterns of interest, for example, the identification of cancerous regions (denoted in purple areas on output images).

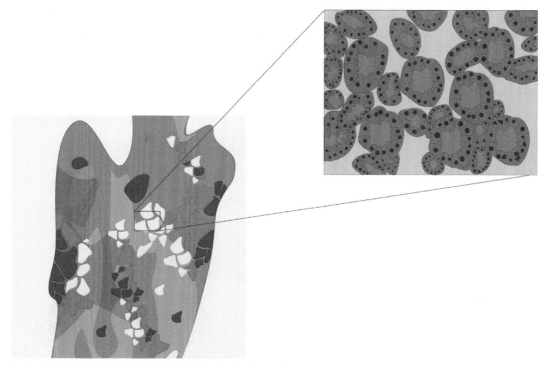

Fig. 6. CNN output with Pattern Identification. Colorized CNN output distinguishing histopathological patch-classified areas within algorithm-identified regions of prostate cancer corresponding to Gleason pattern (GP) score where yellow = GP3, orange = GP4, and red = GP5. GP3 is enlarged to demonstrate CNN recognition, for example, feature extraction, of infiltrative margins indicative of a specific cancerous pattern.

Table 3
Examples of CNN-derived networks useful for computer vision

Inception	Multiple Filters, Lower Computation
Residual Network (ResNet)	deeper networks with less complexity (allowing for less training errors typically associated with deeper networks) (better "explainability" allowing for improved understanding of computer decisions), overcomes "vanishing gradient" barrier arising in deep learning networks
EfficientNet	Efficient scaling of filters, high performance
Visual Geometry Group (VGGNet)	Reduction of training time, improved performance of image recognition

ARTIFICIAL INTELLIGENCE FOR QUALITY CONTROL

The Page Prostate solution also demonstrated value for clinical QC applications in a recent study (**Box 9**).[11]

LIMITATIONS TO THE CLINICAL IMPLEMENTATION OF ARTIFICIAL INTELLIGENCE

Many limitations stymying clinical implementation of ML algorithms stem from data concerns (**Table 5**).

FIT-FOR-USE CLINICAL ARTIFICIAL INTELLIGENCE: EXAMPLES OF INSTITUTIONAL IMPLEMENTATION AND VALIDATION

Core Plus (CorePlus Servicios Clínicos y Patológicos LLC), a high complexity CLIA-certified clinical and anatomic pathology laboratory, holds the distinction as the first US laboratory to implement an AI-based solution for cancer detection in pathology to support accurate pathologist diagnosis as well as for enhanced laboratory efficiency and quality control.[12] The Galen Prostate solution (Ibex Medical Analytics) algorithm was validated for an intended population of interest, predominantly comprising a demographic afflicted by disproportionately high rates of prostate cancer-specific mortality.[13]

101 prostate cancer cases (1279 H&E-stained WSIs) were used to assess clinical validation, a process entailing retrospective evaluation of previously diagnosed prostate core needle biopsy (PCNB) cases via a second-read application offered by the AI-prostate platform. The performance of the AI solution was assessed and compared with pathologist diagnoses used for ground truth, demonstrating promising results (**Table 6**).

Following validation, clinical implementation of the AI-platform for primary use as a QC tool (before sign-out) for 100% of PCNBs has proven to be effective. More than 4000 prostate cases (encompassing more than 54,000 slides and counting) have been analyzed by the AI-platform for adjunctive second-read assistance for pathologists since implementation in June 2020 (**Box 10**).

Box 4
Algorithmic validation and verification: definitions and processes

Validation: The objective of validation is the safe implementation of AI technology, encompassing the process by which an AI model is evaluated to perform as expected for its intended use within its environment before its clinical implementation for patient care. A model may be validated through a series of steps beginning with "qualification," by which a model's output is compared to annotated training data to determine if the model can predict the data back with accuracy. This is followed by the performance assessment with a new "testing set" of slides procured from the same data set used for model training, though not yet introduced to the computer system. The final validatory step involves the incorporation of new data sets from alternate studies or the inclusion of pathologists who are uninvolved with the initial model training process and may create annotations used to assess the degree to which they are matched via computer analysis. Validation processes exclude the assessment of pathologist diagnostic accuracy. Confusion matrixes, dice coefficients, and F score are all methods by which algorithmic accuracy may be evaluated during validation.
Verification: The objective of verification is to establish that an AI model is being used for its intended purpose using evidence-based data to confirm the specified performance requirements have been satisfied.

> **Box 5**
> **Pre-analytical factors important for immunostaining**
>
> - Cold ischemia time
> - Tissue processing parameters (slide thickness, tissue section thickness, and so forth)
> - Immunostaining parameters

The Galen platform (Galen Prostate and Galen Breast) also saw recent routine clinical workflow implementation for second-read/QC purpose sat Maccabi Healthcare Services (Israel), a large health care provider with a centralized pathology institute receiving samples from 350 clinics and hospitals. PCNBs at Maccabi comprise a significant portion of yearly histopathology workload (700 cases per year; >8000 slides) (Table 7).

Alerts from the second-read system were demonstrated by heatmaps focused on specific image areas, resulting in minimal review time (approximately 1% of pathologist FTE). Cancer alerts were raised in 10.1% of slides (583) taken from 232 cases initially given benign diagnoses by pathologists. Gleason 7+ alerts were raised in 5.3% of slides (93) taken from 137 cases initially given diagnoses of Gleason grade 3 + 3.

The AI-prostate solution had previously undergone groundbreaking validation efforts at the University of Pittsburgh Medical Center (UPMC) whereby evaluation against an external validation dataset with different preimaging and scanning parameters demonstrated promising results (Table 8).[14]

The study was the first of its kind to report the deployment and benefits of a multifaceted AI-based algorithm in routine clinical practice for prostate cancer detection, Gleason grading, evaluation of tumor extent, and perineural invasion (PNI)/size, the lattermost feature of which had been neglected in previous AI-based diagnostic research despite bearing substantial clinical and prognostic significance. Using 1627 H&E slides from 100 CNB cases, The AI-solution detected 17 misdiagnosed parts and 6 misdiagnosed cases in the UPMC dataset resulting from pathologist errors in the assessment of cancer detection, grading, and PNI. 12 misdiagnosed prostate cancer cases, including those of high-grade cancer, had been identified by the AI-solution in a previous evaluation study conducted in the largest network of pathology institutes in France (Medipath) tasked with a workload of 5000 annual prostate biopsy cases.[15] Results suggested that the AI-solution demonstrated viability for the automated screening of prostate CNBs for primary diagnosis, QC/second-read, and standardized reporting.

870 H&E slides from 100 PCNBs were used in a subsequent multi-site clinical validation study demonstrating high performance for cancer detection, Gleason grading, and PNI (including high-grade PIN), suggesting the potential for the AI-solution to increase diagnostic objectivity and reproducibility (Table 9).[16]

In the evaluation of Gleason grading and PNI, results demonstrated a higher rate of agreement for the AI-solution with ground truth diagnosis after discrepancy review in comparison to the interobserver agreement between pathologists during the establishment of ground truth.

Table 4
Must-haves" of pre-analytical and analytical quality control during algorithmic development

Pre-analytical QC
Slide-based QC: staining standardization, SOP-driven QC, lab-to-scanner workflow
Scanner-based QC: maintenance and calibration, SOP-driven QC, superusers
Design-based QC: clear objectives, appropriate experimental plan, training and consent

Annotation Quality Control	Model Quality Control	Qualification Quality Control
Documented ground truth	Model screening	Clear objectives
Trained experts	Augmentation tools	Appropriate experimental and statistical plans
Sample heterogeneity	Expert verification	
Peer reviewed annotations		

Box 6
Components of generalizability

Robust generalizability is achievable from a wide range of data variability within 3 primary categories:
1. Patient data, for example, country, institution, ethnicity, age, tumor grade, and size

2. Sample data, for example, preanalytical and analytical variability, file size, image capture magnification

3. User data, for example, pathologists with different experience levels, operating in different settings

---

In addition to seamless QC functionality, pathologists using the Galen platform are also supported by an AI-driven "first read" application for primary diagnosis. AI-based diagnostic tools packaged within the Ibex First Read platform include applications for case prioritization/triage, worklists, slide viewing, IHC pre-ordering, cancer heatmaps, grading, identification of noncancerous findings, sample measurements, and AI-driven reporting. Improved clinical grade accuracy, increased productivity (37%), and shorter turnaround times were noted following the implementation of the first-read solution at Maccabi, driving the business case for full laboratory digitization, further supported by the robust QC capabilities included and easily navigable within the plug-and-play software, sans any additional departmental expenses.

A validation study for the Galen Prostate First Read application using 100 PCNBs demonstrated that pathologists using the AI-application had performed superiorly to those using light microscopy, noting a significant reduction (32%) in major discrepancy rate.[17]

Productivity gains achieved through the use of Galen First Read for primary diagnosis were assessed in another study validating the AI-application against 320 PCNB cases (2411 H&E slides) (**Box 11**).[18]

Advantages of the AI-application were emphasized during case-level discrepancy resolution (**Box 12**).

Box 7
FDA study for the validation of AI-prostate solution

Study Design: Algorithm was assessed on 527 WSIs with data from 5 different countries, $\geq$150 different institutions, a diverse range of patient ethnicities, and differing tumor sizes and grades. 420 WSIs were benign; 190 were malignant. 16 pathologists (14 generalists; 2 uropathology specialists) were used to conduct remote and laboratory readings using different computers. The pathologists selected for the study had a wide range of experience (2–34 years). The same cases were read twice by the same pathologist, once without AI assistance and once using the prostate algorithm.

Study Results:

Statistically significant results pertaining to error reduction when using AI assistance:

• False negative rate for cancer detection reduced by 70%

• False positive rate for cancer detection reduced by 24%

• Pathologists were able to rule out any potential false positives shown to them by the AI system, results reproducible throughout generalist and specialist groups and unaffected by remote or on-site sign out

Pathologists using Paige Prostate in the study increased more than 7% points in sensitivity for correct cancer diagnosis (89.5% to 96.8%)

Results pertaining to efficiency, that is, the use of deferrals, were recorded after the real-life simulation of the clinical scenario. Unnecessary deferrals included slides containing cancer that would have been deferred without AI assistance but were classified as cancer with AI assistance. Necessary deferrals included slides with cancer that would have initially been given a benign diagnosis, which was then sent for deferral with the aid of AI. Results showed:

• 24% decrease in unnecessary deferrals using AI assistance

• 59% increase in necessary deferrals using AI assistance

Box 8

AI for the detection of complex prostate cancer cases in WSIs of PCNB

Study design: multiple-reader, multiple-case study in which pathologists read slides twice, first with and then without AI assistance, with the first read conducted in a different location than the second.

Results:

- 16% improvement in sensitivity, with an overall 60% error reduction when using AI assistance

- The AI-model, within the context of this study, detected prostate cancer with greater sensitivity than the pathologists who did not use AI assistance

- Foci of poorly differentiated and clinically significant prostate adenocarcinoma that was missed by pathologists were identified successfully with the aid of AI.

- With the assistance of Paige Prostate Alpha, pathologists correctly classified smaller, lower grade tumors, with greater frequency than without the aid of the AI-tool. Investigators noted that pathologists also spent less time analyzing each WSI when assisted with AI.

Advantages were also evidenced by decreased case turnaround time (**Box 13**).

These large-scale studies in which pathologists performed complete AI-supported primary diagnoses are the first of their kind, demonstrating promising results suggestive of the positive clinical potential for laboratory-integrated AI-based solutions for GU (**Box 14**).

Algorithms developed for GU-pathology have demonstrated promising results yet are limited to individual studies thereby restricting a truly wholistic evaluation of generalizability (**Table 10**). Clinical relevancy of these endeavors has been obfuscated due to the non-standardization of methods and materials and a lack of consistent or extensive external validation pervading throughout their conglomerate. Tissue sample variations (from microarray, needle biopsy, and radical prostatectomy slides), and variations in image patch size and resolution used to train DL models are some factors impairing true standardized evaluation, notwithstanding instances of neglect to evaluate the correlation between instances of AI-assisted grading and clinical outcome. Many recent investigations have focused on prostate cancer detection from WSIs of needle biopsies,[5,6,9,10,14,19–21,30,31] radical prostatectomies,[32] tissue microarrays,[5,22–24] or from a combination of radical prostatectomy and TMA

slides.[5,33] Recent machine learning developments have focused on the automated detection of cribriform patterns in prostate histology images, demonstrating promising results.[34–36] However, there is a comparative dearth of studies involving the application of machine and deep-learning methods toward the interrogation of other GU foci, for example, urothelial carcinoma,[37–39] sex cord and stromal testicular tumors,[40] and renal tumors.[41–49]

A breakthrough in algorithmic generalization, occurring intercontinentally across different patient populations, laboratories, and reference standards via a diversity of AI-approaches for Gleason grading was demonstrated by results from the most recent PANDA challenge, an exhaustively data-rich histopathology competition for the development of reproducible, AI-driven Gleason grading.[50] The study, though focused solely on algorithmic development for Gleason grading, marked a milestone in computational pathology, with results encouraging further evaluations of AI-tools for Gleason grading in prospective clinical trials (**Box 15**).

Despite not bearing ultimate governance of pathology practice, FDA approval is still of importance for IA tools, as designation may expedite the validation process (FDA-cleared image analysis systems require a minimum of 20 positive/

Box 9

Paige prostate QC value

- Algorithm performance was compared with 3 expert pathologists using 600 transrectal ultrasound-guided PCNB regions from 100 patients.[11]

- Use of the AI-tool yielded a patient-level NPV of 100%, along with a 65.5% reduction of diagnostic time for the material analyzed.

- the algorithm identified malignancy in 4 patients incorrectly recorded as benign by all 3 expert histopathologists on initial reporting, upgrading the cases to malignant after finding small foci of well-differentiated tumors.

Table 5
Limitations to the clinical implementation of AI

Limitation	Overview of Limitation	Current or Prospective Efforts to Address Limitation
Data Transparency, for example, "Black Box" concerns	The obscure nature of deep learning classification pathways is inherently uninterpretable, as output is presented as a zero-knowledge proof whereby steps pertaining to feature the extraction of image objects correlated to clinical endpoints are excluded. An unaddressed burden of proof predisposes to concerns of unreliability.	• 'Rule extraction' techniques, through which hidden information pertaining to histopathologic feature extraction may be revealed, have been devised in attempt to understand the relationship between input parameters and the output of a CNN model. • The emerging field of explainable AI (XAI) seeks to describe the deliberative process of AI-models, including expected impact and potential biases of the algorithmic decision-making process.
Data Quality	High-resolution image reduction techniques used for CNN development, for example, patch extraction, may compromise the quality of CNN training, as higher-level structural information, for example, tumor extent or shape, may only be effectively captured through analysis of larger regions.	Normalization techniques, for example, I. scale normalization compromising for differences in WSI scanning devices and variations in pixel sizes. II. Stain normalization. III. Flexible thresholding techniques compromising for variations in data luminance; in addition to focused spatial correlation amongst patches, multi-level magnification of patches and utilization of larger patch sizes
Data Standardization	A substantial amount of data, potentially derived from multiple WSI scanners using different file formats, may be used for algorithm development. Some scanner-specific formats include "SVS" (Leica Aperio Series) and "MRXS" (Zeiss MIRAX and 3D Histech Panoramic series). Format differences pertain to differences in metadata tags and file compression types. Downstream analysis is dependent upon the capacity of a computational tool to handle a selected image format.	Efforts to achieve a single open-source file format, for example, like DICOM for radiology are necessary. Tagged Image File Format ("TIFF") is a standard image format for WSIs that maintains all image details due to its "lossless" characteristic. "Lossy" compression methods that degrade data may be required to produce smaller file sizes more suitable for easier viewing.

(*continued on next page*)

Table 5
(continued)

Limitation	Overview of Limitation	Current or Prospective Efforts to Address Limitation
Data Availability and Cost	Datasets containing expert-ground-truth annotations for supervised learning techniques is limited. For GU pathology, this paucity is emphasized in immunolabeled WSI datasets containing in situ molecular cell data (multiplexed immunofluorescence). Labeled data are expensive, difficult to acquire, and time-consuming to produce. Data storage cost is a primary impediment to DP implementation, emphasized in small-to-medium-sized departments. Graphical processing units (GPU) are preferred for training and testing of deep neural networks due to their advanced processing power in comparison to central processing units (CPUs), though incur a significantly greater financial expense.	Ultimately, increased utilization of unsupervised learning techniques, not requiring labeled data, will supplant the primary concerns of data availability for supervised training. Currently, open-source data are used to circumvent restrictions levied by data privacy and proprietary measures. Transfer learning techniques using pretrained neural networks, as well as data augmentation techniques are also being used to lessen the pedantic nature of network training and to mitigate shortages in expert-annotated data. However, these techniques are not equivalent to specialist-annotated data.
Data Security	Cloud-based resources used to house DP data are still without a neither fast nor reliable mechanism by which WSIs may be uploaded securely and in a manner compliant with all regulations.	Construction of local AI resources by which security issues may be avoided along with network delays (though currently the construction of such resources is purely speculative)

negative cases for validation, whereas LDT algorithms require 40 positive/negative cases), foster deployment in hospital systems, and encourage practitioner adoption.

FUTURE DIRECTIONS

Digital pathology today remains unliberated from the glass slide. Although devices used for

Table 6
Clinical validation (Ibex Galen prostate solution)

Analysis	AUC	Specificity	Sensitivity
Benign vs Cancer	0.994	96.9%	96.5%
GG1 vs GG2+	0.901	81.1%	82.0%

pathology have evolved since the 17th century, such improvements may be viewed as variations, rather than transformations of traditional pathology practice contingent on physical slides and microscopes. Full laboratory implementation of DP does not substitute any steps involved in conventional 2D histopathology workflows. Rather, additional steps are added which incur extra costs, full-time equivalents for practitioners, and overall time expenditure. Fully digitized histology workflows which forgo the glass slide, a concept still relegated to research forums, offer the potential for instantaneous tissue response speeds in lieu of waiting for histology laboratory results and will likely be operable Table at far cheaper costs than laboratories today. Given the limitations of frozen sections, for example, freezing artifacts exacerbated with lipid-rich tissues, researchers have sought to develop novel slide-free imaging techniques that may foster heightened exploration of

---

Box 10
Impact of AI implementation (Ibex Galen Prostate solution) at CorePlus laboratory

- 1.97% of cases otherwise identified as false negatives were discovered and corrected by the AI-software

- Rate of benign cases identified by AI: 51.04%

- Rate of Gleason grade 1 cases detected by AI: 18.16%;

- Rate of Gleason grade 2+ cases detected by AI: 29.83%

- Rate of technical alerts, for example, controlling for out-of-focus WSIs notified by the Galen Prostate solution: 1.79%

---

molecular studies, as slide-less pathology inherently predisposes to histologically intact tissue specimens unscathed by traditional preanalytical processing techniques. Efforts to develop modalities through which this may be accomplished have demonstrated a powerful capacity for the direct acquisition of molecular-specific images of un-sectioned fresh tissue(Box 16).[51] Model-based pixel value mapping may be used after the application of these techniques to produce pseudo-histologic images from fluorescence signals to H&E staining.

Histopathology for slide-less workflow may commence with slide-less imaging, for example, UV-PAM, followed by virtual deep network staining with final image output. 2D slide-based viewing of complex 3D tissue is inherently prone to time consumption, tissue destruction (during sectioning and slide placement), and sampling errors. 3D visualization of tumor structure has been hypothesized to vastly improve prognostication and treatment decisions.[54] Interpretation of complex 3D glandular architecture using a limited number of 2D histology sections has contributed to the under and over the treatment of patients, pushing researchers to develop workflows that may improve risk assessment and treatment decisions.[55] Using whole slices of prostate tissue, researchers engineered a non-destructive 3D-imaging workflow beginning with the reception of fixed tissue followed by fluorescent staining and transparent tissue configuration. 3D imaging of

the entire tissue occurred using modified "open-top" light sheet microscopy.[54] Physical sectioning was substituted for virtually "sliced" optical sections which were then reconstructed digitally.

Multiple 1-mm diameter human core-needle biopsies were imaged as a whole, with subnuclear features resolved throughout the entire diameter of all benign and malignant prostate gland biopsies. Findings noted inconspicuous epithelial cell nuclei within benign glands and prominent nucleoli within carcinomatous cells of malignant nuclei. The customizable system levied minimal restrictions on specimen size and shape and enabled effective mounting of multiple tissue specimens in individual wells, achieving submicron in-plane resolution at rapid speeds of 1 mm^3min^{-1} per wavelength channel. Prostatectomy samples demonstrated clearing efficacy (refractive index matching of the solvent and tissue) without loss of antigenicity of proteins or any tissue components used for diagnostic or research purposes. Increased nucleic acid yield was noted in comparison to traditional paraffin embedding. This demonstration of high-throughput automated imaging using light-sheet-based 3D microscopy may ultimately lead to broader adoption by clinicians.

3D pathology is ripe with comparatively more data than conventional 2D histology, thereby allowing for a more comprehensive analysis of prognostic 3D microstructures including prostate glands, whereby 3D imaging has demonstrated

---

Table 7
Deployment of AI-solution for prostate clinical workflow (Ibex Galen prostate) at Maccabi healthcare services (from February 2018-September 2020)

	Total	Benign	Adenocarcinoma	Gleason 3 + 3/ASAP	Gleason 7+[A]
Cases	1032	465	567	287	280
Slides (H&E)	12,620	5739	6861	3682	3199

Key: A: Gleason 7+ alert was deployed following February 2019.

Table 8
UPMC AI-algorithm (Ibex Galen prostate) external data set evaluation

Test	Performance
Cancer Detection	AUC = 0.99
Gleason Grade 5	AUC = 0.97
Gleason Grade 7+	AUC = 0.94
PNI	AUC = 0.96
Cancer Size	Correlation Coefficient = 0.88

potential for predicting clinical outcomes in patients with prostate cancer.[56] Core-needle biopsies imaged via open-top light sheet microscopy were digitally reconstructed and stained with computer-simulated H&E. Software was used for 3D visualization of histoarchitecture, detecting overgraded, undergraded, and missed cases of carcinoma and yielding comparatively more precise grading than conventional grading of 2D sections. Such findings present important implications for patient care, for example, in assisting the decision to continue active surveillance versus implementation of intent-to-cure therapy.

Another study evaluating a pipeline for whole prostate biopsies demonstrated the potential for non-destructive, slide-less computational 3D pathology to foster superior prognostic stratification that may guide critical oncology decisions (**Box 17**).[55]

DISCUSSION

Proceeding the 1980s introduction of IHC to pathology practice, histopathological evaluation has advanced through two additional revolutions.[57] The 2010's brought forth molecular pathology, spreading next-generation sequencing (NGS) throughout the entire western world. Clinical implementation of AI marks the third revolution.[57]

Table 9
Multi-site external validation of AI-solution (Ibex Galen prostate)

Test	Performance
Cancer Detection	AUC = 0.997
Gleason Grade 5	AUC = 0.94
Gleason Grade 7+	AUC = 0.99
PNI	AUC = 0.98
HG PIN	AUC = 0.95

Yet, as merely 22% of laboratories enrolled in a 2016 College of American Pathologists (CAP) Histology Quality Improvement Survey reported using QIA tools, a focus on value must first precede efforts to encourage adoption.[58] Positive perspectives fostering AI/QIA implementation may organically cultivate from conditions currently molding the manifold of manual microscopy and the traditional laboratory landscape, one still rearing from workflow incursions foisted on practitioners from the coronavirus-2019 (COVID-19) pandemic. This period has been wrought with challenges catalyzing the clinical implementation of DP tools for WSI-viewing, remote consultations, and work-from-home capabilities, further bolstered by FDA approval for select DP-systems. However, such challenges are exacerbations of those preceding the pandemic, namely pertaining to the management of heavy workloads with efficiency, accuracy, and consistency.

Successful AI deployment accelerated the transformation to a fully digitized pathology laboratory at Maccabi Healthcare Services. The demonstrated value of AI-integration into clinical workflow drove pathologists to support a transition away from traditional microscopy. The necessity of complete digitization has been met with reservations from pathologists who may not approach digital implementation with skepticism, but with a sense of irrelevancy. Doubt marring the utility of digitization is further compounded by daunting expenses for implementation that may appear insurmountable for departments with budget constraints. At Maccabi, the introduction of integrated clinical AI promoted an enticing business case for full laboratory digitization, with AI-implementation at the hospital system providing low risk, high returns, and user-friendly solutions not requiring extensive reconfiguring, investments, or training for appropriate use. These results were further supported by efficiency gains, decreased IHC orders, and an improved work environment achieved through AI-supported primary diagnosis for prostate cancer.

Complete digitization of post-sample preparation histopathology is a prerequisite to exploiting AI tools, as the digitization of a workflow process will lay the foundation for embedding an AI tool within that process. Yet, complete digital workflow for routine primary diagnosis has only seen deployment in few laboratories worldwide.[59] Digitization alone may offer the potential to streamline and improve workflow processes from disease detection, diagnosis, treatment, predictive prognostication, to QC. However, only when partnered with AI will these processes reach their maximum potential.[3]

Box 11
Ibex Galen prostate first read application: productivity improvement

- Marked improvement in diagnostic efficiency was demonstrated, with an overall 27% reduction (32% reduction for benign cases; 25% reduction for prostate cancer cases) in diagnostic time for cases with a valid time measurement (34 benign; 85 cancer) in comparison to standard microscopy.

- Efficiency was slightly higher for benign cases than malignant cases, with an overall gain of 37% in productivity recorded with the use of the AI-application.

- Investigators did not observe diminished accuracy resulting from improvements in efficiency, with case level diagnosis demonstrating the same accuracy as manual microscopy.

Box 12
Ibex Galen prostate first read application: case-level discrepancy resolution

- Ground truth agreement following discrepancy resolution: 97.5% for microscope diagnosis and 97.8% for Galen Prostate AI-solution

- 72% of discrepancies (out of 57 total slides) were identified as small tumors (<3 mm)

- 160 cases (1224 slides) were used to evaluate case level agreement for primary diagnosis

- 95.3% agreement noted between AI and microscopy diagnosis for 378 cancerous and 789 benign slides

- Examples of cases missed by microscopy and detected using AI:
  - A case having only one slide demonstrating findings of prostate cancer
  - A case of high-grade prostate adenocarcinoma (G 4 + 3)

- AI reclassified 3 false-negative slides that were initially classified as benign to that of the correct classification; False negatives for prostate cancer were not elicited with AI assistance.
  - 99.7% of pathologists using Galen Prostate agreed with the classification provided by AI assistance.

Box 13
Ibex Galen prostate first read application: turnaround time (TAT)

- TAT: defined as the total time from first to the last review and sign out of a case by a pathologist

- Evaluation of TAT included 2 arms: microscope arm (238 cases; mean sign out time of 1.8 days) and Galen Prostate/AI-arm (238 cases; mean sign out time of 9.4 minutes).

- 80% of microscopy cases included additional IHC ordering. For the Galen Prostate arm, only 0.6% of cases involved IHCs ordered in addition to those automatically pre-ordered based on AI-classification.

- Final Results: The assistive AI-algorithm was demonstrated to save 1 to 2 days in total TAT while enabling a single review for almost all cases, markedly reducing pathologist TAT

Box 14
Summary of studies evaluating Galen prostate solution for AI-assisted primary diagnosis

- The Galen Prostate platform offers AI-assisted support in the accurate detection and diagnosis of cancer, with features including: Gleason grading, assessment of tumor size, perineural invasion, high-grade PIN, inflammation, and atrophy.

- The Performance of Galen Prostate's AI-based classification and heatmaps detected cancers and other features that were missed by pathologists using a microscope.
  - AI-based classification, heatmaps, and automated measurements significantly improved diagnostic efficiency of prostate biopsy reporting

- Demonstrated that case TAT may be reduced significantly through the clinical integration of an AI-solution into a pathology workflow

- Overall user experience, as reported by surveyed pathologists, was resoundingly positive, with preference indicated toward the use of the AI-platform in comparison to traditional microscopy.

Table 10
Evolution of machine learning for prostate cancer (selected studies 2010-present)[5,6,9,19–29]

Study Year/AI-Model Type	Study Description/Implications	Study Methods, for Example, Training and Evaluation Data	Study Results
2010 Probabilistic Pairwise Markov models (PPMMs)	First system for rapidly detecting prostate cancer regions in a whole-mount (or quarter) histologic section. Increased algorithm sensitivity was necessary to ascertain clinical value; advanced tumors, for example, Gleason grade 5, were poorly identified due to their complete disruption of normal glandular formations	More than 6000 simulations across a dataset of 40 sections from 20 patients.	Detected prostate cancer regions with a sensitivity of 0.87 and a specificity of 0.90.
2012 Boosted Bayesian multiresolution (BBMR) system	Identification of prostate cancer regions from digital biopsy slides, limited by a drop-off in AUC at higher image resolutions due to the lack of fine detail in expert annotations. Study marked the preceding step to the advent of a Gleason grading algorithm capable of scoring the invasiveness and severity of disease.	100 images obtained from 58 patients	AUC of 0.84, 0.83, and 0.76, respectively, at the lowest, intermediate, and highest resolution levels
2013 Machine learning system for automatic prostate cancer detection and grading on H&E-stained tissue images.	First example of automated cancer quantification/superpixel image partitioning for digital prostate histopathology imaging. Designed to address challenges of large data size and the need for high-level tissue information about the locations and grades of tumors for better informed postprostatectomy patient care. Data set was limited in the. Number of images used for cancer classification and restricted to only the sub-images having pure G3 or G4 tissue type, excluding G3+4 and G4+3 sub-images	991 subimages extracted from 50 whole-mount tissue sections from 15 patients with prostatectomy.	Accuracy of 90% for cancer vs noncancer and 85% for high- vs low-grade classification tasks

2016 Deep learning/CNN	First effort to use deep neural networks for prostatic adenocarcinoma detection in H&E-stained needle biopsy tissue slides. Up to 32% of cancer-negative slides could be excluded, indicating the potential for streamlined diagnostic sign-outs.	238 patients, 225 WSIs, 920,000 image patches used for CNN training	Mean ROC for the median analysis: 0.98–0.99 *(90th percentile analysis).
2017 Random forest classifier for automatic Gleason grading	Machine learning classifier using Quantitative Phase Imaging used to discriminate regions with Gleason grade 3 vs 4 in prostatectomy tissue	288 cores from a TMA consisting of 368 prostate cores.	Overall accuracy (AUC): 82% (within the range of human error in the consideration of interobserver variability)
2018 Supervised Deep learning/CNN pipeline for automatic grading of Prostate cancer	First incorporation of a probabilistic approach for supervised learning by multiple experts to account for inter-observer grading variability. A deep learning pipeline was developed for the automated grading of prostate cancer, achieving consistency with literature-reported grading by pathologists.	333 TMA cores from 231 patients and annotated by 6 pathologists for different Gleason grades. $\geq$ 16,000 patch samples used in training. Performance was assessed on an additional 230 WSIs from 56 patients, independent of the training dataset.	Overall grading the agreement of the classifier with the pathologists: unweighted kappa of 0.51; overall agreements between each pathologist and the others: (K = 0.45–0.62). Results suggested that the classifier's performance was within the inter-observer grading variability across the pathologists in this study, consistent with levels reported in the literature.
2018 Deep learning/CNN classifier for automated Gleason Grading of prostate cancer tissue microarrays stained with H&E	First study to train and evaluate the CNN model based on detailed manual expert Gleason annotations of image subregions within each TMA spot image for the applicability of deep learning-based solutions toward more objective and reproducible prostate cancer grading, particularly for cases with heterogeneous Gleason patterns.	Dataset: 5 TMAs each containing 200–300 spots (excluding artifact and nonprostate tissue). Prostate TMA spots were assigned a Gleason pattern of 3, 4 or 5, or benign to each region. training dataset: 641 patients; predictive performance evaluation: separate test cohort of 245 patients	Inter-annotator agreements between the model and each pathologist: kappa = 0.75 and 0.71, respectively; comparable with the inter-pathologist agreement (kappa = 0.71).

(continued on next page)

Table 10
(continued)

Study Year/AI-Model Type	Study Description/Implications	Study Methods, for Example, Training and Evaluation Data	Study Results
2018 Deep learning/Residual network system for SPOP mutation detection	Quantitative model to predict whether or not SPOP is mutated in prostate cancer; first pipeline to predict gene mutation probability in cancer from digitized H&E-stained microscopy slides (WSIs with H&E staining)	177 patients with prostate cancer, 20 having mutant SPOP; evaluation on independent test cohort of 152 patients, 19 having mutant SPOP	distinguishing SPOP mutant from SPOP nonmutant patients during training (test AUROC = 0.74, P = .0007 Fisher's Exact Test) Validation: Mutants and nonmutants were accurately distinguished despite TCGA slides being frozen sections and MSK-IMPACT slides being formalin-fixed paraffin-embedded sections (AUROC = 0.86, P = .0038).
2019 Deep learning/CNN-based system for automated Gleason grading	Comparison of cross-validation (CV) approaches to evaluate the performance of a classifier model for the automated grading of prostate cancer. The study evaluated performance of an AI model to facilitate the adoption of deep learning techniques for image analysis by health care systems and regulatory bodies. Investigators concluded that studies should evaluate the performance of AI-models using patient-based CV and multi-expert data for reproducibility and generalizability that may extend to other machine learning applications.	TMA (333 cores) from 231 patients who underwent radical prostatectomy Digitized images of tissue cores were annotated by 6 pathologists for 4 classes (benign and Gleason grades 3, 4, and 5)	20-fold leave-patches-out CV resulted in mean (SD) accuracy of 97.8% (1.2%), sensitivity of 98.5% (1.0%), and specificity of 97.5% (1.2%) for classifying benign patches vs cancerous patches. 20-fold leave-patients-out CV resulted in mean (SD) accuracy of 85.8% (4.3%), sensitivity of 86.3% (7.2%), and specificity of 85.5% (7.2%). 20-fold leave-cores-out CV resulted in mean (SD) accuracy of 86.7% (3.7%), sensitivity of 87.2% (4.0%), and specificity of 87.7% (5.5%)

| 2019 Deep learning/CNN-based system for automatic Gleason pattern classification | Digitized prostate biopsies were used to evaluate automatic Gleason pattern classification for the grade group determination of prostate biopsies. The Inception-v3 CNN was used to demonstrate the potential for deep learning to improve histopathological grading and treatment selection for prostate cancer. | 96 prostate biopsies from 38 patients are annotated on pixel-level. | Differentiation between nonatypical and malignant (GP $\geq$ 3) areas resulted in an accuracy of 92% with a sensitivity and specificity of 90% and 93%, respectively. The differentiation between GP $\geq$ 4 and GP $\leq$ 3 resulted in an accuracy of 90%, with a sensitivity and specificity of 77% and 94%, respectively. Concordance of our automated GG determination method with a genitourinary pathologist was obtained in 65% (κ = 0.70), indicating substantial agreement. |
| 2019 Multiple instance learning-based deep learning system | Multiple instance learning system developed in response to requirements for large, manually annotated training datasets for highly supervised learning that have hindered the deployment of deep learning systems in clinical practice. System used only the reported diagnosis of WSIs as targeted labels for training to avoid expensive and time-consuming pixel-wise annotations. Demonstrated the unprecedented scale of training for classification models that may accurately detect and grade prostate cancer from PCNB WSIs. | 44,732 whole slide images from 15,187 patients without any form of data curation. | Tests on prostate cancer, basal cell carcinoma, and breast cancer metastases to axillary lymph nodes resulted in AUCs above 0.98 for all cancer types. For the prostate model, 3 of the 12 false negatives were correctly predicted as negative by the algorithm. Three other slides displayed atypical morphologic features insufficient to diagnose carcinoma. Confirmed 6 false negatives contained very low tumor volume. AUC for the prostate test set improved from 0.991 to 0.994 after accounting for ground truth corrections. |

(continued on next page)

Table 10
(continued)

Study Year/AI-Model Type	Study Description/Implications	Study Methods, for Example, Training and Evaluation Data	Study Results
2019 Shallow and Deep Gaussian Processes for the classification of prostate histology	Novel Optical density Granulometry-based descriptors (a technique based on mathematical morphology) were fashioned to extract complex histologic prostate images, demonstrating the potential to improve early prostate cancer diagnosis when evaluated in comparison to patch-based shallow classification methods and high-performing derivatives of CNN-architecture, that is, VGG19, Inception v3, and Xception.	Training dataset of 60 WSIs. Models were compared on 17 WSIs. Malignant regions of the pathologic images were given manual pixel-wise annotations by a team of expert pathologists.	5-fold CV: AUC values ≥ 0.98 for both shallow and deep Gaussian Processes, outperforming current state of the art patch-based shallow classifiers and very competitive in comparison to high-performing CNN-architecture derivatives. The one-layer Gaussian process identified annotated areas of cancer with 83.87% sensitivity. Investigators noted that no more than a layer was needed to achieve excellent generalization results, in comparison to more complex, multi-layered CNNs.
2021 Deep learning/residual CNN	A deep residual CNN was developed for patch classification at coarse, for example, benign vs malignant, and fine, for example, benign vs Gleason 3 vs 4 vs 5, levels.	WSIs containing 85 prostate core biopsy specimens from 25 patients were annotated for Gleason 3, 4, and 5 prostate adenocarcinomas by a urologic pathologist. 14,803 image patches were sampled from the WSIs for model training.	The model demonstrated 91.5% accuracy ($P<.001$) for the coarse-level classification of image patches as benign vs malignant (0.93 sensitivity, 0.90 specificity, and 0.95 average precision). The model demonstrated 85.4% accuracy ($P<.001$) for the fine-level classification of image patches as benign vs Gleason 3 vs Gleason 4 vs Gleason 5 (0.83 sensitivity, 0.94 specificity, and 0.83 average precision), with the greatest number of confusions occurring during distinction between adenocarcinomas Gleason 3 and 4, and Gleason 4 and 5

Box 15
PANDA challenge for generalizable AI-assisted diagnosis and Gleason grading of prostate cancer

Study Design:

A total of 12,625 WSIs of prostate biopsies were collected from 6 different sites for algorithm development, "tuning," for example, performance evaluation in competition, and independent validation. Cases for development, tuning, and internal validation were sourced from 2 institutions (Netherlands/Sweden). Cases for external validation contained data from the US (741 cases obtained from 2 independent medical laboratories and a tertiary teaching hospital) and the EU (330 cases obtained from the Karolinska University Hospital in Sweden). Histologic preparation and scanning of data used for external validation were performed by different laboratories. All selected algorithms were fashioned using deep-learning methods, primarily CNN-based end-to-end training using case-level information only (ISUP GG of a specimen used as the target label for an entire WSI).

Study Data:

Model development set: 10,616 WSIs

Performance evaluation set: 393 WSIs

Internal validation set (postcompetition): 545 WSIs

External validation set: 1071 WSIs

Reference standards for datasets:

Training/Model development: pathology reports from routine clinical practice (Netherlands); one uropathologist following routine clinical workflow (Sweden)

Internal validation set: consensus of 3 uropathologists from 2 institutions with 19 to 28 years (mean of 22 years) of clinical experience after residency (Netherlands); four uropathologists from 4 institutions all with greater than 25 years of clinical experience after residency

External validation set (US): panel of six US or Canadian uropathologists from six institutions with 18 to 34 years (mean of 25 years) of clinical experience after residency

External validation set (EU): reviewed by a single uropathologist

1010 teams of 1290 developers from 65 countries

Total number of algorithms submitted: 34,262

Total number of algorithmic predictions: 32,137,756

Methods:

Most leading teams, including the competition winner, used patch-extraction techniques to collect a series of smaller images sampled from a WSI which were then used for end-to-end training of a CNN used to predict the ISUP GG of a WSI in a computationally efficient manner.

Findings:

On the United States and European external validation sets, the algorithms achieved agreements of 0.862 (quadratically weighted κ, 95% confidence interval (CI), 0.840 to 0.884) and 0.868 (95% CI, 0.835–0.900) with expert uropathologists.

This principle retains merit in reverse, as demonstrated by recent efforts to mitigate high workload burden at the Gravina Hospital in Caltagirone (Sicily), leading to the deployment of a fully digital, LIS-centric laboratory.[59] Digitization was inclusive of fluorescence applications and frozen sections for intraoperative assessment, facilitating the interconnectivity of all workflow steps via the LIS resulting in an easier, streamlined workflow. Digital implementation facilitated the introduction of AI-tools for prostate pathology into the workflow (Context Vision INIFY Prostate solution), fostering better diagnostic concordance among pathologists. Increased WSI quality was also observed after AI-implementation, as AI-utilization drew attention to workflow quality as paramount to the successful achievement of optimal AI output. The Caltagirone example demonstrated that the potential to advance DP is not limited to newfound improvements in accuracy and efficiency brought

---

Box 16
Slide-free technologies/optical technologies

Confocal Microscopy

- Superior image resolution and contrast

Nonlinear Microscopy

- Has enabled several new types of optical contrast for slide-free histopathology, including label-free contrasts useful for identifying specific tissue microstructures of great importance in pathology.[52]

- Has demonstrated greater efficacy in delineating medical kidney features requiring special staining, for example, silver stain for glomerulonephritis (visualization of tram track sign), but are difficult to visualize with WSI. Reduces the need for special staining by using thin optical sectioning for high-quality images otherwise obscured by physical slides

- Ability to recognize fine features such as mitochondria damage and swelling.

Optical Coherence Tomography(OCT)[53]

- Qualitative comparison between OCT and histopathology images shows that structural details resolved by OCT are in good agreement with histology

- Ability of OCT in showing relevant microstructures without tissue sectioning can be used in guiding surgical procedure

Structured Illumination

- For super-resolution/depth sectioning

Light-Sheet Microscopy

- Not ideal for clinical samples due to geometric constraints and tedious sample preparation

- Open-top light sheet microscopy has enabled whole-tissue 3D imaging suitable for clinical specimens

Photoacoustic microscopy (UV-PAM)

- Combines light and sound to achieve subcellular imaging via transmission of pulsed beams of light which are then absorbed by tissues that heat to expand, creating a sound wave detected by a microphone.

- Visualizes molecules at ultraviolet levels whereby proteins and nucleic acids are absorbed

- Label-free imaging modality that can generate histologic images of biological tissue surface without physical sectioning, yet is able to provide a similar contrast as H&E labeling used in conventional histology

MUSE (ultra-violet light-based imaging)

- Wide-field illumination significantly improves imaging speed

---

forth directly through AI-solutions, rather through issues otherwise overlooked if not for their implementation.

Prostate pathology has been the primary focus of algorithmic development for GU applications, as evidenced by65% of 112 studies featured within a recent literature review update for urologic AI, most of which involved algorithm development for prostate cancer detection/diagnostics and related applications.[60] Most studies pertaining to the algorithmic development of other GU systems are still relegated to academia and should be explored for further clinical applicability.

SUMMARY

As machine learning (ML) solutions for genitourinary pathology image analysis are fostered by a progressively digitized laboratory landscape, these integrable modalities usher in a revolution in histopathological diagnosis. As technology advances, limitations stymying clinical artificial intelligence (AI) will not be extinguished without thorough validation and interrogation of ML tools by pathologists and regulatory bodies alike. ML-solutions deployed in clinical settings for applications in prostate pathology yield promising results. Recent breakthroughs in clinical artificial intelligence for

> **Box 17**
> **Risk stratification of prostate cancer using 3D glandular features**
>
> - 3D glandular features extracted from FFPE blocks (with a known outcome) were used to predict biochemical recurrence of prostate cancer, with findings demonstrating 3D glandular features superior to their 2D-counterparts for the risk stratification of patients with aggressive versus indolent disease.
>
> - 3D imaging of whole prostate biopsies was conducted in addition to co-staining of tissue with pseudo-H&E (fluorescent H&E analog) and a replica CK8 immunofluorescence stain (specific for luminal epithelial cells in all prostate glands). A generative adversarial network (GAN) was used to digitally replicate the antibody.
>
> - Segmentation of the gland lumen, epithelium, and surrounding stroma was effectively and easily executed without the need for manual annotations or "real" immunolabelling.
>
> - Digital removal of stroma occurred following segmentation, revealing glandular skeletons whereby features such as tortuosity and branching (unmeasurable in 2D), inferred to have disease association, were extracted and used to predict biochemical recurrence.
>
> - 3D elicitation of such findings led to a statistically significant prediction of disease.
>
> - The model demonstrated superior accuracy in predicting manually annotated glandular regions than 2D deep learning or standard 3D segmentation techniques.

genitourinary pathology demonstrate unprecedented generalizability, heralding prospects for a future in which AI-driven assistive solutions may be seen as laboratory faculty, rather than novelty.

- Generalizability of an algorithmic model is tantamount to its clinical implementation.

- AI solutions can buttress the capabilities of digitized workflow processes.

- Extensive external validation must precede the clinical implementation of an AI-tool.

CLINICS CARE POINTS

- AI assistance can help improve diagnostic accuracy and efficiency.

- For clinicians, the deep-learning subtype of AI has demonstrated vast potential for rapid and accurate image interpretation, quality control for error reduction, and workflow improvement.[61]

- Deep neural networks have emerged as the gold standard for accurate image classification.

- AI can serve as a valuable QC tool for digital or microscopy diagnosed cases.

- Multiple instances and weakly supervised learning for AI model training is superior to highly supervised techniques.

- Models trained under full supervision on small, curated datasets do not translate well to clinical practice.[9]

DISCLOSURE

The authors have nothing to disclose.

REFERENCES

1. Park S, Parwani AV, Aller RD, et al. The history of pathology informatics: A global perspective. J Pathol Inform 2013;4:7.
2. Pantanowitz L, Sharma A, Carter AB, et al. Twenty years of digital pathology: An overview of the road travelled, what is on the horizon, and the emergence of vendor-neutral archives. J Pathol Inform 2018;9:40.
3. Eloy C, Bychkov A, Pantanowitz L, et al. DPA–ESDIP–JSDP task force for worldwide adoption of digital pathology. J Pathol Inform 2021;12:51.
4. Dangott B. Whole slide image analysis. In: Parwani AV, editor. Whole slide imaging. Switzerland: Springer; 2022. p. 203–21.
5. Nir G, Hor S, Karimi D, et al. Automatic grading of prostate cancer in digitized histopathology images: Learning from multiple experts. Med Image Anal 2018;50:167–80.

6. Litjens G, Sanchez CI, Timofeeva N, et al. Deep learning as a tool for increased accuracy and efficiency of histopathological diagnosis. Sci Rep 2016;6:26286.

7. Li C, Li X, Rahaman M, et al. A comprehensive review of computer-aided whole-slide image analysis: From datasets to feature extraction, segmentation, classification, and detection approaches. arXiv. Preprint posted online February 21, 2021. Available at: https://arxiv.org/abs/2102.10553. Accessed January 7, 2022.

8. Paige Receives First Ever FDA Approval for AI Product in Digital Pathology. 2021. Available at: https://www. businesswire.com/news/home/20210922005369/en/ Paige-Receives-First-Ever-FDA-Approval-for-AI-Product-in-Digital-Pathology.

9. Campanella G, Hanna MG, Geneslaw L, et al. Clinical-grade computational pathology using weakly supervised deep learning on whole slide images. Nat Med 2019;25(8):1301–9.

10. Raciti P, Sue J, Ceballos R, et al. Novel artificial intelligence system increases the detection of prostate cancer in whole slide images of core needle biopsies. Mod Pathol 2020;33(10):2058–66.

11. da Silva LM, Pereira EM, Salles PG, et al. Independent real-world application of a clinical-grade automated prostate cancer detection system. J Pathol 2021;254(2):147–58.

12. Ibex Medical Analytics. First U.S. Lab implements AI-based solution for cancer detection in pathology. PR Newswire. Updated September 1. Available at: https://www.prnewswire.com/il/news-releases/first--us-lab-implements-ai-based-solution-for-cancer-detection-in-pathology-301121728.html. Accessed January 30, 2022.

13. Miller KD, Goding Sauer A, Ortiz AP, et al. Cancer Statistics for Hispanics/Latinos, 2018. CA Cancer J Clin 2018;68(6):425–45.

14. Pantanowitz L, Quiroga-Garza GM, Bien L, et al. An artificial intelligence algorithm for prostate cancer diagnosis in whole slide images of core needle biopsies: a blinded clinical validation and deployment study. The Lancet Digital Health 2020;2(8): e407–16.

15. Laifenfeld D, Sandbank J, Linhart C, et al. Performance of an AI-based cancer diagnosis system in France's largest network of pathology institutes. 2019:S177-S178.

16. Laifenfeld D, Vecsler M, Raoux D, et al. AI-Based Solution for Cancer Diagnosis in Prostate Core Needle Biopsies: A Prospective Blinded Multi-Site Clinical Study. Lab Invest 2021;101(Suppl 1):580–1.

17. Comperat E, Rioux-Leclercq N, Levrel O, et al. Clinical level AI-based solution for primary diagnosis and reporting of prostate biopsies in routine use: a prospective reader study. Virchows Archiv 2021; 479(Suppl 1):S60–1.

18. Raoux D, Sebag G, Yazbin I, et al. Novel AI based solution for supporting primary diagnosis of prostate cancer increases the accuracy and efficiency of reporting in clinical routine presented at: USCP 2021; 2021. Available at: https://uscap.econference.io/public/fYV-k0yI/main/sessions/9644/31166. Accessed January 15, 2021.

19. Lucas M, Jansen I, Savci-Heijink CD, et al. Deep learning for automatic Gleason pattern classification for grade group determination of prostate biopsies. Virchows Arch 2019;475(1):77–83.

20. Esteban AE, Lopez-Perez M, Colomer A, et al. A new optical density granulometry-based descriptor for the classification of prostate histological images using shallow and deep Gaussian processes. Comput Methods Programs Biomed 2019; 178:303–17.

21. Kott O, Linsley D, Amin A, et al. Development of a deep learning algorithm for the histopathologic diagnosis and gleason grading of prostate cancer biopsies: A pilot study. Eur Urol Focus 2021;7(2): 347–51.

22. Nguyen TH, Sridharan S, Macias V, et al. Automatic Gleason grading of prostate cancer using quantitative phase imaging and machine learning. J Biomed Opt 2017;22(3):36015.

23. Arvaniti E, Fricker KS, Moret M, et al. Automated Gleason grading of prostate cancer tissue microarrays via deep learning. Sci Rep 2018;8(1): 12054.

24. Nir G, Karimi D, Goldenberg SL, et al. Comparison of Artificial Intelligence Techniques to Evaluate Performance of a Classifier for Automatic Grading of Prostate Cancer From Digitized Histopathologic Images. JAMA Netw Open 2019;2(3):e190442.

25. Doyle S, Feldman M, Tomaszewski J, et al. A boosted Bayesian multiresolution classifier for prostate cancer detection from digitized needle biopsies. IEEE Trans Biomed Eng 2012;59(5):1205–18.

26. Monaco JP, Tomaszewski JE, Feldman MD, et al. High-throughput detection of prostate cancer in histological sections using probabilistic pairwise Markov models. Med Image Anal 2010;14(4):617–29.

27. Gorelick L, Veksler O, Gaed M, et al. Prostate histopathology: learning tissue component histograms for cancer detection and classification. IEEE Trans Med Imaging 2013;32(10):1804–18.

28. Kothari S, Phan JH, Stokes TH, et al. Pathology imaging informatics for quantitative analysis of whole-slide images. J Am Med Inform Assoc 2013;20(6): 1099–108.

29. Schaumberg A, Rubin M, Fuchs T. H&E-stained Whole Slide Image Deep Learning Predicts SPOP Mutation State in Prostate Cancer. 2018.

30. Somanchi S, Neill DB, Parwani AV. Discovering anomalous patterns in large digital pathology images. Stat Med 2018;37(25):3599–615.

31. Strom P, Kartasalo K, Olsson H, et al. Artificial intelligence for diagnosis and grading of prostate cancer in biopsies: a population-based, diagnostic study. Lancet Oncol 2020;21(2):222–32.

32. Han W, Johnson C, Gaed M, et al. Histologic tissue components provide major cues for machine learning-based prostate cancer detection and grading on prostatectomy specimens. Sci Rep 2020;10(1):9911.

33. Tolkach Y, Dohmgörgen T, Toma M, et al. High-accuracy prostate cancer pathology using deep learning. Nat Machine Intelligence 2020;2(7):411–8.

34. Zelic R, Giunchi F, Lianas L, et al. Interchangeability of light and virtual microscopy for histopathological evaluation of prostate cancer. Sci Rep 2021;11(1): 3257.

35. Singh M, Kalaw EM, Jie W, et al. Cribriform pattern detection in prostate histopathological images using deep learning models. arXiv 2019;1910:04030.

36. Leo P, Chandramouli S, Farre X, et al. Computationally derived cribriform area index from prostate cancer hematoxylin and eosin images is associated with biochemical recurrence following radical prostatectomy and is most prognostic in gleason grade group 2. Eur Urol Focus 2021;7(4):722–32.

37. Choi HK, Jarkrans T, Bengtsson E, et al. Image analysis based grading of bladder carcinoma. Comparison of object, texture and graph based methods and their reproducibility. Anal Cell Pathol 1997; 15(1):1–18.

38. Spyridonos P, Cavouras D, Ravazoula P, et al. Neural network-based segmentation and classification system for automated grading of histologic sections of bladder carcinoma. Anal Quant Cytol Histol 2002; 24(6):317–24.

39. Jansen I, Lucas M, Bosschieter J, et al. Automated Detection and Grading of Non-Muscle-Invasive Urothelial Cell Carcinoma of the Bladder. Am J Pathol 2020;190(7):1483–90.

40. Linder N, Taylor JC, Colling R, et al. Deep learning for detecting tumour-infiltrating lymphocytes in testicular germ cell tumours. J Clin Pathol 2019; 72(2):157–64.

41. Bhalla S, Chaudhary K, Kumar R, et al. Gene expression-based biomarkers for discriminating early and late stage of clear cell renal cancer. Sci Rep 2017;7(1):44997.

42. Li F, Yang M, Li Y, et al. An improved clear cell renal cell carcinoma stage prediction model based on gene sets. BMC Bioinformatics 2020;21(1):232.

43. Giulietti M, Cecati M, Sabanovic B, et al. The role of artificial intelligence in the diagnosis and prognosis of renal cell tumors. Diagnostics (Basel) 2021; 11(2):206.

44. Fenstermaker M, Tomlins SA, Singh K, et al. Development and validation of a deep-learning model to assist with renal cell carcinoma histopathologic interpretation. Urology 2020;144:152–7.

45. Tabibu S, Vinod PK, Jawahar CV. Pan-renal cell carcinoma classification and survival prediction from histopathology images using deep learning. Sci Rep 2019;9(1):10509.

46. Singh NP, Bapi RS, Vinod PK. Machine learning models to predict the progression from early to late stages of papillary renal cell carcinoma. Comput Biol Med 2018;100:92–9.

47. Singh NP, Vinod PK. Integrative analysis of DNA methylation and gene expression in papillary renal cell carcinoma. Mol Genet Genomics 2020;295(3): 807–24.

48. Kim H, Lee SJ, Park SJ, et al. Machine learning approach to predict the probability of recurrence of renal cell carcinoma after surgery: Prediction model development study. JMIR Med Inform 2021; 9(3):e25635.

49. Cheng J, Han Z, Mehra R, et al. Computational analysis of pathological images enables a better diagnosis of TFE3 Xp11.2 translocation renal cell carcinoma. Nat Commun 2020;11(1):1778.

50. Bulten W, Kartasalo K, Chen P-HC, et al. Artificial intelligence for diagnosis and Gleason grading of prostate cancer: the PANDA challenge. Nat Med 2022;28(1):154–63.

51. Kang L, Li X, Zhang Y, et al. Deep learning enables ultraviolet photoacoustic microscopy based histological imaging with near real-time virtual staining. Photoacoustics 2022;25:100308.

52. Liu Y, Levenson RM, Jenkins MW. Slide over: Advances in slide-free optical microscopy as drivers of diagnostic pathology. Am J Pathol 2022. https:// doi.org/10.1016/j.ajpath.2021.10.010.

53. Tampu IE, Maintz M, Koller D, et al. Optical coherence tomography for thyroid pathology: 3D analysis of tissue microstructure. Biomed Opt Express 2020; 11(8):4130–49.

54. Glaser AK, Reder NP, Chen Y, et al. Multi-immersion open-top light-sheet microscope for high-throughput imaging of cleared tissues. Nat Commun 2019;10(1):2781.

55. Xie W, Reder NP, Koyuncu C, et al. Prostate cancer risk stratification via non-destructive 3D pathology with annotation-free gland segmentation and analysis. medRxiv 2021. https://doi.org/10.1101/2021. 08.30.21262847.

56. Glaser AK, Reder NP, Chen Y, et al. Light-sheet microscopy for slide-free non-destructive pathology of large clinical specimens. Nat Biomed Eng 2017; 1(7):0084.

57. Salto-Tellez M, Maxwell P, Hamilton P. Artificial intelligence—the third revolution in pathology. Histopathology 2019;74(3):372–6.

58. Paxton A. Quantitative image analysis: In guideline, preliminary rules for pathology's third revolution. Cap Today2019.

59. Fraggetta F, Caputo A, Guglielmino R, et al. A Survival Guide for the Rapid Transition to a Fully Digital Workflow: The "Caltagirone Example. Diagnostics (Basel) 2021;(10):11. https://doi.org/10.3390/diagnostics11101916.

60. Chen AB, Haque T, Roberts S, et al. Artificial intelligence applications in urology: Reporting standards to achieve fluency for urologists. Urol Clin North Am 2022;49(1):65–117.

61. Topol EJ. High-performance medicine: the convergence of human and artificial intelligence. Nat Med 2019;25(1):44–56.

UNITED STATES POSTAL SERVICE®
Statement of Ownership, Management, and Circulation (All Periodicals Publications Except Requester Publications)

1. Publication Title	2. Publication Number		3. Filing Date
SURGICAL PATHOLOGY CLINICS	025 – 478		9/18/2022

4. Issue Frequency	5. Number of Issues Published Annually	6. Annual Subscription Price
MAR, JUN, SEP, DEC	4	$237.00

7. Complete Mailing Address of Known Office of Publication *(Not printer) (Street, city, county, state, and ZIP+4®)*

ELSEVIER INC.
230 Park Avenue, Suite 800
New York, NY 10169

Contact Person
Malathi Samayan

Telephone *(Include area code)*
215-239-3688

8. Complete Mailing Address of Headquarters or General Business Office of Publisher *(Not printer)*

ELSEVIER INC.
230 Park Avenue, Suite 800
New York, NY 10169

9. Full Names and Complete Mailing Addresses of Publisher, Editor, and Managing Editor *(Do not leave blank)*

Publisher *(Name and complete mailing address)*

DOLORES MELONI, ELSEVIER INC.
1600 JOHN F KENNEDY BLVD. SUITE 1800
PHILADELPHIA, PA 19103-2899

Editor *(Name and complete mailing address)*

TAYLOR HAYES, ELSEVIER INC.
1600 JOHN F KENNEDY BLVD. SUITE 1800
PHILADELPHIA, PA 19103-2899

Managing Editor *(Name and complete mailing address)*

PATRICK MANLEY, ELSEVIER INC.
1600 JOHN F KENNEDY BLVD. SUITE 1800
PHILADELPHIA, PA 19103-2899

10. Owner *(Do not leave blank. If the publication is owned by a corporation, give the name and address of the corporation immediately followed by the names and addresses of all stockholders owning or holding 1 percent or more of the total amount of stock. If not owned by a corporation, give the names and addresses of the individual owners. If owned by a partnership or other unincorporated firm, give its name and address as well as those of each individual owner. If the publication is published by a nonprofit organization, give its name and address.)*

Full Name	Complete Mailing Address
WHOLLY OWNED SUBSIDIARY OF REED/ELSEVIER, US HOLDINGS	1600 JOHN F KENNEDY BLVD. SUITE 1800 PHILADELPHIA, PA 19103-2899

11. Known Bondholders, Mortgagees, and Other Security Holders Owning or Holding 1 Percent or More of Total Amount of Bonds, Mortgages, or Other Securities. If none, check box ▶ ☐ None

Full Name	Complete Mailing Address
N/A	

12. Tax Status *(For completion by nonprofit organizations authorized to mail at nonprofit rates) (Check one)*
The purpose, function, and nonprofit status of this organization and the exempt status for federal income tax purposes:
☒ Has Not Changed During Preceding 12 Months
☐ Has Changed During Preceding 12 Months *(Publisher must submit explanation of change with this statement)*

PS Form **3526**, July 2014 *(Page 1 of 4) (see instructions page 4)]* PSN: 7530-01-000-9931 **PRIVACY NOTICE:** See our privacy policy on www.usps.com.

---

13. Publication Title	14. Issue Date for Circulation Data Below
SURGICAL PATHOLOGY CLINICS	JUNE 2022

15. Extent and Nature of Circulation

			Average No. Copies Each Issue During Preceding 12 Months	No. Copies of Single Issue Published Nearest to Filing Date
a. Total Number of Copies *(Net press run)*			319	306
b. Paid Circulation (By Mail and Outside the Mail)	(1)	Mailed Outside-County Paid Subscriptions Stated on PS Form 3541 (Include paid distribution above nominal rate, advertiser's proof copies, and exchange copies)	228	226
	(2)	Mailed In-County Paid Subscriptions Stated on PS Form 3541 (Include paid distribution above nominal rate, advertiser's proof copies, and exchange copies)	0	0
	(3)	Paid Distribution Outside the Mails Including Sales Through Dealers and Carriers, Street Vendors, Counter Sales, and Other Paid Distribution Outside USPS®	68	67
	(4)	Paid Distribution by Other Classes of Mail Through the USPS (e.g. First-Class Mail®)	0	0
c. Total Paid Distribution *(Sum of 15b (1), (2), (3), and (4))*			296	293
d. Free or Nominal Rate Distribution (By Mail and Outside the Mail)	(1)	Free or Nominal Rate Outside-County Copies included on PS Form 3541	23	13
	(2)	Free or Nominal Rate In-County Copies Included on PS Form 3541	0	0
	(3)	Free or Nominal Rate Copies Mailed at Other Classes Through the USPS (e.g. First-Class Mail)	0	0
	(4)	Free or Nominal Rate Distribution Outside the Mail (Carriers or other means)	0	0
e. Total Free or Nominal Rate Distribution *(Sum of 15d (1), (2), (3) and (4))*			23	13
f. Total Distribution *(Sum of 15c and 15e)*			319	306
g. Copies not Distributed *(See Instructions to Publishers #4 (page 4)*)			0	0
h. Total *(Sum of 15f and g)*			319	306
i. Percent Paid *(15c divided by 15f times 100)*			92.79%	95.75%

* If you are claiming electronic copies, go to line 16 on page 3. If you are not claiming electronic copies, skip to line 17 on page 3.

16. Electronic Copy Circulation

	Average No. Copies Each Issue During Preceding 12 Months	No. Copies of Single Issue Published Nearest to Filing Date
a. Paid Electronic Copies ▶		
b. Total Paid Print Copies (Line 15c) + Paid Electronic Copies (Line 16a) ▶		
c. Total Print Distribution (Line 15f) + Paid Electronic Copies (Line 16a) ▶		
d. Percent Paid (Both Print & Electronic Copies) (16b divided by 16c × 100) ▶		

☒ I certify that 50% of all my distributed copies (electronic and print) are paid above a nominal price.

17. Publication of Statement of Ownership

☒ If the publication is a general publication, publication of this statement is required. Will be printed in the DECEMBER 2022 issue of this publication. ☐ Publication not required.

18. Signature and Title of Editor, Publisher, Business Manager, or Owner

Malathi Samayan - Distribution Controller

Malathi Samayan

Date 9/18/2022

I certify that all information furnished on this form is true and complete. I understand that anyone who furnishes false or misleading information on this form or who omits material or information requested on the form may be subject to criminal sanctions (including fines and imprisonment) and/or civil sanctions (including civil penalties).

PS Form **3526**, July 2014 *(Page 3 of 4)* **PRIVACY NOTICE:** See our privacy policy on www.usps.com

Moving?

Make sure your subscription moves with you!

To notify us of your new address, find your **Clinics Account Number** (located on your mailing label above your name), and contact customer service at:

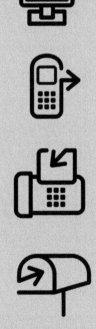

Email: journalscustomerservice-usa@elsevier.com

800-654-2452 (subscribers in the U.S. & Canada)
314-447-8871 (subscribers outside of the U.S. & Canada)

Fax number: 314-447-8029

Elsevier Health Sciences Division
Subscription Customer Service
3251 Riverport Lane
Maryland Heights, MO 63043

*To ensure uninterrupted delivery of your subscription, please notify us at least 4 weeks in advance of move.